ENDING THE WAR METAPHOR

The Changing Agenda for Unraveling the Host-Microbe Relationship

Workshop Summary

Forum on Microbial Threats
Board on Global Health

INSTITUTE OF MEDICINE
OF THE NATIONAL ACADEMIES

THE NATIONAL ACADEMIES PRESS
Washington, D.C.
www.nap.edu

THE NATIONAL ACADEMIES PRESS   500 Fifth Street, N.W.   Washington, DC 20001

NOTICE: The project that is the subject of this report was approved by the Governing Board of the National Research Council, whose members are drawn from the councils of the National Academy of Sciences, the National Academy of Engineering, and the Institute of Medicine.

This project was supported by the American Society for Microbiology; Burroughs Wellcome Fund; Defense Threat Reduction Agency; GlaxoSmithKline; Infectious Disease Society of America; Lawrence Livermore National Laboratory; Merck; Pfizer; Sanofi Pasteur; U.S. Department of Health and Human Services' National Institutes of Health/National Institute for Allergies and Infectious Disease and Centers for Disease Control and Prevention; U.S. Department of Defense/Global Emerging Infections Surveillance/Walter Reed Army Institute of Research; U.S. Department of Homeland Security; U.S. Department of State; and U.S. Department of Veterans Affairs. The views presented in this report are those of the editors and attributed authors and are not necessarily those of the funding agencies.

This report is based on the proceedings of a workshop that was sponsored by the Forum on Microbial Threats. It is prepared in the form of a workshop summary by and in the name of the editors, with the assistance of staff and consultants, as an individually authored document. Sections of the workshop summary not specifically attributed to an individual reflect the views of the editors and not those of the Forum on Microbial Threats. The content of those sections is based on the presentations and the discussions that took place during the workshop.

Library of Congress Cataloging-in-Publication Data

Ending the war metaphor : the changing agenda for unraveling the host-
   microbe relationship : workshop summary / Forum on Microbial
   Threats, Board on Global Health.
      p. ; cm.
   Includes bibliographical references.
   ISBN 0-309-09601-4 (pbk.)
   1. Host-parasite relationships—Congresses. 2. Communicable diseases
—Transmission—Congresses. 3. Microbiology—Congresses.
   I. Institute of Medicine (U.S.). Forum on Microbial Threats.
      [DNLM: 1. Host-Parasite Relations—Congresses. 2. Communicable
   Diseases, Emerging—microbiology—Congresses. 3. Communicable
   Diseases, Emerging—prevention & control—Congresses. 4. Drug
   Resistance, Microbial—Congresses.   QX 45 E56 2006]
   RB153.E53 2006
   616.9'041—dc22
                                                    2006012949

Additional copies of this report are available from the National Academies Press, 500 Fifth Street, N.W., Lockbox 285, Washington, DC 20055; (800) 624-6242 or (202) 334-3313 (in the Washington metropolitan area); Internet, http://www.nap.edu.

For more information about the Institute of Medicine, visit the IOM home page at: **www.iom.edu.**

Copyright 2006 by the National Academy of Sciences. All rights reserved.

Printed in the United States of America.

The serpent has been a symbol of long life, healing, and knowledge among almost all cultures and religions since the beginning of recorded history. The serpent adopted as a logotype by the Institute of Medicine is a relief carving from ancient Greece, now held by the Staatliche Museen in Berlin.

COVER: A detailed section of a stained glass window 21 × 56″ depicting the natural history of influenza viruses and zoonotic exchange in the emergence of new strains was used to design the front cover. Based on the work done at St. Jude Children's Research Hospital supported by American Lebanese Syrian Associated Charities (ALSAC) and the National Institute of Allergy and Infectious Diseases (NIAID). Artist: Jenny Hammond, Highgreenleycleugh, Northumberland, England.

*"Knowing is not enough; we must apply.
Willing is not enough; we must do."*
—Goethe

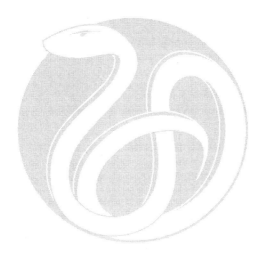

INSTITUTE OF MEDICINE
OF THE NATIONAL ACADEMIES

Advising the Nation. Improving Health.

THE NATIONAL ACADEMIES
Advisers to the Nation on Science, Engineering, and Medicine

The **National Academy of Sciences** is a private, nonprofit, self-perpetuating society of distinguished scholars engaged in scientific and engineering research, dedicated to the furtherance of science and technology and to their use for the general welfare. Upon the authority of the charter granted to it by the Congress in 1863, the Academy has a mandate that requires it to advise the federal government on scientific and technical matters. Dr. Ralph J. Cicerone is president of the National Academy of Sciences.

The **National Academy of Engineering** was established in 1964, under the charter of the National Academy of Sciences, as a parallel organization of outstanding engineers. It is autonomous in its administration and in the selection of its members, sharing with the National Academy of Sciences the responsibility for advising the federal government. The National Academy of Engineering also sponsors engineering programs aimed at meeting national needs, encourages education and research, and recognizes the superior achievements of engineers. Dr. Wm. A. Wulf is president of the National Academy of Engineering.

The **Institute of Medicine** was established in 1970 by the National Academy of Sciences to secure the services of eminent members of appropriate professions in the examination of policy matters pertaining to the health of the public. The Institute acts under the responsibility given to the National Academy of Sciences by its congressional charter to be an adviser to the federal government and, upon its own initiative, to identify issues of medical care, research, and education. Dr. Harvey V. Fineberg is president of the Institute of Medicine.

The **National Research Council** was organized by the National Academy of Sciences in 1916 to associate the broad community of science and technology with the Academy's purposes of furthering knowledge and advising the federal government. Functioning in accordance with general policies determined by the Academy, the Council has become the principal operating agency of both the National Academy of Sciences and the National Academy of Engineering in providing services to the government, the public, and the scientific and engineering communities. The Council is administered jointly by both Academies and the Institute of Medicine. Dr. Ralph J. Cicerone and Dr. Wm. A. Wulf are chair and vice chair, respectively, of the National Research Council.

www.national-academies.org

FORUM ON MICROBIAL THREATS

Stanley M. Lemon (*Chair*), School of Medicine, University of Texas Medical Branch, Galveston
P. Frederick Sparling (*Vice-chair*), University of North Carolina, Chapel Hill
Margaret A. Hamburg (*Vice-chair*), Nuclear Threat Initiative/Global Health & Security Initiative, Washington, D.C.
David Acheson, Center for Food Safety and Applied Nutrition, Food and Drug Administration, Rockville, Maryland
Ruth Berkelman, Emory University, Center for Public Health Preparedness and Research, Rollins School of Public Health, Atlanta, Georgia
Roger Breeze, Centaur Science Group, Washington, D.C.
Steven J. Brickner, Pfizer Global Research and Development, Pfizer Inc., Groton, Connecticut
Joseph Bryan, Office of Medical Services, Department of State, Washington, D.C.
Nancy Carter-Foster, Program for Emerging Infections and HIV/AIDS, U.S. Department of State, Washington, D.C.
Mark Feinberg, Merck Vaccine Division, Merck & Co., West Point, Pennsylvania
J. Patrick Fitch, Lawrence Livermore National Laboratory, Livermore, California
S. Elizabeth George, Biological and Chemical Countermeasures Program, Department of Homeland Security, Washington, D.C.
Jesse L. Goodman, Center for Biologics Evaluation and Research, Food and Drug Administration, Rockville, Maryland
Eduardo Gotuzzo, Instituto de Medicina Tropical–Alexander von Humbolt, Universidad Peruana Cayetano Heredia, Lima, Peru
Jo Handelsman, College of Agricultural and Life Sciences, University of Wisconsin, Madison
Carole A. Heilman, Division of Microbiology and Infectious Diseases, National Institute of Allergy and Infectious Diseases, National Institutes of Health, Bethesda, Maryland
David L. Heymann, Polio Eradication, World Health Organization, Geneva, Switzerland
Phil Hosbach, New Products and Immunization Policy, Sanofi Pasteur, Swiftwater, Pennsylvania
James M. Hughes, Global Infectious Diseases Program, Emory University, Atlanta, Georgia
Stephen Johnston, University of Texas Southwestern Medical Center, Dallas
Gerald T. Keusch, Boston University School of Medicine and Boston University School of Public Health, Massachusetts
Lonnie King, College of Veterinary Medicine, Michigan State University, East Lansing

George Korch, United States Army Medical Research Institute for Infectious Diseases, Ft. Detrick, Maryland
Joshua Lederberg, The Rockefeller University, New York
Joseph Malone, Department of Defense Global Emerging Infections System, Walter Reed Army Institute of Research, Silver Spring, Maryland
Lynn Marks, Medicine Development Center, GlaxoSmithKline, Collegeville, Pennsylvania
Stephen S. Morse, Center for Public Health Preparedness, Columbia University, New York
Michael T. Osterholm, Center for Infectious Disease Research and Policy, School of Public Health, University of Minnesota, Minneapolis
George Poste, Arizona BioDesign Institute, Arizona State University, Tempe
David A. Relman, Stanford University, Palo Alto, California
Gary A. Roselle, Central Office, Veterans Health Administration, Department of Veterans Affairs, Washington, D.C.
Anne Schuchat, National Center for Infectious Diseases, Centers for Disease Control and Prevention, Atlanta, Georgia
Janet Shoemaker, Office of Public Affairs, American Society for Microbiology, Washington, D.C.
Brian Staskawicz, Department of Plant and Microbial Biology, University of California, Berkeley
Terence Taylor, International Institute for Strategic Studies, Washington, D.C.

Liaisons

Enriqueta Bond, Burroughs Wellcome Fund, Research Triangle Park, North Carolina
Nancy Carter-Foster, Program for Emerging Infections and HIV/AIDS, U.S. Department of State, Washington, D.C.
Edward McSweegan, National Institute of Allergy and Infectious Diseases, National Institutes of Health, Bethesda, Maryland

Staff

Eileen Choffnes, Forum Director
Stacey Knobler, Former Forum Director*
Elizabeth Kitchens, Research Associate**
Kim Lundberg, Research Associate
Allison Mack, Science Writer
Muhammad Salaam, Project Assistant
Kate Skoczdopole, Research Associate

---

*Until December 2004
**Until March 2005

Reviewers

This report has been reviewed in draft form by individuals chosen for their diverse perspectives and technical expertise, in accordance with procedures approved by the National Research Council's Report Review Committee. The purpose of this independent review is to provide candid and critical comments that will assist the institution in making its published report as sound as possible and to ensure that the report meets institutional standards for objectivity, evidence, and responsiveness to the study charge. The review comments and draft manuscript remain confidential to protect the integrity of the deliberative process. We wish to thank the following individuals for their review of this report:

John Bailar, University of Chicago, Illinois
Ruth Berkelman, Center for Public Health Preparedness and Research, Rollings School of Public Health, Emory University, Atlanta, Georgia
Lora Hooper, Center for Immunology, University of Texas Southwestern Medical Center, Dallas
Stephen S. Morse, Center for Public Health Preparedness, School of Public Health, Columbia University, New York

The review of this report was overseen by **Melvin Worth,** Scholar-in-Residence, National Academies, who was responsible for making certain that an independent examination of this report was carried out in accordance with institutional procedures and that all review comments were carefully considered. Responsibility for the final content of this report rests entirely with the authoring committee and the institution.

Preface

The Forum on Emerging Infections was created in 1996 in response to a request from the Centers for Disease Control and Prevention and the National Institutes of Health. It was established by the Institute of Medicine (IOM) to provide structured opportunities for leaders from government, academia, and industry to meet and examine issues of shared concern regarding research, prevention, detection, and management of emerging or reemerging infectious diseases. In pursuing this task, the Forum provides a venue to foster the exchange of information and ideas, identify areas in need of greater attention, clarify policy issues by enhancing knowledge and identifying points of agreement, and inform decision makers about science and policy issues. The Forum seeks to illuminate issues rather than resolve them directly; for this reason, it does not provide advice or recommendations on any specific policy initiative pending before any agency or organization. Rather, its strengths are embodied in the diversity of its membership and the contributions of individual members expressed throughout the activities of the Forum. In September 2003, the Forum changed its name to the Forum on Microbial Threats.

ABOUT THE WORKSHOP

In the mid-1970s, the U.S. Surgeon General claimed that infectious diseases had been conquered through the development and use of antibiotics and vaccines and that therefore it was time to shift the U.S. government's attention and resources to the "War on Cancer." The ensuing years have brought us Legionnaire's disease, toxic shock syndrome, an awareness of Lyme disease, outbreaks of hantavirus throughout the southwestern United States, SARS, and of course, HIV. The discovery that infection with *Helicobacter pylori* is associated with peptic ulcer and gastric cancer has led to an increasing search for the infectious nature of other "noninfectious" diseases such as atherosclerosis.

Infectious diseases remain the leading causes of death and morbidity on our planet. For these reasons, the IOM's Forum on Microbial Threats hosted a public workshop: "Ending the War Metaphor: The Future Agenda for Unraveling the Host-Microbe Relationship." Through invited presentations and discussion, this workshop aimed to inform the Forum, the public, and policymakers of the dynamic host-microbe-environment relationships and to explore the issues that must be resolved to better prepare and protect the global community from infectious disease threats.

Resistance in microbes—bacterial, viral, or protozoan—to therapeutics is not surprising or new. It is, however, an increasing challenge as drug resistance accumulates and accelerates, even as the drugs for combating infections are reduced in power and number. Today some strains of bacterial and viral infections are treatable with only a single drug, some no longer have effective treatments. The disease burden from multidrug-resistant strains of tuberculosis, malaria, hepatitis, and HIV is growing in both developed and developing countries.

The challenges of resistance are compounded by growing concerns about the possible use of biological weapons leading to large-scale disease outbreak or exposure. The ability to respond effectively to such exposures could be significantly compromised by the introduction of drug-resistant pathogens. The use of prophylactic drugs or therapies on large populations may also contribute to the development of drug resistance and thus increase both the immediate and longer-term challenges of treating infectious diseases.

With such evidence of a dwindling armamentarium to wage our wars against infectious diseases, it has been suggested that a paradigm shift is warranted in how we address the threats posed by pathogens. In an attempt for the Forum to understand how such a new lens might be devised through which the challenges of disease should be viewed, the presentations and discussions of the workshop were structured to explore the existing knowledge and unanswered questions indicated by (but not limited to) the following topics:

- host-pathogen interactions: defining the concepts of pathogenicity, virulence, colonization, commensalism, and symbiosis;
- the ecology of host-microbe interactions;
- understanding the dynamic relationships of host-microbe interactions;
- novel approaches for mitigating or minimizing the development of antimicrobial resistance; and
- challenges and opportunities for developing a new paradigm to replace the "war metaphor" of the host-microbial relationship.

The issues pertaining to these topical areas were addressed through invited presentations and subsequent discussions that highlighted the complexity and incompleteness of our appreciation of the dynamic interplay between a host and its associated microbial flora and fauna, and identified areas for research collaborations within and between the clinical medicine, veterinary medicine, and plant pathology communities.

ACKNOWLEDGMENTS

The Forum on Microbial Threats and the IOM wish to express their warmest appreciation to the individuals and organizations who gave valuable time to provide information and advice to the Forum through their participation in the workshop. A full list of presenters can be found in Appendix A.

The Forum is indebted to the IOM staff who contributed during the course of the workshop and the production of this workshop summary. On behalf of the Forum, we gratefully acknowledge the efforts led by Eileen Choffnes, director of the Forum, Kim Lundberg, research associate, and Kate Skoczdopole, research associate, who dedicated much effort and time to developing this workshop's agenda, and for their thoughtful and insightful approach and skill in translating the workshop proceedings and discussion into this workshop summary. We would also like to thank our science writer, Alison Mack, for her thoughtful and insightful approach and skill in translating the workshop proceedings and discussion into this workshop summary.

Finally, the Forum also thanks sponsors that supported this activity. Financial support for this project was provided by the American Society for Microbiology; Burroughs Wellcome Fund; Defense Threat Reduction Agency; GlaxoSmithKline; Infectious Disease Society of America; Lawrence Livermore National Laboratory; Merck; Pfizer; Sanofi Pasteur; U.S. Department of Health and Human Services' National Institutes of Health/National Institute for Allergies and Infectious Disease and Centers for Disease Control and Prevention; U.S. Department of Defense/Global Emerging Infections Surveillance/Walter Reed Army Institute of Research; U.S. Department of Homeland Security; U.S. Department of State; and U.S. Department of Veterans Affairs. The views presented in this workshop summary are those of the editors and workshop participants and are not necessarily those of the funding organizations.

Stanley M. Lemon, *Chair*
P. Frederick Sparling, *Vice-chair*
Margaret Hamburg, *Vice-chair*
Forum on Microbial Threats

Contents

	SUMMARY AND ASSESSMENT	1
1	MICROBIAL COMMUNITIES OF THE GUT	35

The Role of the Indigenous Microbiota in Zebrafish
Gastrointestinal Tract Development, 36
    Karen Guillemin
Host-Bacterial Mutualism in the Human Intestine, 41
    Fredrik Bäckhed, Ruth E. Ley, Justin L. Sonnenburg,
    Daniel A. Peterson, Jeffrey I. Gordon
Activities of Human Colonic Microbes, 52
    Abigail A. Salyers

2	BEYOND THE GUT: INSIGHTS FROM OTHER HOST-MICROBE SYSTEMS	80

It Takes a Village: Role of Indigenous Microbial Communities in
Infectious Disease, 81
    Christina Matta and Jo Handelsman
The Molecular Basis of Bacterial Innate Immunity in
Arabidopsis thaliana, 91
    Brian Staskawicz

3	THE ECOLOGY OF PATHOGENESIS	102

The Zen of Pathogenicity, 103
    Stanley Falkow

Pathogenicity and Symbiosis: Human Gastric Colonization by
Helicobacter pylori as a Model System of Amphibiosis, 115
  Martin J. Blaser
Induction of Pathogenic Immune Responses in Susceptible Hosts
by Commensal Enteric Bacteria, 131
  R. Balfour Sartor
How Do Changes in Microecology Affect the Human Host?, 140
  María G. Domínguez-Bello

4   THE HOST RESPONSE TO PATHOGENS   **159**
The Intestinal Epithelium: An Interactive Barrier Between Host
and Microbe, 160
  Marian Neutra
How the Host "Sees" and Responds to Pathogens, 167
  David A. Relman

**5   ADDRESSING COMPLEXITY IN MICROBIAL AND HOST
COMMUNITIES**   **175**
DNA Microarrays as Salivary Diagnostic Tools for Characterizing
the Oral Cavity's Microbial Community, 176
  *Laura M. Smoot, James C. Smoot, Hauke Smidt, Peter A. Noble,
  Martin Könneke, Z.A. McMurry, and David A. Stahl*
Population Biology of Multiple Hosts and Multiple Pathogens, 185
  Mark E.J. Woolhouse and Sonya Gowtage-Sequeira
Host Range and Emerging and Reemerging Pathogens, 192
  Mark E.J. Woolhouse and Sonya Gowtage-Sequeira

**6   MANIPULATING HOST-MICROBE INTERACTIONS:
PROBIOTIC RESEARCH AND REGULATIONS**   **207**
Molecular Analysis of Probiotic-Host Interactions in the
Gastrointestinal Tract, 209
  Michiel Kleerebezem
Role of Probiotics in Modulation of Host Immune Response, 220
  *Susanna Cunningham-Rundles, Siv Ahrne, John Peoples,
  Francesca Tatad, Mohamed Mohamed, and Mirjana Nesin*
Regulating Pre- and Probiotics: A U.S. FDA Perspective, 229
  Julienne Vaillancourt
From Research in Microbiology to Guidelines, 237
  Lorenzo Morelli and Elena Bessi

APPENDIXES

A   AGENDA   261

B   ACRONYMS   265

C   FORUM MEMBER BIOGRAPHIES   268

Tables and Figures

TABLES

1-1 Comparison of the Glycoside Hydrolase and Polysaccharide Lyases in the Human, Mouse, and *B thetaiotaomicron* Genomes, 63

1-2 Effects of the Microbiota on Host Biology, Defined by Comparing Germ-Free (GF) and Conventionally-Raised (CONV-R) Rodents, 69

1-3 Six Ways Environmental Engineers Improve Bioreactor Efficiency, 73

3-1 Genes Associated with IBD and Experimental Colitis, 138

5-1 Counts of All, Emerging or Reemerging and Zoonotic Species of Human Pathogens and Comparison of the Relative Risks of Emergence for Zoonotic and Nonzoonotic Species for Each of the Major Pathogen Groups, 186

5-2 Main Categories of Drivers Associated with Emergence and Reemergence of Human Pathogens, 194

6-1 Overview of Genome Sequences of Food-Grade Bacteria, 213

6-2 Functional Classification of Predicted *ivi* Gene Functions in *L. plantarum* and Pathogenic Bacteria, 216

6-3 *Lactobacillus* Species Recovered and Genetically Identified from Biopsies of Seven Adults, 242

6-4 Host Specificity of the *Lactobacillus* Species, 244

FIGURES

S-1   The Convergence Model, 5

1-1   Important events in zebrafish development, 37
1-2   Representation of the diversity of bacteria in the human intestine, 44
1-3   Taxon richness estimates for bacteria in the human GI tract, 46
1-4   Lessons about adaptive foraging for glycans obtained from
      B. thetaiotaomicron, 48
1-5   The flow of contents through the small intestine and colon, 54
1-6   Flow of antibiotic resistance genes (hypothetical), 60

2-1   Ferdinand Julius Cohn (1828–1898), Heinrich Anton De Bary
      (1832–1888), and Robert Koch (1843–1910), 83
2-2   Schematic depiction of the first strategies to select in vivo for
      promoters that are induced by plant (left panel) or animal
      (right panel) hosts, 86
2-3   A rice plant (left) and *Arabidopsis thaliana* (right), a model plant
      for host-pathogen interactions, 92
2-4   Phenotypes of bacterial disease resistance, 95
2-5   *Arabidopsis* disease resistance genes, 96
2-6   Representative protein motifs found in immune receptors of plants
      and animals, 97
2-7   Model for RPS2-mediated innate immunity, 98
2-8   Model of RPS2-mediated immunity in *Arabidopsis*, 99

3-1   Host macrophage engulfing the plague bacillus (*Yersinia pestis*), 104
3-2   Infectious diseases were, and still are, the most common cause of
      death worldwide, 105
3-3   Illustration of the old rhyme (based on a poem by Jonathan Swift,
      author of *Gulliver's Travels*), "Big fleas have little fleas upon their
      backs to bite them, and little fleas have lesser fleas and, so on,
      ad infinitum.", 114
3-4   Modern and ancient *H. pylori* populations, 116
3-5   Who are we?, 118
3-6   Schematic of the natural history of *H. pylori* populations and host
      characteristics in colonized individuals over their lifetime, 119
3-7   Equilibrium relationships between coevolved persistent microbes and
      their hosts, 120
3-8   Prevalence of *H. pylori* in human populations in developing and
      developed countries, 121
3-9   Potential pathways by which *H. pylori* colonization increases risk of
      gastric cancer, 125

TABLES AND FIGURES   xviii

3-10 Proposed reciprocal relationship between adenocarcinomas of the stomach and esophagus, 127
3-11 Schematic of *H pylori* variation in a single host, 130
3-12 Induction of homeostatic or pathogenic immune responses by commensal bacteria, 132
3-13 Immune activation and chronic intestinal inflammation depends on the presence of commensal luminal bacteria in multiple animal models, 134
3-14 Interaction of genetic, environmental, and microbial factors in the pathogenesis of IBD, 136
3-15 Fate of dietary products in the rumen, providing microbial products and biomass for the nutrition of the host, 142
3-16 Model of modulation of adaptive and innate immunity by indigenous bacteria, showing the unknown effect of other microbes on mucosal immunity, 144
3-17 Evolution of human societies and their diseases, 146
3-18 Host-microbial interactions shape health and disease, 147

4-1 The follicle-associated epithelium and MALT: a close collaboration, 161
4-2 Reovirus has access to carbohydrate receptors on M cells, 163
4-3 The "backpack" hybridoma tumor protocol, 165
4-4 Variation in gene expression in health and disease, 171

5-1 Phylogenetic tree generated from small subunit rRNA sequences of oral microorganisms, 178
5-2 Description of the MAGIChip DNA oligonucleotide microarray technology used in the Stahl Laboratory, 182
5-3 Numbers of species of zoonotic pathogens associated with different types of nonhuman host, 197
5-4 Relationship between breadth of host range and the fraction of pathogen species regarded as emerging or reemerging, 198
5-5 Expected relationship between outbreak size and two key epidemiologic parameters, 201

6-1 Schematic representation of pure culture genomics in relation to GI tract behavior, and corresponding molecular analyses of host responses, 212
6-2 Response of CD8+ naive (CD45RA+) and CD8+ memory (CD45 RO+) cord blood T cells to bacterial antigens, 226
6-3 Intracellular cytokine response of cord blood monocytes from term infants to bacterial antigens, 227

6-4 Differential response of T cells (CD3+) and natural killer (NK) subpopulations defined as NK (CD3–CD56+), NK bright (CD3–CD56+bright), and NKT (CD56+CD3+) lymphocytes from HIV-positive children to bacterial antigens, 228
6-5 Stages of premarket review and regulation for live biotherapeutics, 235
6-6 Guidelines for the evaluation of probiotics for food use, 249

Summary and Assessment

ENDING THE WAR METAPHOR: THE CHANGING AGENDA FOR UNRAVELING THE HOST-MICROBE RELATIONSHIP

The History of Medicine

2000 B.C.—Here, eat this root.
1000 A.D.—That root is heathen. Here, say this prayer.
1850 A.D.—That prayer is superstition. Here, drink this potion.
1920 A.D.—That potion is snake oil. Here, swallow this pill.
1945 A.D.—That pill is ineffective. Here, take this penicillin.
1955 A.D.—Oops . . . bugs mutated. Here, take this tetracycline.
1960–1999—39 more "oops." Here, take this more powerful antibiotic.
2000 A.D.—The bugs have won! Here, eat this root.

—Anonymous (WHO, 2000)

In 1967, U.S. Surgeon General William H. Stewart told a White House gathering of health officers that "it was time to close the book on infectious diseases and shift all national attention (and dollars) to what he termed 'the New Dimensions' of health: chronic diseases" (Garrett, 1994; Stewart, 1967). In the ensuing years, Americans became intimately acquainted with a range of emerging infections including Legionnaire's disease, toxic shock syndrome, AIDS, Lyme disease, West Nile encephalitis, and SARS. Complacency has given way to concern regarding a spectrum of microbial threats—including antimicrobial-resistant pathogens, emergent and reemergent diseases with pandemic potential, and outbreaks of exotic viruses such as monkeypox—propelled by a seemingly inevitable convergence of biological, environmental, ecological, and socioeconomic factors (IOM, 2003a,b). At the same time, the association of various chronic diseases with microbial infection (e.g, peptic ulcer with *Helicobacter pylori*, liver cancer with hepatitis B and C viruses, and Lyme arthritis with *Borrelia burgdorferi*) has deepened respect for the destructive potential of infectious agents (IOM, 2004).

Infectious diseases continue to cause high morbidity and mortality throughout the world, particularly in developing countries. In 2001, infectious diseases accounted for an estimated 26 percent of deaths worldwide (Kindhauser, 2003). Moreover, there are indications that the tide of human conquest over microbial pathogens is turning. Over the last 30 years, 37 new pathogens have been identified as human disease threats, and an estimated 12 percent of known human pathogens have been recognized as either emerging or reemerging (Merell and Falkow, 2004). Having fallen steadily since the turn of the century, the number of deaths attributable to infection in the United States began to increase in the early 1980s, due in large part to the HIV/AIDS pandemic (Armstrong et al., 1999; Lederberg, 2000).

In the face of these challenges, the metaphor of "war" on infectious diseases—characterized by the systematic search for the microbial "cause" of each disease, followed by the development of antimicrobial therapies—can no longer guide biomedical science or clinical medicine. A new paradigm is needed that incorporates a more realistic and detailed picture of the dynamic interactions among and between host organisms and their diverse populations of microbes, only a fraction of which act as pathogens. To explore the crafting of a new metaphor for host-microbe relationships, and to consider how such a new perspective might inform and prioritize biomedical research, the Forum on Microbial Threats of the Institute of Medicine (IOM) convened the workshop, *Ending the War Metaphor: The Changing Agenda for Unraveling the Host-Microbe Relationship* on March 16 and 17, 2005.

Workshop participants reviewed current knowledge and approaches to studying the best-known host-microbe system—the bacterial inhabitants of the human gut—as well as key findings from studies of microbial communities associated with other mammals, fish, plants, soil, and insects. Participants and discussants also considered the evolutionary and environmental origins of pathogenesis and reviewed recent findings describing how hosts recognize and respond to pathogens. Additional presentations and discussions addressed the complexity of microbial communities and ecological relationships among pathogens, such as zoonoses, that infect multiple hosts. Finally, participants examined the prospects for manipulating host-microbe relationships to promote health and mitigate disease.

The workshop's primary goal of replacing the war metaphor for infectious disease intervention represents an expansion of the Forum's focus on microbial threats to health. The perspective adopted herein is one that recognizes the breadth and diversity of host-microbe relationships beyond those relative few that result in overt disease.

ORGANIZATION OF WORKSHOP SUMMARY

This workshop summary report is prepared for the Forum membership in the name of the editors as a collection of individually authored papers and commentary. Sections of the workshop summary not specifically attributed to an individual reflect the views of the editors and not those of the Forum on Microbial Threats, its sponsors, or the Institute of Medicine (IOM). The contents of the unattributed sections are based on the presentations and discussions that took place during the workshop.

The workshop summary is organized within chapters as a topic-by-topic description of the presentations and discussions. Its purpose is to present lessons from relevant experience, delineate a range of pivotal issues and their respective problems, and put forth some potential responses as described by the workshop participants.

Although this workshop summary provides an account of the individual presentations, it also reflects an important aspect of the Forum philosophy. The workshop functions as a dialogue among representatives from different sectors and presents their beliefs on which areas may merit further attention. However, the reader should be aware that the material presented here expresses the views and opinions of the individuals participating in the workshop and not the deliberations of a formally constituted IOM study committee. These proceedings summarize only what participants stated in the workshop and are not intended to be an exhaustive exploration of the subject matter or a representation of consensus evaluation.

THE RISE AND FALL OF THE WAR METAPHOR

More than a century of research, sparked by the germ theory of disease and rooted in historic notions of contagion that long precede Pasteur and Koch's 19th-century research and intellectual synthesis, underlies current knowledge of microbe-host interactions (Lederberg, 2000). This pathogen-centered understanding attributed disease entirely to the actions of "invading" microorganisms, thereby drawing the lines of battle between "them" and "us," the injured hosts (Casadevall and Pirofski, 1999). Although it was recognized in Koch's time that some microbes did not cause disease in previously exposed hosts (e.g., milkmaids who had been exposed to cowpox did not become infected with smallpox), the fact that his postulates[1] could not account for microbes that did not cause

---

[1] Koch's postulates include the following: (1) the bacteria must be present in every case of the disease, (2) the bacteria must be isolated from the host with the disease and grown in pure culture, (3) the specific disease must be reproduced when a pure culture of the bacteria is inoculated into a healthy susceptible host, and (4) the bacteria must be recoverable from the experimentally infected host.

disease in all hosts was not generally appreciated until the advent of vaccines and the subsequent introduction of immunosuppressive therapies in the 20th century (Casadevall and Pirofski, 1999; Isenberg, 1988). By then, the paradigm of the systematized search for the microbial causes of disease, followed by the development of antimicrobial and other therapies to eradicate them, had been firmly established in clinical practice.

The considerable impact of this approach, further enabled by improvements in sanitation, diet, and living conditions in the industrialized world, served to cement the belief that humanity was engaged in a war against pathogenic microbes, and that we were winning (Lederberg, 2000). By the mid-1960s, experts opined that, since infectious disease was all but controlled, researchers should focus their attention on other difficult medical challenges, such as heart disease, cancer, and psychiatric disorders. This optimism and complacency was shaken with the appearance of HIV/AIDS in the early 1980s, and was dealt a further blow with the emergence and spread of multidrug-resistant bacteria. As these experiences began to lead researchers to reexamine the host-microbe relationship, additional reasons to do so began to accumulate: pandemic threats from newly emergent (e.g., SARS) and reemergent (e.g., influenza) infectious diseases; lethal outbreaks of Ebola, hantavirus, and other such exotic viruses; and a new appreciation for the associations of various chronic diseases with prior microbial infections, as noted above.

Forum member Joshua Lederberg has envisioned the future of humanity and microbes as "episodes of a suspense thriller that could be entitled, *Our Wits Versus Their Genes*" (Lederberg, 2000). Our wits have so far afforded us increased longevity and reduced mortality from infectious disease, but the defenses we have mounted to make these gains are no match, over the long run, for the rapidly changing and adaptable genomes of microbial pathogens. We are vulnerable not only to emerging infectious diseases, but also to less treatable strains of pathogens (e.g., *Staphylococcus aureus*, *Streptococcus pneumoniae*) once seemingly conquered. The global health threat and economic burden posed by microbial resistance to therapeutics was highlighted in a recent Forum workshop, in which participants concluded that the management of microbial resistance over the long term would require "a sea of change…in how we view the ecology and evolution of infection" and the recognition of resistance "as an integral part—not an aberrant part—of the ecology of microbial life" (IOM, 2003b). However, doing so will require a far greater understanding of the evolutionary processes that underlie the development of resistance.

Changes in global ecology, climate, and weather are also increasing human vulnerability and exposure to microbial threats, as are more localized factors such as economic development, land use, travel, poverty, and war. A convergence of biological, environmental, sociopolitical, and ecological factors, depicted in Figure S-1, can be seen to influence the host-microbe relationships that lie at the core of disease emergence.

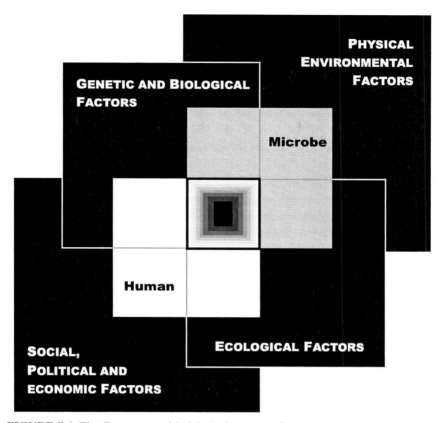

FIGURE S-1 The Convergence Model. At the center of the model is a box representing the convergence of factors leading to the emergence of an infectious disease. The interior of the box is a gradient flowing from white to black; the white outer edges represent what is known about the factors in emergence, and the black center represents the unknown (similar to the theoretical construct of the "black box" with its unknown constituents and means of operation). Interlocking with the center box are the two focal players in a microbial threat to health—the human and the microbe. The microbe-host interaction is influenced by the interlocking domains of the determinants of the emergence of infection: genetic and biological factors; physical environmental factors; ecological factors; and social, political, and economic factors.
SOURCE: IOM (2003a).

PATHOGENESIS REVISITED

The vast majority of microbes do not produce overt illness in their hosts, but instead establish themselves as persistent colonists that can be described as either low-impact parasites (e.g., causes of asymptomatic infection), commensals (organisms that "eat from the same table," deriving benefit without harming their hosts), or symbionts (establishing a mutually beneficial relationship with the host) (Blaser, 1997; Merrell and Falkow, 2004). These states, while separate, represent part of a continuum—one that extends to pathogenesis and disease—that may be occupied at any point by a specific microbial species through the influence of environmental and genetic factors (Casadevall and Pirofski, 2000, 2002, 2003). Persistent colonization of a host by a microbe is rarely a random event; such coexistence depends upon a relationship between host and microbe that can be characterized as a stable equilibrium (Blaser, 1997). In the case of microbes that cause persistent, asymptomatic infection, physiological or genetic changes in either host or microbe may disrupt this equilibrium and shift the relationship toward pathogenesis, resulting in illness and possibly death for the host (Merrell and Falkow, 2004).

Early views of pathogenesis and virulence were based on the assumption that these characteristics were intrinsic properties of microorganisms, although it was recognized that pathogenesis was neither invariant nor absolute (Casadevall and Pirofski, 1999). Over the course of the last century, the identification of increasing numbers of microbial pathogens and the characterization of the diseases they cause has begun to reveal the extraordinary complexity and individuality of host-pathogen relationships. As a result, it has become exceedingly difficult to identify what makes a microbe a pathogen. One response to this dilemma has been to define pathogenesis from the perspective of the host, who experiences disease only when the presence of a microbe (whether protozoan, bacterial, or viral) results in damage—whether that damage is actually mediated by the pathogen itself, or by the host's immune response to it (Casadevall and Pirofski, 1999, 2003).

A broader view, reflected in many workshop presentations and discussions, considers how pathogens coexist within host-microbial communities and places infectious disease within an ecological context. This perspective acknowledges the ecological and evolutionary impact of advancing civilization—and particularly the "war on disease"—on host-microbe systems, and promotes a more realistic, deeper, and nuanced understanding of the relationships upon which these systems depend (Lederberg, 2000). The time has come to abandon notions that put host against microbe in favor of an ecological view that recognizes the interdependence of hosts with their microbial flora and fauna and the importance of each for the other's survival. Such a paradigm shift would advance efforts to domesticate and subvert potential pathogens and to explore and exploit the vast potential of nonpathogenic microbial communities to improve health.[2]

---

[2] Refer to p. 27 first paragraph under the section "Raising Awareness of the Host-Microbe Relationship" for further information on the paradigm shift.

IT'S A SMALL WORLD: MICROBIAL COMMUNITIES OF THE GUT

The gastrointestinal (GI) tract represents an important and challenging system for exploring how microbial communities become established within their hosts, how their members maintain stable ecological niches, and how these dynamics relate to host health and disease (see Chapter 1). The complex, dynamic, and spatially diversified microbial community, or *microbiota*, of the human gut is believed to be comprised of at least 10^{13} microorganisms (Xu and Gordon, 2003). This estimation includes more than 800 species of bacteria (Bäckhed et al., 2005; Gordon, 2005) (most of which have not yet been successfully cultured in the laboratory), fungi, numerous viral species including bacteriophages, (Breitbart et al., 2003) archaea (e.g., methanogens), and eukaryotes (e.g., helminths and protozoa) (Dominguez-Bello, 2005; Fagarasan et al., 2002; Hylemon and Harder, 1998; Xu and Gordon, 2003). The collective genomes of the microbiota in the human gut, known as the *microbiome*, is approximately one hundred-fold larger than that of its host (Bäckhed et al., 2004; Savage, 1977; Xu and Gordon, 2003). Therefore, as Bäckhed et al. have recently argued, "It seems appropriate to view ourselves as a composite of many species and our genetic landscape as an amalgam" of the human genome and the microbiome (2005).

The complexity of the human gut microbiota has been studied using culture-based assays and, more recently, a variety of molecular methods. These include fluorescent in situ hybridization, terminal restriction fragment length polymorphisms, microarrays, and direct sequencing of 16S libraries (Breitbart et al., 2003). The latter has revealed the presence of only 8 of 55 known bacterial divisions in the human gut, but great diversity among them at the strain and subspecies level exists (Bäckhed et al., 2005; Winter et al, 2004). This pattern suggests strong selection pressure on these microbes and coevolution between them and their host—a conclusion supported by findings that reveal how *Bacteroides thetaiotaomicron*, a prominent intestinal anaerobe, maintains a stable ecological niche despite dietary shifts and attacks by bacteriophage and the human immune system (see Gordon in Chapter 1). Knowledge of the viral components of the gut microbiota is comparatively limited; however, a recent study of viral genotypes in human feces (Breitbart et al., 2003) suggests that bacteriophages play an important role in shaping the gut microbiome (Bäckhed et al., 2005). Methanogenic archaea in the gut appear to orchestrate the final step in processing plant polysaccharides, but their role in determining the structural and functional stability and diversity of the gut microbiota is largely unexplored (Bäckhed et al., 2005; Gordon, 2005).

The Molecular Basis of Mutualism

The gut microbiota acts as an exquisitely tuned metabolic "organ" within the host, according to presenter Jeffrey Gordon (see Chapter 1) (Bäckhed et al., 2004;

Casadevall and Pirofski, 2000; Xu and Gordon, 2003). Microbes and mammals have coevolved mutually beneficial (symbiotic) relationships, typically based on nutrient sharing, in which the microbiota perform functions that their hosts have not evolved. For example, mammals are inherently limited in their ability to break down polysaccharides, which represent an abundant energy source in a plant-based diet (Hooper et al., 2002). Instead of producing the enzymes for carbohydrate hydrolysis, mammals recruit a diverse community of microorganisms that allow them to make efficient use of a broad range of foodstuffs; the microbes, in turn, gain access to abundant, readily fermentable carbon sources. An especially complex version of this exchange occurs among ruminants, who obtain nutrients solely by digesting the bacteria that feed upon the grass and other fodder swallowed by their mammalian hosts, as described by presenter Maria Dominguez-Bello (see Chapter 3). Thus over the course of evolution, symbiotic gut bacteria have become master physiological chemists, employing a broad range of strategies to manipulate host genomes, Gordon observed.

Identifying the host genes targeted by gut microbes and the mechanisms by which they manipulate host gene expression could lead to novel approaches for preventing and controlling a variety of diseases and promoting human health. To explore such host-microbe interactions at a molecular level, researchers have introduced genetically mutable components of the human intestinal microbiota into germ-free animals (Bäckhed et al., 2004; Hooper et al., 1998, 2001, 2002; Rawls et al., 2004; Xu and Gordon, 2003); several such studies are described in Chapter 1. Examination of the transcriptional response of germ-free mice to colonization with *B. thetaiotaomicron* reveal that the bacterium modulates the expression of host genes known to influence a wide range of intestinal functions in addition to nutrient absorption, including mucosal barrier formation, xenobiotic metabolism, angiogenesis, and postnatal intestinal maturation (Hooper et al., 2001; Xu and Gordon, 2003). Related studies show that in addition to mediating energy harvest from the diet, the gut microbiota also influences energy storage by the host, and thereby, individual predisposition toward obesity (see Gordon in Chapter 1) (Bäckhed et al., 2004).

Additional research being performed in germ-free animals involves the initial establishment of microbiota in the gut (in humans, during the early days of infancy), its influence on host development (e.g., immunity), and the mechanisms by which hosts perceive and respond to the presence of colonizing microbes. Presenter Karen Guillemin (see Chapter 1) pursues these fundamental questions in germ-free zebrafish, an experimental system that simplifies analyses of microbial influence on host development while closely approximating GI tract and immune system maturation, as well as gut microbiota diversity, in mammals. Although this approach has demonstrated the pervasive influence of the microbiota over a variety of events in the maturation of the GI tract, it raises further questions regarding the potential for individual developmental variation arising from differences in microbiota from one member of a species to another. In humans, such variation could accrue among contemporaries who live in different environments, as well as over the course of history.

Microbe-Microbe Interactions

The complex web of interactions that must occur among the denizens of the gut is even less well studied than those that take place between microbe and host, but undoubtedly no less important to gut function and development. Microbe-microbe relationships include nutritional interactions—such as the previously described metabolism of the end products of bacterial fermentation by archaea—and genetic exchanges that occur through transformation, phage transduction, and conjugation (see Salyers in Chapter 1). For example, *Bacteroides* species recently have been shown to acquire and transfer antibiotic resistance genes among distantly related bacteria (e.g., *Escherichia coli*) that colonize the same ecological niche (Whittle et al., 2002; Wilson and Salyers, 2003). While important as a mechanism in the spread of antibiotic resistance, with its attendant impact on public health, Salyers emphasized it as merely an indicator, the "tip of the iceberg" of pervasive genetic exchange among members of endogenous microbial communities.

In light of this discovery, further study of the gut as a "cauldron of microevolution" is clearly warranted (Gordon, 2005; Salyers, 2005; Wilson and Salyers, 2003). Key questions to be investigated include how and where microbial gene transfers occur, the extent to which such transfers have contributed to the evolution of pathogens, and the potential for such transfers to influence phenomena other than antibiotic resistance, such as host metabolism and microbial virulence.

IT'S A SMALL UNIVERSE:
INSIGHTS FROM OTHER HOST-MICROBE SYSTEMS

The host-microbe environment of the human gut is complex, compelling, and likely to yield important scientific and medical insights, but the same can be said for microbial communities in plants, insects, and the soil (dubbed "nature's GI tract" by presenter Jeffrey Gordon) that have received considerably less attention. One workshop contributor highlighted recent findings in these systems that suggest the importance of inter-microbe communication (see Handelsman in Chapter 2); another noted similarity between the strategies used by plant and animal pathogens and compared the defenses mounted against them by their disparate hosts (see Staskewicz in Chapter 2). Moreover, the gut is but one site of microbial colonization in mammals; recent studies of oral microbial communities in humans (Smoot et al., 2005) are discussed later in this summary and in Chapter 5 (see Relman), and new data are emerging rapidly on the microbial communities of the human female genital tract.

Camouflage and Communication in Microbial Communities

Many momentous discoveries in microbiology—the germ theory of disease, the discovery and characterization of viruses, the techniques of cell culture, and the analysis of cell differentiation—were first achieved by plant biologists, but were not recognized at the time by their peers in other disciplines (Handelsman, 2005). Thus, while it is not surprising that studies of plants and their associated microbial communities have added considerably to knowledge of host-microbe relationships, these findings have not been widely appreciated nor have they been well integrated with current understanding of the human gut microbiota. There is a need to take a broader view to include perspectives from other biological systems. Many significant biological control processes were originally recognized in plants—such as RNA silencing—only to be demonstrated decades later to be conserved and operational in mammalian systems as well.

Research by presenter Jo Handelsman offers a new opportunity to apply insights derived from host-microbe studies in plants, in this case, toward a new understanding of the importance of microbial signaling to host health. Handelsman and coworkers demonstrated that inter-microbe communications that lead to disease could be disrupted, and that beneficial lines of communication could be protected against pathogenic saboteurs (see Chapter 2). For example, they observed that plant diseases can be suppressed by treatments that modify the microbial community of the root to make it more like the community in the soil, a conclusion which they have dubbed the "camouflage hypothesis" (Gilbert et al., 1994).

These studies have led to further examinations of the interactions between endogenous microbes and disease outcomes in other host-microbe systems, with the most recent example being the gut of the gypsy moth caterpillar (Broderick et al., 2004). In the relatively simple gypsy moth system, the Handelsman lab has begun to explore how signaling within microbial communities influences their ability to protect their hosts from disease and other perturbations (Handelsman, 2005). Among their discoveries in examining the gypsy moth "metagenome"—a representative collection of genomic clones derived from its gut microflora—is the presence of at least one gene associated with quorum sensing (also known as autoinduction), a bacterial system that monitors population density and coordinates gene expression with population growth (Bassler 1999; Dunn and Handelsman, 2002; Greenberg 1997; Handelsman, 2005; Hastings and Greenberg, 1999). The researchers are currently pursuing experiments to gauge the impact of this gene on gut community structure and robustness.

Microbial Disease in Plants and Animals

Research presented by Brian Staskawicz (see Chapter 2) suggests that microbial pathogens that colonize in animals share common strategies with those that infect plants (Staskawicz et al., 2001). Both sorts of pathogens can deliver proteins into host cells that mimic, suppress, or modulate host defense signaling pathways and enhance pathogen fitness, and both are recognized by similarly sophisticated host surveillance systems. Striking architectural similarities between surface appendages of plant and animal pathogenic bacteria suggest common mechanisms of infection, while structural differences reflect the profound differences between plant and animal cells, most notably the presence or absence of a cell wall.

Plants lack the mobilized immune surveillance system and capacity for adaptive immunity present in animals. However, the form of innate immunity evident in plants, which responds to the presence of pathogen effector proteins, is in many ways comparable to innate mammalian mechanisms that recognize conserved molecular patterns on microbial surfaces (Staskawicz, 2005). Host surveillance proteins in plants, encoded by resistance (R) genes, are thought to mediate pathogen recognition by functioning as receptors for specific phytopathogen effector proteins (Baker et al., 1997). Interaction between these components triggers a rapid defensive reaction, known as the hypersensitive response, characterized by tissue death at the site of infection (Baker et al., 1997). This localized reaction limits the spread of infection and often precedes the development of nonspecific resistance throughout the plant, a phenomenon known as systemic acquired resistance. Striking structural similarities have been noted among R genes derived from several plant species that confer resistance to diverse bacterial, fungal, viral, and nematode pathogens. This suggests common patterns of defensive signaling among plants (Baker et al., 1997).

Conserved cellular defense responses in plants may also be analogous to certain innate immune responses to pathogens in vertebrates and insects, suggesting that these defense pathways are highly conserved and may be inherited from a common ancestor (Baker et al., 1997). Animals, plants, and yeast have been found to share structural (and in the case of plants and animals, functional) homology in a key enzyme (caspase) that regulates programmed cell death upon infection with a pathogen (Rojo et al., 2004). A prevalent protein class involved in plant disease resistance, the nucleotide-binding/leucine-rich repeat (NB/LRR) proteins, contains significant homology with Toll-like receptor (TLR) proteins associated with innate immunity in insects and mammals; more specifically, plant NB/LRR disease resistance proteins share homology with mammalian intracellular protein receptors NOD1[3] and NOD2, which function as intracellular receptors of bacterial peptidoglycan and which participate in the inflammatory cascade that causes Crohn's disease (Staskawicz, 2005; Staskawicz et al., 2001). The prepon-

---

[3]NOD proteins are defined as proteins carrying Nucleotide-Oligomerization Domains (NODs) that are involved in the regulation of immune responses and apoptosis. NOD1 and NOD2 are involved in host recognition of small molecules that are components of bacterial peptidoglycan and activate nuclear factor kappa-B (NF-κB) in response to sensing these molecules.

derance of conserved motifs and, presumably, mechanisms among plant and animal proteins involved with innate immunity has encouraged communication and even collaboration among the scientists who study these systems in widely different species—an unfortunately rare occurrence that may yield significant insights on the structure, function, and evolution of innate immunity.

THE ECOLOGY OF PATHOGENESIS

An ecological view of pathogenesis recognizes it as a strategy for microbial survival that reflects ongoing evolution between a microbe and its host (Falkow, 2005; Merrell and Falkow, 2004). Pathogenic microbes acquire genes that enable them to exploit their hosts through relationships that, under conditions of adaptation, tend toward persistence. Deadly disease may result if this delicate equilibrium is upset by genetic or physiological changes (in either the host or the microbe), or by ecological changes that result in infection of a host that is not part of a microbe's established transmission cycle (e.g., Lyme disease in humans) (Falkow, 2005; IOM, 2003a). As contributor Stanley Falkow (see Chapter 3) and others—including Jared Diamond in his Pulitzer Prize-winning book *Guns, Germs, and Steel* (Diamond, 1999)—have observed, the advent of infectious disease adapted to humans is a relatively recent phenomenon, made possible by the existence of large host populations in close contact with one another and abetted by poor hygiene, malnutrition, and the opportunity for zoonotic transmission afforded by animal domestication (Falkow, 2005; McNeill, 1976).

Applying the ecological model to the distinction between commensal and pathogen, Falkow proposed that true pathogens—microbes that depend upon a pathogenic relationship with their hosts for survival—use their invasive properties, such as toxins and virulence factors, to establish a niche that is devoid of competition from other (noninvasive, and therefore nonpathogenic) microbes (Falkow, 2005). He compared the diverse and elaborate means by which true pathogens cross anatomical barriers and breach defenses in their hosts with the claws and fangs of eukaryotic predators. In addition to these obligate invaders, Falkow also ascribed significant human morbidity and mortality to both "accidental" pathogens, which can infect us but are not dependent upon our species for survival, and "opportunistic" microbes, which cause disease only in patients with immune system defects. He noted that while overt clinical disease frequently results from these encounters, it is not a necessary outcome of the host-pathogen interaction. Thus, he concluded, "the focus on clinical disease may distract us from understanding the actual mechanisms of the host-pathogen relationship."

Pathogenesis in Context: The Dual Nature of *Helicobacter pylori*

The human stomach bacterium *Helicobacter pylori* is an exemplar of those microbes that confer both costs and benefits upon their hosts (Blaser, 1997, 2005).

While strongly associated with increased risk for peptic ulcer disease and gastric cancer, recent evidence suggests that *H. pylori* reduces the risk of esophageal diseases (e.g., severe gastric reflux and esophageal cancer), and possibly also of obesity and childhood diarrheal diseases (Blaser, 2005; Blaser and Atherton, 2004; Domínguez-Bello, 2005). In the model of this host-microbe interaction presented by Martin Blaser (see Chapter 3), the persistence of *H. pylori* in the stomach depends upon a precisely balanced equilibrium between bacterial effectors and host responses. Rather than causing acute harm, colonization gradually and subtly increases the host's vulnerability to serious health risks (Blaser, 2005; Blaser and Atherton, 2004).

Considerable evidence shows that *H. pylori* has inhabited the human stomach for at least 60,000 years and that the course of coevolution between microbe and host has spanned millions of years (Blaser, 2005; Blaser and Atherton, 2004). Blaser described the basis for this prototypical mammalian-microbe partnership as an elaborate, bidirectional interplay of signals: microbes communicating with their host via metabolites and toxins, and hosts communicating with their microbes via metabolites and defense molecules. However, recent changes in human ecology (e.g., reduced transmission resulting from improved hygiene and smaller family size; decreased host advantage from colonization, increased use of antibiotics) have apparently led to a decline in prevalence of *H. pylori* among people in developed countries—a trend that suggests the possible eventual disappearance of the microbe from the human microbiota.

What consequences will result from this loss? Blaser presented a range of evidence suggesting that one might expect a decline in cases of gastric cancer and peptic ulcer, as well as an increase in cases of esophageal cancer—and, in fact, these opposing trends appear to be under way in populations in developed countries (Blaser, 2005). He also characterized the disappearance of *H. pylori* as an indicator of the probable fate of other members of the human microbiota, each of which occupies a distinct niche by exchanging signals with its host. Thus, in addition to monitoring the specific effects of the retreat of *H. pylori* from human populations, workshop participants echoed the conclusions of Blaser and Atherton (2004) in urging investigation of the general phenomenon of extinction among members of our microflora (Blaser, 2005). Such losses, which are likely to alter physiological signaling, may contribute to the increasing prevalence of diseases such as gastroesophageal reflux, obesity, diabetes, asthma, and various malignancies.

Further support for this notion was provided by presenter Maria Domínguez-Bello (see Chapter 3), whose studies of indigenous American Indians determined that the presence of multiple intestinal parasites was not correlated with reduced lean body mass in this population. Indeed, Domínguez-Bello found that the presence of *H. pylori* in the GI tracts of American Indian children was associated with higher lean body mass and better nutritional status. To understand the importance of microbiome diversity to human health, and therefore, the consequences of los-ing that diversity, Dominguez-Bello argues that we must study host-microbe relationships in primitive societies as well as in industrialized populations.

Microbial and Host Factors in Disease

Additional workshop presentations and discussions considered intricate host-microbe interactions associated with a variety of diseases, most notably inflammatory bowel diseases (IBDs) such as Crohn's disease and ulcerative colitis (Sartor, 2005). Such conditions highlight the inadequacy of the war metaphor, with its "us versus them" paradigm for pathogenesis. Workshop presenters also support Falkow's observation that the innate immune system (which provides nonspecific protection against microbes, in contrast to the agent-specific defenses mounted by the adaptive immune system) has largely evolved "to keep the commensals in their place," rather than to defend against primary pathogens (Falkow, 2005).

An apt description of the interplay between the innate immune system and commensal flora in the human gut appears in a recent review by MacDonald and Monteleone, who describe this relationship as "precarious," given the mounting evidence that perturbations in this finely balanced ecosystem can lead to inflammation (MacDonald and Monteleone, 2005). When that balance is upset, the authors observe, "the commensal flora appears to act as a surrogate bacterial pathogen, and it is thought that lifelong inflammation ensues because the host response is incapable of eliminating the flora." The cause of this imbalance remains to be determined, but a prevailing explanation implicates improvements in hygiene and readily available antibiotics in the developed world, where IBD and related inflammatory diseases, as well as allergies and asthma, are on the rise (MacDonald and Monteleone, 2005). These developments have drastically reduced human exposure to overt infection, and perhaps more importantly, to harmless gut microbes that somehow influence the maturation and regulation of host immunity.

Multiple factors apparently contribute to the host-microbe disequilibrium that underlies IBDs, according to Balfour Sartor (see Chapter 3). Genetic susceptibility predisposes some hosts to mount an overly hostile immune response to luminal commensal bacteria, but it also appears that the relative balance of injurious versus protective bacterial species is altered in affected individuals (Sartor, 2004, 2005.) Promising modes of therapy for IBD may therefore employ selective antibiotics to reduce the populations of injurious species, and conversely, introduce beneficial bacterial species (probiotics; see subsequent discussion and Chapter 6) and/or dietary supplements, known as prebiotics, that stimulate the growth or activity of beneficial species. However, Sartor observed, this promising picture is complicated by striking host and bacterial species specificity in the production of colitis. Since the definition of a "bad" bacterium depends upon the context, antibiotic, probiotic, or prebiotic therapeutic regimens for IBD need to be tailored to patients' genetic profiles and microbiota.

THE HOST RESPONSE

Recent insights on the complex etiologies of IBDs and related inflammatory diseases reveal limitations in our ability, as host organisms, to appropriately react to the microbes we encounter. Thus, it is clear that a complete understanding of pathogenesis must consider not only how microorganisms inflict damage—the primary focus of research under the war metaphor—but also the mechanisms by which hosts discriminate among microbes and convert that information into an immune response. This expanded field of inquiry is yielding intriguing results, as described in workshop presentations and discussions on the following topics: the identification in mammalian epithelial cells of pattern recognition receptors (PRRs) and their previously mentioned counterparts in plants (MacDonald and Monteleone, 2005; Querishi and Medzhitov, 2003; Staskawicz, 2005; Staskawicz et al., 2001); the characterization of host-microbe interactions that establish mucosal immunity in the gut (Neutra, 2005; Neutra et al., 2001); and the analysis of patterns of global host gene expression in response to infection (Manger and Relman, 2000; Relman, 2005).

Host Recognition of Microbe-Associated Molecular Patterns

PRRs are a broad class of host molecules that activate innate immune responses upon encountering certain conserved molecules and structures[4] common to pathogenic bacteria, viruses, and fungi (but not, apparently, to multicellular parasites) (Kopp and Medzhitov, 2003; Querishi and Medzhitov, 2003). Among the features recognized by PRRs are peptidoglycans and lipoproteins found in most bacteria, CpG sequence strings in DNA, lipopolysaccharides associated with gram-negative bacteria, teichoic acids associated with gram-positive bacteria, and double-stranded RNA replication intermediates of viruses (Didierlaurent et al., 2002). PRRs have been implicated in triggering a variety of innate immune responses, including the opsonization of foreign antigens and the induction of host complement, coagulation, phagocytic, and proinflammatory signaling cascades. Cytokines, interferons, chemokines, and other proinflammatory effectors induced as part of the innate immune response to microbial invasion in turn help to stimulate and shape the adaptive immune response (mediated primarily through B and T lymphocytes) to specific antigens on invading microbes.

PRRs include cytosolic proteins such as NOD2 and RIG-1, proteins such as TLRs expressed on the cell surface or within cytoplasmic vesicles, and extracel-

---

[4]The cornerstone of innate host defense mechanisms is based on specific recognition of signature molecules of microorganisms. These are frequently referred to as pathogen-associated molecular patterns (PAMPs); however, as some innocuous and endogenous microbes share similar signature molecules with their pathogenic counterparts, a more appropriate name for them is microbe-associated molecular patterns (MAMPs) (Aderem and Ulevitch, 2000; Didierlaurent et al., 2001).

lular proteins such as C-reactive protein (Querishi and Medzhitov, 2003). Recent findings associate three major polymorphisms in the NOD2 protein of gut epithelial cells with increased risk for Crohn's disease (see Sartor in Chapter 3) (Hugot et al., 2001; Kobayashi et al., 2005; Maeda et al., 2005; Ogura et al., 2001). Individuals bearing these mutant forms of NOD2 are impaired in their ability to clear bacteria from the intestinal mucosal surface or from infected epithelial cells.

Knowledge of the diverse microbial signatures recognized by PRRs has expanded rapidly, but recent findings indicate that there is much more to be learned about the various means by which hosts detect the microbes in their midst. For example, presenter David Relman raised the question of whether mammalian hosts recognize endogenous archaea, since these organisms do not display any of the known molecular patterns recognized by PRRs (Relman, 2005). As he and coworkers have recently discovered, methanogenic archaea play a central role in some cases of gingivitis by removing molecular hydrogen from their environment, thereby benefiting the bacteria that actually damage gum tissue. In other patients, microbes other than archaea have been found to serve as hydrogen scavengers; thus, the "pathogen" that causes gingivitis is not a single microbe, but a microbial community. It remains to be determined whether archaea are detected by their mammalian hosts, and if so, what sort of disease response their presence might arouse.

The Intestinal Epithelium: An Interactive Barrier

Epithelial cells raise daunting barriers to microbial invasion. Tight junctions, apical surface coats, the secretion of protective substances (e.g., mucins), and antimicrobial agents (e.g., defensins, cecropins, lactoferrin, and lysozyme) provide broad protection against microorganisms to which hosts have not been previously exposed (Boman, 2000; Corfield et al., 2000; Didierlaurrent et al., 2001; Frey et al., 1996; Madara et al., 1990). Much of the intestinal epithelium features a combination of these innate defenses, but they are reduced in cells that lie between lymphoid follicles and the intestinal lumen (Neutra, 2005). The follicle-associated epithelium serves as a key interchange in signaling between luminal microbes (both pathogens and commensals) on one side of the epithelial barrier, and host immune and inflammatory cells on the other (see Neutra in Chapter 4) (Kagnoff and Eckmann, 1997). These specialized sites permit selective sampling of the microbial contents of the lumen and delivery of microbes and antigens to the mucosa-associated lymphoid tissues. This occurs without provoking the sort of massive intestinal inflammation typified by IBDs, which harms both host and beneficial microbes.

Lymphoid follicles are not widely distributed along the path of the gut, but are collected in relatively rare locations known as immune induction sites (Neutra, 2005). In humans, immune induction sites such as Peyer's patches are most numerous in the colon and rectum, and are also found in the oral cavities, tonsils, and adenoids. According to workshop presenter Marian Neutra, this makes sense, as these locations represent areas of greatest exposure to microbes. Also, because sampling microbes exposes the host to the risk of infection, it is best confined to a fraction of the otherwise well-defended epithelium. The cells responsible for transporting pathogens and antigens from the lumen to the lymphoid tissue, known as epithelial M cells, are unique to immune induction sites (Neutra, 2005; Neutra et al., 2001). These immunological "gatekeepers" collaborate closely with memory (and probably naive) B and T cells, as well as dendritic cells.

Neutra described a variety of recent discoveries regarding the workings of M cells (see Chapter 4). Understanding the molecular means by which M cells fulfill their gatekeeping role could inform the design of mucosal vaccines to prevent infection by pathogens such as HIV and provide insights on the prevention and treatment of IBDs and associated immune disorders (Kozlowski and Neutra, 2003; Neutra, 2005). Similarly, knowing how certain pathogens exploit immune induction sites in order to gain entry to a protected niche within their hosts could lead to novel preventive strategies against a variety of microbial threats, including *Salmonella*, *Shigella*, poliovirus, and reoviruses (Neutra and Kraehenbuhl, 1994).

Variability in Host Responses to Pathogens

Using molecular techniques such as complete genome sequences, DNA microarrays, and advanced proteomics to monitor microbial and host cell gene expression, researchers have greatly expanded our understanding of the complexities of host-microbe interactions (Chang et al., 1994; Cummings and Relman, 2000; Dalwadi et al., 2001; Gao and Moore, 1996; Hemmer et al., 1999; Kroes et al., 1999; Relman 2002; Relman et al., 1990, 1992; Sutton et al., 2000). David Relman described a variety of studies he and coworkers have conducted using DNA microarrays to examine transcript abundance in white blood cells following exposure to known bacterial and viral pathogens (see Chapter 4). Their findings illustrate the range of host transcriptional response to infection, identify recurring patterns, and suggest sources of variability.

One factor that has *not* been found to produce significant differences in host gene expression is the distinction between pathogen- versus commensal-associated stimuli (Relman, 2005). A considerable literature of in vitro studies of cultured human cells exposed to various microbes and microbial components, as well as in vivo experiments conducted by Relman and coworkers in nonhuman primates infected with viral or bacterial pathogens (see Chapter 4) suggests that the host transcriptional response to such stimuli is to a large extent stereotypical. Several genetic loci involved in this response have been identified; many control common mechanisms by which hosts recognize and respond to microbes, such as genes encoding PRRs (e.g., TLRs, NOD) and elements of immune response systems (e.g., the NF-kappa-B regulon).

But if the host cannot distinguish between pathogenic and commensal microbes, what initiates the disease response? Relman suggests that hosts react when they detect microbial stimuli in a location, or at a time, or in a concentration different from the normal parameters of their microbiota. In this scenario, lifelong stimulation of the host by commensal microbes establishes a dynamic homeostasis which, when disturbed by the unusual behavior of pathogens, alerts the host to mount a disease response.

Detailed comparisons of host transcriptional responses to various pathogens over time are, however, revealing subtle transcriptional signatures upon the host response. Such variability—which is thought to result from pathogen-specific mechanisms that co-opt, subvert, or modify the stereotypical host response to microbial stimuli—could be exploited for diagnostic purposes. Some promising initial efforts toward this goal were described, including the use of host transcriptional patterns to identify infants with Kawasaki syndrome, which in its symptomatology resembles several other pediatric infectious diseases (Relman, 2005), and also to distinguish among patients with dengue, malaria, and typhoid (Falkow, 2005). More generally, workshop participants reflected on the promise of using the tools of molecular genetics (which, it was noted, will continue to improve with time) to better understand host-microbe relationships—both individually and in the context of microbial communities—by examining gene expression patterns in both hosts and microbes over time.

ADDRESSING COMPLEXITY IN MICROBIAL AND HOST COMMUNITIES

The task of placing host-microbe relationships within an ecological context was undertaken by workshop presentations on two major sources of complexity in host-microbe ecosystems: the biodiversity of endogenous microbial communities, and the networks of host-microbe relationships among pathogens that typically infect multiple hosts (which are in turn infected by multiple pathogens).

Microbial ecologist David Stahl (see Chapter 5) set the stage for this session by asserting that a better understanding of the natural history of microbes—their diversity, as well as their phylogenetic and ecological relationships to each other and to other living things—will improve our ability to develop questions and hypotheses that probe host-microbe relationships at the molecular level. Unlike other biological disciplines concerned with higher organisms (e.g., botany, herpetology, primatology), microbiology did not experience a comparable period of natural history, due in large part to the difficulty of culturing most microbes. With the advent of genomic technologies, however, researchers are no longer limited to surveying the mere fraction of microbial diversity represented by culturable organisms, and are beginning to discover, in Stahl's words, our "planet of the microbes."

Diversity and Dynamics in Microbial Ecosystems

The same technologies that enable researchers to recover molecular information directly from the environment also permit them to deduce phylogenetic relationships and assess the dynamics of complex microbial systems over time (Stahl, 2005). Stahl described how he and coworkers have employed these methods to investigate a variety of host-microbe systems, including microbial fermentation in the cow, the community structure of human oral microbiota and its relationship to local and systemic disease, and the relationship between gut microflora composition and fiber (cellulose) digestion in pigs.

The pig study was intended to shed light on the larger question of whether gut function in mammals—and especially humans—could be modified by altering the structure of the endogenous microbial community (Stahl, 2005). After initial sampling and characterization of the microflora via 16S ribosomal RNA fingerprinting in both experimental and control animals, the researchers increased the cellulose content in the experimental animals' feed over an 8-week period. During this time, they sampled the microbial community in both control and experimental animals on a weekly basis. Initial analyses of these samples revealed a dramatic increase in one bacterial species—*Prevotella*—in the microbiota of pigs with the highest fiber content in their diet. A similar shift in community composition occurred across two separate groups of experimental animals, suggesting that the microbial response to this dietary change is reproducible.

Population Biology of Multiple Hosts and Multiple Pathogens

Veterinary biologist Mark Woolhouse (see Chapter 5) enlarged the ecological perspective beyond microbial ecosystems within individual hosts to address the relationships among all hosts colonized by the same microbial species. In particular, he addressed the web of relationships surrounding the transmission and survival of zoonotic pathogens in novel hosts. These organisms make up more than half of all known pathogens and, when compared with nonzoonotic pathogens, are twice as likely to be associated with emerging diseases (Cleaveland et al., 2001; Woolhouse, 2002, 2005).

The population biology approach to examining multihost-pathogen relationships taken by Woolhouse and colleagues has afforded several important insights regarding pathogen emergence and evolution. For example:

- Pathogens "jump" between species quite rapidly—on an ecological, rather than evolutionary, time scale—and frequently jump into unrelated host species.
- Single-stranded RNA viruses jump between hosts more frequently than other pathogenic microbes in part because they are more genetically unstable and prone to mutation, and therefore more adaptable.
- Transmission efficiency for many zoonoses—including H5N1 influenza,

sleeping sickness, and verocytotoxigenic *E. coli* (VTEC)[5]—is such that a relatively small ecological change (in the host) or a genetic change (in the pathogen) could spark an epidemic.

• Newly emerged pathogens are not subject to historical evolutionary constraints; therefore, the best evolutionary strategy for a pathogen population coexisting in two or more host species may be to become more virulent in one host species.

• Constraints on susceptibility and pathogenicity imposed by coevolution may no longer hold when new host-pathogen associations emerge or ancient associations are disrupted, affecting both the magnitude and severity of disease outbreaks (Woolhouse and Dye, 2001; Woolhouse et al., 2002).

These findings suggest that coevolution between hosts and pathogens plays an important role in disease emergence and reemergence. Demonstrating this influence requires the integration of research on the population biology of microbes and hosts with molecular biological and genetic analyses of host-microbe interactions (Woolhouse and Dye, 2001; Woolhouse et al., 2002). Workshop participants noted that an important first step toward achieving such a synthesis would be to forge connections among diverse scientific disciplines. Collaborations among researchers in the medical, veterinary, plant science, and microbiology research communities, who currently study host-microbe interactions in relative isolation, represent a promising engine of advancement for this crucial field of scientific inquiry.

MANIPULATING HOST-MICROBE INTERACTIONS: PROBIOTIC RESEARCH AND REGULATION

The concept that ingesting certain microbes could prevent or even treat intestinal disease was introduced more than a century ago (Metchnikoff, 1901; Nowak-Wegryzn, 2005). However, despite far-reaching health claims associated with daily consumption of foods containing live bacterial cultures, the biological effects of such products have been demonstrated only under extremely limited

---

[5]Verocytotoxigenic *E. coli* (VTEC) cause serious diarrheal disease. In 10 to 15 percent of cases, hemolytic uremic syndrome (which can result in kidney failure or even death) develops as a complication. The most frequent serotype isolated is O157, but other serotypes, such as O139, have been reported. VTEC is a common commensal organism in cattle, sheep, and other farm animals, The infectious dose is very low, about 10–100 organisms, and thus often causes waterborne outbreaks when animal feces-contaminated material gains access to water supplies post-treatment or where treatment is inadequate. Source: Lightfoot NF. 2003. Bacteria of potential health concern. In Bartram J, Cotruvo J, Exner M, Fricker C, Glasmacher A, eds. *Heterotrophic Plate Counts and Drinking-Water Safety*. London, UK: IWA Publishing. Available: www.who.int/entity/water_sanitation_health/dwq/HPC5.pdf.

conditions. Indeed, as several workshop participants pointed out, even the general term for such ingested microbial products, *probiotics*, is subject to broad interpretation.

As defined by an expert panel convened in 2002 by the Food and Agriculture Organization (FAO) of the United Nations and the World Health Organization (WHO), probiotics are "live microorganisms administered in adequate amounts which confer a beneficial health effect on the host" (Joint FAO/WHO Working Group, 2002). Currently, the main sources of probiotics are dairy foods containing live cultures of *Lactobacillus* and/or *Bifidobacterium*; however, more expansive definitions of probiotics have included microbial components and nonviable or killed microorganisms (Vaillancourt, 2005). Prebiotics, a related concept, are generally considered to be nondigestible substances (e.g., oligosaccharides) added to the diet with the intent of selectively stimulating growth or activity of beneficial indigenous intestinal bacteria (ISAPP, 2005). Synbiotics, according to presenter Lorenzo Morelli, are defined as "mixtures of probiotics and prebiotics that beneficially affect the host by improving the survival and implantation of live microbial dietary supplements in the GI tract of the host" (Andersson et al., 2001).

The central question of what is meant by "beneficial health effects" in this context, and more importantly, how such overtly qualitative notions can be replaced by quantifiable variables, dominated workshop discussion on this topic. The most convincing evidence of probiotic efficacy concerns the treatment of acute infectious diarrhea and the prevention of antibiotic-associated diarrhea (Cremonini et al., 2002; D'Souza et al., 2002; Szajewska and Mrukowicz, 2001; Van Niel et al., 2002). Other conditions potentially treatable by microbes include chronic diarrhea (Xiao et al., 2003), IBD (Schultz et al., 2004), irritable bowel syndrome (Saggioro, 2004), food allergy (Majamaa and Isolauri, 1997). and cancer (Agrawal et al., 2004; Bettegowda et al., 2003; Dang et al., 2001, 2004; Peyromaure and Zerbib, 2004; Wiemann and Starnes, 1994). Conditions that could potentially be prevented with probiotics include travelers' diarrhea (Hilton et al., 1997), necrotizing enterocolitis (Dani et al., 2002), urogenital infections (Cadieux et al., 2002), atopic diseases (e.g., asthma, atopic dermatitis, allergic rhinitis) (Kalliomaki et al., 2001), and dental caries (Nase et al., 2001). Some researchers have also envisioned the use of probiotics to prevent infectious complications of cystic fibrosis, rheumatoid arthritis, and cancer (Vanderhoof, 2001). However, very few double blind, placebo-controlled clinical trials have been conducted to monitor any of these potential effects.

In addition to exploring the potential of probiotic bacteria to promote a variety of specific beneficial changes in their human hosts and how such benefits might be measured, workshop participants considered the regulation of probiotic products. Current FAO/WHO guidelines for the evaluation of probiotics in food and relevant United States Food and Drug Administration (FDA) regulations were presented, along with several unresolved issues that need to be addressed in order to keep pace with this fast-moving and promising field.

Genomic Assessment of Probiotic Activity

Recently developed genomic technologies provide a promising route to evaluating the effects of probiotics on the host-microbe relationship, according to presenter Michiel Kleerebezem of the Wageningen Centre for Food Sciences in the Netherlands. He described the use of bioinformatics techniques to identify, in a single probiotic strain (WCFS1) of the bacterium *Lactobacillus plantarum*, genes that are transcriptionally activated upon introduction into the host, to monitor host gene expression following colonization with *L. plantarum*, and to reveal candidate genes associated with specific beneficial probiotic phenotypes (see Chapter 6).

Kleerebezem and coworkers discovered that of the 72 genes in *L. plantarum* WCFS1 they found were induced upon introduction to a mouse GI tract model, 30 had previously been identified as having been induced in pathogenic bacteria introduced into the same model. These commonly induced genes would, therefore, seem to be associated with microbial survival, rather than virulence—an idea that was further explored by introducing individual deletion mutants of *L. plantarum* WCFS1, each of which lacked a candidate "survival" gene, into the mouse model. These experiments identified a subset of genes essential to microbial persistence in the host, although their actual function remains unknown. Taking this strategy to a human model, the researchers collaborated with colleagues at Lund University in Sweden to examine the activity of a closely related strain, *L. plantarum* 299V, in the human colon. Despite limitations in the detection of bacterial gene expression in this host system, they found increased activity in several genes known to be associated with metabolic and biosynthetic pathways.

Kleerebezem and colleagues have also established in vitro and in vivo human models to monitor the interaction with probiotic bacteria from the host's perspective, revealing distinct changes in transcriptional activity upon stimulation with the *L. plantarum* WCFS1 probiotic strain. The responding host genes were found to encode fatty acid metabolism and lipid transfer factors, as well as cytoskeletal factors that suggest an increased turnover of epithelial cells.

In a further attempt to find clues to identify specific probiotic functions at the molecular level, Kleerebezem's group is using gene chips to compare *L. plantarum* strains. By correlating phenotypic and genotypic data, they have identified candidate genes associated with probiotic properties that include reduced risk of VTEC infection and protection against inflammatory disease. If these genotype-phenotype links are confirmed, it may be possible to engineer the overexpression of such protective loci in second-generation probiotic bacterial strains.

Immune Regulation by Probiotics: Evidence and Application

Do probiotic bacteria actually regulate the mucosal immune response? This central question was approached through a series of related queries posed by presenter Suzanne Cunningham-Rundles. She reviewed progress to date toward providing answers, describing studies that support the following conclusions (see Chapter 6):

- Probiotic microbes have short-term regulatory effects on immune response.
- Specific immune mechanisms are selectively affected by commensal (probiotic) microbes.
- Although host immune response to commensals is to a great extent stereotyped (as is the host response to pathogens, as previously discussed), there is enough specificity to permit manipulation of the immune response by probiotics.
- Commensal bacteria influence the priming of the immune response, probably through the action of T regulatory cells.
- Oral consumption of probiotic bacteria can have a therapeutic effect by improving gut flora richness and barrier function and by down-regulating inflammation.

Research in Cunningham-Rundles' lab, concerning the possible role of commensal bacteria in the priming of the immune response, has led to a series of studies that explore the possibility that microbial colonization could be manipulated. The primary goal of this effort is to encourage colonization by commensal strains known to reduce inflammation, and its associated risks for neonatal development, in vulnerable preterm and other low birth-weight infants. In collaboration with the aforementioned Swedish developers of *L. plantarum* 299V, Cunningham-Rundles and coworkers have also conducted a trial in which HIV positive children with failure to thrive, a condition linked to chronic inflammation, were treated with juice fortified with the probiotic bacterium. Although the results were mixed, those children who gained height and weight also showed a dramatically improved immune response. Based on the results of this study, the group is preparing an investigational new drug (IND) application (see subsequent discussion of regulatory issues) for probiotic-fortified formula intended for use in low birth-weight infants.

Regulatory Approaches and Future Challenges

Both FAO/WHO joint guidelines on the evaluation of probiotics in food (see Morelli in Chapter 6) and U.S. FDA regulations (see Vaillancourt in Chapter 6) distinguish between microbes delivered as food and those that are used for a specific therapeutic purpose, such as to mitigate a pathological condition (Morelli, 2005; Vaillancourt, 2005). However, FDA regulations do not include or define the terms *probiotic* or *prebiotic*. The FDA's Office of Vaccine Research and Review in the Center for Biologics Evaluation and Research (OVRR/CBER) uses the term *live biotherapeutics* to describe the probiotics it regulates; this category encompasses bacteria, yeast, or live virus used in prevention or treatment.

Because intended use determines how a probiotic is regulated, another FDA entity, the Center for Food Safety and Applied Nutrition (CFSAN), regulates probiotics and prebiotics marketed as dietary supplements or food ingredients.

Most prebiotics fit the FDA definition of a dietary supplement ("a product taken by mouth that contains a dietary ingredient intended to supplement the diet"), and to date, so do all probiotic products on the market. Although this situation is expected to change, workshop participants noted, there is little incentive for manufacturers of probiotics currently marketed as dietary supplements to develop them as biotherapeutics, given the rigors and expense of the associated review and regulation process. This situation confuses many consumers, who struggle to understand the vague health claims associated with probiotics and other dietary supplements, and who may (especially if they are ill) misinterpret such claims as proof of therapeutic efficacy. But unless serious adverse events can be shown to result from the use of a dietary supplement, the FDA cannot remove the product from the market. It was noted that a similarly confusing situation currently exists for European consumers, but that many countries in Europe are currently considering legislation to require proof for all health claims.

Although the dietary supplement/biotherapeutic dichotomy may remain a part of U.S. regulation of probiotics for some time, presenter Julienne Vaillancourt of OVRR/CBER expects the regulatory process for biotherapeutics to expand and change to reflect new knowledge. In fact, she identified several issues that need to be addressed in revisions to current regulations; these include the need to define and set guidelines for the evaluation of colonization and potency as they relate to biotherapeutics, and also to establish protocols for investigating the potential pathogenicity of probiotic strains. In addition, it was observed that although the most promising populations of beneficial microbes adhere to mucosal surfaces, most probiotics currently on the market have been isolated from stool samples that contain very few mucosal-adherent bacteria. Moreover, the vast majority of probiotic efficacy trials are conducted on the basis of the analysis of stool samples.

Thus, it is not only clear that guidelines and regulations governing probiotics must be revised to reflect recent research findings, but also that this goal is a fast-moving target. Lorenzo Morelli predicted the advent, within two to three years, of new products such as targeted probiotics or biotherapeutics that enhance production of specific cytokine or suppress specific pathogens, as well as new genotype-based methods of surveying microbial populations and assessing host-microbe interactions. By their very nature, such innovations will demand adjustments to current regulatory practices for probiotics.

PURSUING A NEW PARADIGM

With the development of genomic and bioinformatic tools, and with the expectation that the future will bring even more powerful technologies for resolving the vast diversity of microbial communities, researchers can at last begin to study host-microbe relationships in their complexity. There is much to be discovered about the composition of microbial communities, how they assemble and self-regulate, and the means by which their members communicate with each other and with their hosts. Even in the relatively familiar and well-studied territory of the human gut, many basic questions remain unanswered. The following list of such queries, posed by David Relman and elaborated upon by several workshop participants, could equally be applied to a variety of other endogenous microbial communities and host-microbe ecosystems including, but not limited to:

1. How variable is the composition of the gut microbiota among human populations?
2. What is the role of timing in determining the acquisition and composition of the gut microbiota, and how does initial exposure and host genetics influence this process?
3. What drives the development of the immune response with respect to the temporal exposure to different pathogens?
4. How variable is the gut microbiota across space? Is the gut an assembly of microhabitats? Is it continuously variable?
5. What is the role of the individual host or host species in dictating the nature of the commensal microflora? Will this specificity permit the manipulation of either host or microbial community to benefit both?
6. How do microbial communities self-regulate?
7. What mechanisms enable endogenous communities to exchange information with their hosts, and vice versa?
8. How can the presence of phages, viruses, and archaea in the gut microbiota be characterized in terms of diversity and population sizes? What ecological roles do these organisms play in this and other microbial communities?
9. What is the role of polymicrobial interactions, biofilms, and other communities of indigenous microbes (e.g., skin)?
10. What do microbial community members do? What do pathogens do when they are not being pathogens (e.g., do their toxins have an ecological role)?

Interdisciplinary Research on Host-Microbe Interactions

Participants noted that the understanding of host-microbe relationships could be greatly advanced by the expansion and implementation of key recommendations of the IOM report, *Microbial Threats to Health* (2003a), that encourage an integrated and cooperative research effort by human and animal health communities on infectious disease threats. It was recognized that these goals would be furthered by engaging the plant research community and that the collaborative research agenda on infectious disease should incorporate host-microbe ecology. Interdisciplinary infectious disease centers such as those proposed in the *Micro-*

bial Threats to Health report could support research on such topics as the ecology of microbial communities across species and among multiple hosts and the response of microbial communities to novel ecological pressures and opportunities for host colonization. Much more needs to be learned about the roles of eukaryotic viruses in these processes—discussion of the possible roles played by DNA or RNA viruses were virtually absent in this workshop, reflecting a major gap in our understanding.

Connection among such centers on an international scale would further advance research goals by providing a "critical mass" of researchers to address the extreme complexity of scientific inquiry at the community and ecosystem level. A logical partner for international collaboration (as well as an example upon which to base U.S. programs) is the European network for research on the prevention and control of zoonoses, Med-Vet-Net (Med-Vet-Net, 2005). Founded in 2004, Med-Vet-Net comprises 300 scientists from 8 veterinary and 7 public health institutes, along with the Society for Applied Microbiology (UK), who are linked by a variety of structures intended to improve scientific collaboration and the dissemination of knowledge.

Opportunities for Global Survey of the Gut Microbiome

Workshop presentations and discussions clearly demonstrated both the feasibility and promise of conducting a microbial survey of human and animal microbiota. As noted by Bäckhed et al. (2005), "experimental and computational tools are now in hand to comprehensively characterize the nature of microbial diversity in the gut, the genomic features of its keystone members, the operating principles that underlie the nutrient foraging and sharing behaviors of these organisms, the mechanisms that ensure the adaptability and robustness of this systems, and the physiological benefits we accrue from this mutualistic relationship." The technical feasibility of microbial genomic surveillance now makes it possible to conduct global surveys of gut microbiota and also to monitor how these microbial communities respond (in terms of structure and composition) to environmental change. Indeed, it was observed, the collection of this data could be viewed as an extension of the human genome project to encompass the "organismal metagenome." In addition to advancing understanding of the etiology and epidemiology of infectious disease, this project may shed light on microbial influence on a host of chronic disorders, including GI conditions, allergy, asthma, diabetes, and obesity.

Participants also considered the collection, organization, and analysis of survey data on the gut microbiome. To assemble an encyclopedic representation, samples must be obtained from humans and animals across a broad range of geographic, nutritional, and health environments, as well as from several anatomical microenvironments. Standards for sampling methods would need to be established, and it was agreed that attempts should be made to identify and obtain appropriate samples that may already exist in clinical and research communities—an effort that, in addition to reducing the time and expense of data collection, could also strengthen ties among potential collaborators in studies of host-microbe interactions. Finally, participants emphasized the importance of archiving sample material so that trends can be followed over time, and also to permit future analyses based on improved technologies.

RAISING AWARENESS OF THE HOST-MICROBE RELATIONSHIP

Our "war" on infectious microbes has restricted the spread of several pathogens and drastically reduced the burden of human disease, but the metaphor appears to be reaching the end of its usefulness. Recent findings on host-microbe interactions in a variety of settings, which highlight the many benefits of some microbes—as well as the potential for exploiting those benefits to further advantage—reveal the limitations of pure antagonism toward the microbes among us. At best, the war metaphor is a limiting mental shortcut that distracts from abundant opportunities to improve human and animal health. At worst, it represents a dangerous influence on disease control practices that have accelerated the development of antimicrobial resistance among human and animal pathogens, and perhaps also increased virulence in some pathogens. Put simply, the war metaphor must be replaced or, as comically (yet ominously) predicted in the epigraph to this summary, the bugs will win. We hosts are far better served by recognizing microbes as the allies they (mostly) are, and by making the best of our intimate alliances with them.

Such a message, which does not invoke the threat of catastrophe, will be difficult to send. The notion of microbes as the "enemy" will not fade quickly, especially given the relative complexity of the ecological perspective that would supplant the "us vs. them" paradigm. The most optimistic scenario for changing this opinion may be to begin within the infectious disease research community, where scientists who tend to focus on interactions between individual microbes and hosts could be encouraged to better understand and incorporate the concepts of community and ecosystem dynamics in their studies. A better-informed research community could then help to influence governmental and other funding agencies to recognize the importance of studying and funding proposals to examine host-microbe relationships to human health. Recognition of the commercial potential of probiotics could also encourage federal support for research, regulation, and the development of strain collections, reagents, and good manufacturing practices.

A similar "sea change" could occur if medical professionals encourage their patients to appreciate the benefits associated with the microbial flora and fauna that exist on and in us, and indeed to recognize that without these microbes, life as we know it would not exist. Many physicians are exercising new caution in prescribing antibiotics and some are able to explain their reasons for doing so to their patients, but far more must be done—and said—to promote public understanding and support of the largely beneficial role that microbes play in their lives. If advances in the understanding of the specific actions of microbes in the development of immunity and protection from chronic disease can be translated into clinical practice, people may be able to declare a truce in the war on germs.

REFERENCES

Aderem A, Ulevitch RJ. 2000. Toll-like receptors in the induction of the innate immune response. *Nature* 406(6797):782–787.

Agrawal N, Bettegowda C, Cheong I, Geschwind JF, Drake CG, Hipkiss EL, Tatsumi M, Dang LH, Diaz LA Jr, Pomper M, Abusedera M, Wahl RL, Kinzer KW, Zhou S, Huso DL, Vogelstein B. 2004. Bacteriolytic therapy can generate a potent immune response against experimental tumors. *Proceedings of the National Academy of Sciences* 101(42):15172–15177.

Andersson H, Asp NG, Bruce A, Roos S, Wadstrom T, Wold AE. 2001. Health affects of probiotics and prebiotics: A literature review on human studies. *Scandanavian Journal of Nutrition* 45: 58–75.

Armstrong GL, Conn LA, Pinner RW. 1999. Trends in infectious disease mortality in the United States during the 20th century. *Journal of the American Medical Association* 281(1):61–66.

Bäckhed F, Ding H, Wang T, Hooper LV, Koh GY, Nagy A, Semenkovich CF, Gordon JI. 2004. The gut microbiota as an environmental factor that regulates fat storage. *Proceedings of the National Academy of Sciences* 101(44):15718-15723.

Bäckhed F, Ley RE, Sonnenburg JL, Peterson DA, Gordon JI. 2005. Host-bacterial mutualism in the human intestine. *Science* 307(5717):1915–1920.

Baker B, Zambryski P, Staskawicz B, Dinesh-Kumar SP. 1997. Signaling in plant-microbe interactions. *Science* 276(5313):726–733.

Bassler BL. 1999. How bacteria talk to each other: Regulation of gene expression by quorum sensing. *Current Opinion in Microbiology* 2(6):582–587.

Bettegowda C, Dang LH, Abrams R, Huso DL, Dillehay L, Cheong I, Agrawal N, Borzillary S, McCaffery JM, Watson EL, Lin KS, Bunz F, Baidoo K, Pomper MG, Kinzler KW, Vogelstein B, Zhou S. 2003. Overcoming the hypoxic barrier to radiation therapy with anaerobic bacteria. *Proceedings of the National Academy of Sciences USA* 100(25):15083–15088.

Blaser M. 1997. Ecology of *Helicobacter pylori* in the human stomach. *Journal of Clinical Investigation* 100(4):759–762.

Blaser MJ. 2005 (March 16). *Session I: Host-Pathogen Interactions: Defining the Concepts of Pathogenicity, Virulence, Colonization, Commensalism, and Symbiosis.* Presentation at the Forum on Microbial Threats Workshop Ending the War Metaphor: The Changing Agenda for Unraveling the Host-Microbe Relationship, Washington, D.C., Institute of Medicine, Forum on Microbial Threats.

Blaser MJ, Atherton JC. 2004. *Helicobacter pylori* persistence: Biology and disease. *Journal of Clinical Investigation* 113(3):321–333.

Boman HG. 2000. Innate immunity and the normal microflora. *Immunology Review* 173:5–16.

Breitbart M, Hewson I, Mahaffy JM, Nulton J, Salamon P, Rohwer F. 2003. Metagenomic analysis of an uncultured viral community from human feces. *Journal of Bacteriology* 185(20):6220–6223.

Broderick NA, Raffa KF, Goodman RM, Handelsman J. 2004. Census of the bacterial community of the gypsy moth larval midgut by using culturing and culture-independent methods. *Applied Environmental Microbiology* 70(1):293–300.

Cadieux P, Burton J, Gardiner G, Braunstein L, Bruce AW, Kang CY, Reid G. 2002. Lactobacillus strains and vaginal ecology. *Journal of the American Medical Association* 287(15):1940–1941.

Casadevall A, Pirofski LA. 1999. Host-pathogen interactions: Redefining the basic concepts of virulence and pathogenicity. *Infection and Immunity* 67(8):3703–3713.

Casadevell A, Pirofski LA. 2000. Host-pathogen interactions: Basic concepts of microbial commensalism, colonization, infection, and disease. *Infection and Immunity* 68(12):6511–6518.

Casadevell A, Pirofski LA. 2002. The meaning of microbial exposure, infection, colonization, and disease in clinical practice. *Lancet Infectious Diseases* 2(10):628–635.

Casadevell A, Pirofski LA. 2003. The damage-response framework of microbial pathogenesis. *Nature Reviews Microbiology* 1(1):17–24.

Chang Y, Cesarman E, Pessin MS, Lee F, Culpepper J, Knowles DM, Moore PS. 1994. Identification of herpesvirus-like DNA sequences in AIDS-associated Kaposi's sarcoma. *Science* 266(5192): 1865–1869.

Cleaveland S, Laurenson MK, Taylor LH. 2001. Diseases of humans and their domestic mammals: Pathogen characteristics, host range and the risk of emergence. *Philosophical Transactions of the Royal Society of London Series B* 365(1411):991–999.

Corfield AP, Myerscough N, Longman R, Sylvester P, Arul S, Pignatelli M. 2000. Mucins and mucosal protection in the gastrointestinal tract: New prospects for mucins in the pathology of gastrointestinal disease. *Gut* 47(4):589–594.

Cremonini F, Di Caro S, Nista EC, Bartolozzi F, Capelli G, Gasbarrini G, Gasbarrini A. 2002. Meta-analysis: The effect of probiotic administration on antibiotic-associated diarrhoea. *Alimentary Pharmacology and Therapeutics* 16(8):1461–1467.

Cummings CA, Relman DA. 2000. Using DNA microarrays to study host-microbe interactions. *Emerging Infectious Diseases* 6(5):513–525.

Dalwadi H, Wei B, Kronenberg M, Sutton CL, Braun J. 2001. The Crohn's disease-associated bacterial protein I2 is a novel enteric T cell superantigen. *Immunity* 15(1):149–158.

Dang LH, Bettegowda C, Huso DL, Kinzler KW, Vogelstein B. 2001. Combination bacteriolytic therapy for the treatment of experimental tumors. *Proceedings of the National Academy of Sciences USA* 98(26):15155–15160.

Dang LH, Bettegowda C, Agrawal N, Cheong I, Huso DL, Frost P, Loganzo F, Greenberger L, Barkoczy J, Pettit GR, Smith AB 3rd, Gurulingappa H, Khan S, Parmigiani G, Kinzler KW, Zhou S, Vogelstein B. 2004. Targeting vascular and avascular compartments of tumors with C. novyi-NT and anti-microtubule agents. *Cancer Biology and Therapy* 3(3):326–337.

Dani C, Biadaioli R, Bertini G, Martelli E, Rubaltelli FF. 2002. Probiotics feeding in prevention of urinary tract infection, bacterial sepsis and necrotizing enterocolitis in preterm infants. A prospective double-blind study. *Biology of the Neonate* 82(2):103–108.

Diamond, J. 1999. *Guns, Germs, and Steel: The Fates of Human Societies*. New York: W.W. Norton & Company.

Didierlaurent A, Sirard JC, Kraehenbuhl JP, Neutra MR. 2001. How the gut senses its content. *Cellular Microbiology* 4(2):61–72.

Didierlaurent A, Sirard JC, Kraehenbuhl JP, Neutra MR. 2002 (February). How the gut senses its content. *Cellular Microbiology* 4(2):61–72.

Dominguez-Bello. 2005 (March 16). *Session I: Host-Pathogen Interactions: Defining the Concepts of Pathogenicity, Virulence, Colonization, Commensalism, and Symbiosis*. Presentation at the Forum on Microbial Threats Workshop Ending the War Metaphor: The Changing Agenda for Unraveling the Host-Microbe Relationship, Washington, D.C., Institute of Medicine, Forum on Microbial Threats.

D'Souza AL, Rajkumar C, Cooke J, Bulpitt CJ. 2002. Probiotics in prevention of antibiotic associated diarrhoea: Meta-analysis. *British Medical Journal* 324(7350):1361.

Dunn AK, Handelsman J. 2002. Toward an understanding of microbial communities through analysis of communication networks. *Antonie Van Leeuwenhoek* 81(1–4):565–574.

Fagarasan S, Muramatsu M, Suzuki K, Nagaoka H, Hiai H, Honjo T. 2002. Critical roles of activation-induced cytidine deaminase in the homeostasis of gut flora. *Science* 298(5597):1424–1427.

Falkow S. 2005 (March 17). *Session III: Understanding the Dynamic Relationships of Host-Microbe Interactions*. Presentation at the Forum on Microbial Threats Workshop Ending the War Metaphor: The Changing for Unraveling the Host-Microbe Relationship, Washington, D.C., Institute of Medicine, Forum on Microbial Threats.

Frey A, Giannasca KT, Weltzin R, Giannasca PJ, Reggio H, Lencer WI, Neutra MR. 1996. Role of the glycocalyx in regulating access of microparticles to apical plasma membranes of intestinal epithelial cells—implications for microbial attachment and oral vaccine targeting. *Journal of Experimental Medicine* 184(3):1045–1059.

Gao SJ, Moore PS. 1996. Molecular approaches to the identification of unculturable infectious agents. *Emerging Infectious Diseases* 2(3):159–167.

Gilbert GS, Handelsman J, Parke JL. 1994. Root camouflage and disease control. *Phytopathology* 84(3):222–225.

Gordon J. 2005 (March 16). *Session I: Host-Pathogen Interactions: Defining the Concepts of Pathogenicity, Virulence, Colonization, Commensalism, and Symbiosis*. Presentation at the Forum on Microbial Threats Workshop Ending the War Metaphor: The Changing Agenda for Unraveling the Host-Microbe Relationship, Washington, D.C., Institute of Medicine, Forum on Microbial Threats.

Greenberg EP. 1997. Quorum sensing in gram-negative bacteria: Cell density-dependent gene expression controls luminescence in marine bacteria and virulence in several pathogens. *American Society of Microbiology News* 63:371–377.

Handelsman J. 2005 (March 16). *Session I: Host-Pathogen Interactions: Defining the Concepts of Pathogenicity, Virulence, Colonization, Commensalism, and Symbiosis*. Presentation at the Forum on Microbial Threats Workshop Ending the War Metaphor: The Changing Agenda for Unraveling the Host-Microbe Relationship. Washington, D.C., Institute of Medicine, Forum on Microbial Threats.

Hastings JW, Greenberg EP. 1999. Quorum sensing: The explanation of a curious phenomenon reveals a common characteristic of bacteria. *Journal of Bacteriology* 181(9):2667–2668.

Hemmer B, Gran B, Zhao Y, Marques A, Pascal J, Tzou A, Kondo T, Cortese I, Bielekova B, Straus SE, McFarland HF, Houghten R, Simon R, Pinilla C, Martin R. 1999. Identification of candidate T-cell epitopes and molecular mimics in chronic Lyme disease. *Nature Medicine* 5(12):1375–1382.

Hilton E, Kolawowski P, Singer C, Smith M. 1997. Efficacy of *Lactobacillus* GG as a diarrheal preventive in travelers. *Journal of Travel Medicine* 4:41–43.

Hooper LV, Wong MH, Thelin A, Hansson L, Falk PG, Gordon JI. 2001. Molecular analysis of commensal host-microbial relationships in the intestine. *Science* 291(5505):881–884.

Hooper LV, Midtvedt T, Gordon JI. 2002. How host-microbial interactions shape the nutrient environment of the mammalian intestine. *Annual Review of Nutrition* 22:283-307.

Hooper TL, Hopkinson DN, Bhabra MS. 1998. Pulmonary graft preservation: A worldwide survey of current clinical practice. *Journal of Heart and Lung Transplantation* 17(5):525–531.

Hugot JP, Chamaillard M, Zouali H, Lesage S, Cezard JP, Belaiche J, Almer S, Tysk C, O'Morain CA, Gassull M, Binder V, Finkel Y, Cortot A, Modigliani R, Laurent-Puig P, Gower-Rousseau C, Macry J, Colombel JF, Sahbatou M, Thomas G. 2001. Association of NOD2 leucine-rich repeat variants with susceptibility to Crohn's disease. *Nature* 411(6837):599–603.

Hylemon PB, Harder J. 1998. Biotransformation of monoterpenes, bile acids, and other isoprenoids in anaerobic ecosystems. *FEMS Microbiology Reviews* 22(5):475–488.

IOM (Institute of Medicine). 2003a. *Microbial Threats to Health: Emergence, Detection, and Response*. Washington, DC: The National Academies Press.

IOM. 2003b. *The Resistance Phenomenon in Microbes and Infectious Disease Vectors.* Washington, DC: The National Academies Press.
IOM. 2004. *The Infectious Etiology of Chronic Diseases.* Washington, DC: The National Academies Press.
ISAPP (International Scientific Association for Probiotics and Prebiotics). 2005. About ISAPP. [Online]. Available: http://www.isapp.net/IS_about.htm [accessed on December 19, 2005].
Isenberg HD. 1988. Pathogenicity and virulence: Another view. *Clinical Microbiology Reviews* 1(1):40–53.
Joint FAO/WHO Working Group. 2002. Guidelines for the evaluation of probiotics in food. [Online]. Available: http://www.fao.org/es/ESN/food/foodandfood_probio_en.stm [accessed December 19, 2005].
Kagnoff MF, Eckmann L. 1997. Epithelial cells as sensors for microbial infection. *Journal of Clinical Investigation* 100(1):6–10.
Kalliomaki M, Salminen S, Arvilommi H, Kero P, Koskinen P, Isolauri E. 2001. Probiotics in primary prevention of atopic disease: A randomized placebo-controlled trial. *Lancet* 357(9262):1076–1079.
Kindhauser MK. 2003. *Communicable Diseases 2002: Global Defense Against the Infectious Disease Threat.* Geneva, Switzerland: WHO.
Kobayashi KS, Chamaillard M, Ogura Y, Henegariu O, Inohara N, Nunez G, Flavell RA. 2005. Nod2-dependent regulation of innate and adaptive immunity in the intestinal tract. *Science* 307(5710):731–734.
Kopp E, Medzhitov R. 2003. Recognition of microbial infection by Toll-like receptors. *Current Opinion in Immunology* 15(4):396–401.
Kozlowski PA, Neutra MR. 2003. The role of mucosal immunity in prevention of HIV transmission. *Current Molecular Medicine* 3(3):217–228.
Kroes I, Lepp PW, Relman DA. 1999. Bacterial diversity within the human subgingival crevice. *Proceedings of the National Academy of Sciences USA* 96(25):14547–14552.
Lederberg J. 2000. Infectious history. *Science* 288(5464):287–293.
MacDonald TT, Monteleone G. 2005. Immunity, inflammation and allergy in the gut. *Science* 307(5717):1920–1925.
Madara JL, Nash S, Moore R, Atisook K. 1990. Structure and function of the intestinal epithelial barrier in health and disease. *Monographs in Pathology* 31:306–324.
Maeda S, Hsu LC, Liu H, Bankston LA, Iimura M, Kagnoff MF, Eckmann L, Karin M. 2005. Nod2 mutation in Crohn's disease potentiates NF-kappaB activity and IL-1beta processing. *Science* 307(5710):734–738.
Majamaa H, Isolauri E. 1997. Probiotics: A novel approach in the management of food allergy. *Journal of Allergy and Clinical Immunology* 99(2):179–185.
Manger ID, Relman DA. 2000. How the host "sees" pathogens: Global gene expression responses to infection. *Current Opinion in Immunology* 12(2):215–218.
McNeill WH. 1976. *Plagues and Peoples.* New York: Anchor Books. P. 369.
Med-Vet-Net. 2005. MedVetNet Homepage. [Online]. Available: http://www.medvetnet.org/cms/ [accessed December 19, 2005].
Merell DS, Falkow S. 2004. Frontal and stealth attack strategies in microbial pathogenesis. *Nature* 430(6996):250–256.
Metchnikoff E. 1901. Sur la flore du corps humain. *Manchester Literary and Philosophical Society* 45:1–38.
Morelli L. 2005 (March 17). *Session IV: Novel Approaches for Mitigating the Development of Resistance.* Presentation at the Forum on Microbial Threats Workshop Ending the War Metaphor: The Changing Agenda for Unraveling the Host-Microbe Relationship, Washington, D.C., Institute of Medicine, Forum on Microbial Threats.

Nase L, Hatakka K, Savilahti E, Saxelin M, Ponka A, Poussa T, Korpela R, Meurman JH. 2001. Effect of long-term consumption of a probiotic bacterium, *Lactobacillus rhamnosus* GG, in milk on dental caries and caries risk in children. *Caries Research* 35(6):412–420.

Neutra MR. 2005 (March 17). *Session II: Ecology of Host-Microbe Interactions*. Presentation at the Forum on Microbial Threats Workshop Ending the War Metaphor: The Changing Agenda for Unraveling the Host-Microbe Relationship, Washington, D.C., Institute of Medicine, Forum on Microbial Threats.

Neutra MR, Kraehenbuhl JP. 1994. Cellular and molecular basis for antigen transport in the intestinal epithelium. In: Ogra PL, Mestecky J, Lamm ME, Strober W, McGhee JR, Bienstock J, eds. *Handbook of Mucosal Immunology*. Boston, MA: Academic Press, Inc. Pp. 27–39.

Neutra MR, Mantis NJ, Kraehenbuhl JP. 2001. Collaboration of epithelial cells with organized mucosal lymphoid tissues. *Nature Immunology* 2(11):1004–1009.

Nowak-Wegryzn A. 2005. Future approaches to food allergy. *Pediatrics* 111(6):1672–1680.

Ogura Y, Bonen DK, Inohara N, Nicolae DL, Chen FF, Ramos R, Britton H, Moran T, Karaliuskas R, Duerr RH, Achkar JP, Brant SR, Bayless TM, Kirschner BS, Hanauer SB, Nunez G, Cho JH. 2001. A frameshift mutation in NOD2 associated with susceptibility to Crohn's disease. *Nature* 411(6837):603–606.

Peyromaure M, Zerbib M. 2004. T1G3 transitional cell carcinoma of the bladder: Recurrence, progression and survival. *BJU International* 93(1):60–63.

Querishi ST, Medzhitov R. 2003. Toll-like receptors and microbial infection. *Genes and Immunity* 4(2):87–94.

Rawls JF, Samuel BS, Gordon JI. 2004. Gnotobiotic zebrafish reveal evolutionarily conserved responses to the gut microbiota. *Proceedings of the National Academy of Sciences USA* 101(13): 4596–4601.

Relman DA. 2002. New technologies, human-microbe interactions, and the search for previously unrecognized pathogens. *Journal of Infectious Diseases* 186(Suppl 2):S254–S258.

Relman DA. 2005 (March 17). *Session II: Ecology of Host-Microbe Interactions*. Presentation at the Forum on Microbial Threats Workshop Ending the War Metaphor: The Changing Agenda for Unraveling the Host-Microbe Relationship, Washington, D.C., Institute of Medicine, Forum on Microbial Threats.

Relman DA, Loutit JS, Schmidt TM, Falkow S, Tompkins LS. 1990. The agent of bacillary angiomatosis. An approach to the identification of uncultured pathogens. *New England Journal of Medicine* 323(23):1573–1580.

Relman DA, Schmidt TM, MacDermott RP, Falkow S. 1992. Identification of the uncultured bacillus of Whipple's disease. *New England Journal of Medicine* 327(5):293–301.

Rojo E, Martin R, Carter C, Zouhar J, Pan S, Plotnikova J, Jin H, Paneque M, Sanchez-Serrano JJ, Baker B, Ausubel FM, Raikhel NV. 2004. VPE-gamma exhibits a caspase-like activity that contributes to defense against pathogens. *Current Biology* 14(21):1897–1906.

Saggioro A. 2004. Probiotics in the treatment of irritable bowel syndrome. *Journal of Clinical Gastroenterolgy* 38(Suppl 6):S104–S106.

Salyers A. 2005 (March 16). *Session I: Host-Pathogen Interactions: Defining the Concepts of Pathogenicity, Virulence, Colonization, Commensalism, and Symbiosis*. Presentation at the Forum on Microbial Threats Workshop Ending the War Metaphor: The Changing Agenda for Unraveling the Host-Microbe Relationship, Washington, D.C., Institute of Medicine, Forum on Microbial Threats.

Sartor RB. 2004. Therapeutic manipulation of the enteric microflora in inflammatory bowel diseases: Antibiotics, probiotics, and prebiotics. *Gastroenterology* 126(6):1620–1633.

Sartor RB. 2005 (March 16). *Session I: Host-Pathogen Interactions: Defining the Concepts of Pathogenicity, Virulence, Colonization, Commensalism, and Symbiosis*. Presentation at the Forum on Microbial Threats Workshop Ending the War Metaphor: The Changing Agenda for Unraveling the Host-Microbe Relationship, Washington, D.C., Institute of Medicine, Forum on Microbial Threats.

Savage DC. 1977. Microbial ecology of the gastrointestinal tract. *Annual Reviews in Microbiology* 31:107–133.

Schultz M, Timmer A, Herfarth HH, Sartor RB, Vanderhoof JA, Rath HC. 2004. Lactobacillus GG in inducing and maintaining remission of Crohn's disease. *BMC Gastroenterology* 4:5.

Smoot LM, Smoot JC, Smidt H, Noble PA, Konneke M, McMurry ZA, Stahl DA. 2005. DNA microarrays as salivary diagnostic tools for characterizing the oral cavity's microbial community. *Advances in Dental Research* 18(1):6–11.

Stahl D. 2005 (March 17). *Session II: Ecology of Host-Microbe Interactions*. Presentation at the Forum on Microbial Threats Workshop Ending the War Metaphor: The Changing Agenda for Unraveling the Host-Microbe Relationship, Washington, D.C., Institute of Medicine, Forum on Microbial Threats.

Staskawicz BJ. 2005 (March 16). *Session I: Host-Pathogen Interactions: Defining the Concepts of Pathogenicity, Virulence, Colonization, Commensalism, and Symbiosis*. Presentation at the Forum on Microbial Threats Workshop Ending the War Metaphor: The Changing Agenda for Unraveling the Host-Microbe Relationship, Washington, D.C., Institute of Medicine, Forum on Microbial Threats.

Staskawicz BJ, Mudgett MB, Dangl JL, Galan JE. 2001. Common and contrasting themes of plant and animal diseases. *Science* 292(22):2285–2289.

Stewart WH. 1967. "A Mandate for State Action," presented at the Association of State and Territorial Health Officers, Washington, D.C., Dec. 4, 1967. Taken from: Garrett L. 1994. *The Coming Plague: Newly Emerging Diseases in a World Out of Balance*. New York: Penguin Books. P. 33, footnote 9.

Sutton CL, Kim J, Yamane A, Dalwadi H, Wei B, Landers C, Targan SR, Braun J. 2000. Identification of a novel bacterial sequence associated with Crohn's disease. *Gastroenterology* 119(1): 23–31.

Szajewska H, Mrukowicz JZ. 2001. Probiotics in the treatment and prevention of acute infectious diarrhea in infants and children: A systematic review of published randomized, double-blinded, placebo-controlled trials. *Journal of Pediatric Gastroenterology and Nutrition* 33(Suppl 2): S17–S25.

Vaillancourt R. 2005 (March 17). *Session IV: Novel Approaches for Mitigating the Development of Resistance*. Presentation at the Forum on Microbial Threats Workshop Ending the War Metaphor: The Changing Agenda for Unraveling the Host-Microbe Relationship, Washington, D.C., Institute of Medicine, Forum on Microbial Threats.

Van Niel CW, Feudtner C, Garrison MM, Christakis DA. 2002. Lactobacillus therapy for acute infectious diarrhea in children: A meta-analysis. *Pediatrics* 109(4):678–684.

Vanderhoof JA. 2001. Probiotics: Future directions. *American Journal of Clinical Nutrition* 73(6): 1152S–1155S.

Whittle G, Shoemaker NB, Salyers AA. 2002. The role of Bacteroides conjugative transposons in the dissemination of antibiotic resistance genes. *Cellular and Molecular Life Sciences* 59(12):2044–2054.

WHO (World Health Organization). 2000. Factors contributing to resistance. In: *World Health Organization Report on Infectious Diseases 2000: Overcoming Antimicrobial Resistance*. [Online]. Available: http://www.who.int/infectious-disease-report/2000/ [accessed January 6, 2005].

Wiemann B, Starnes CO. 1994. Coley's toxins, tumor necrosis factor and cancer research: A historical perspective. *Pharmacology and Therapeutics* 64(3):529–564.

Wilson B, Salyers AA. 2003. Is the evolution of bacterial pathogens an out-of-body experience? *Trends in Microbiology* 11(8):347–350.

Winter C, Smit A, Herndl GJ, Weinbauer MG. 2004. Impact of virioplankton on archaeal and bacterial community richness as assessed in seawater batch cultures. *Applied Environmental Microbiology* 70(2):804–813.

Woolhouse ME. 2002. Population biology of emerging and re-emerging pathogens. *Trends in Microbiology* 10(Suppl 10):S3–S7.

Woolhouse M. 2005 (March 17). *Session II: Ecology of Host-Microbe Interactions.* Presentation at the Forum on Microbial Threats Workshop Ending the War Metaphor: The Changing Agenda for Unraveling the Host-Microbe Relationship, Washington, D.C., Institute of Medicine, Forum on Microbial Threats.

Woolhouse M, Dye C. 2001. Population biology of emerging and re-emerging pathogens. *Philosophical Transactions of the Royal Societies of London Series B Biological Sciences* 356:979–1106.

Woolhouse M, Webster JP, Domingo E, Charlesworth B, Levin B. 2002. Biological and biomedical implications of the co-evolution of pathogens and their hosts. *Nature Genetics* 32(4):569–577.

Xiao SD, Zhang de Z, Liu HY, Wang GS, Xu GM, Zhang ZB, Lin GJ, Wang GL. 2003. Multicenter, randomized, controlled trial of heat-killed *Lactobacillus acidophilus* LB in patients with chronic diarrhea. *Advances in Therapy* 20(5):253–260.

Xu J, Gordon JI. 2003. Inaugural article: Honor thy symbionts. *Proceedings of the National Academy of Sciences USA* 100(18):10452–10459.

1

Microbial Communities of the Gut

OVERVIEW

The gastrointestinal tract represents an important and challenging system for exploring how microbial communities become established within their hosts, how their members maintain stable ecological niches, and how these dynamics relate to host health and disease. The complex, dynamic, and spatially diversified microbial community of the human gut is believed to be composed of at least 10^{13} microorganisms, including more than 800 species of bacteria (most of which have not yet been successfully cultured in the laboratory), numerous viral species including bacteriophages, archaea (e.g., methanogens), and eukaryotes (e.g., helminths and protozoa). The collective genome of the microbiota in the human gut is approximately one hundred-fold larger than that of its host. Therefore, as Bäckhed et al. (2005) state in their contribution to this chapter, "It seems appropriate to view ourselves as a composite of many species and our genetic landscape as an amalgam of genes embedded in our *Homo sapiens* genome and in the genomes of our affiliated microbial partners."

The first paper in this chapter, contributed by workshop presenter Karen Guillemin, focuses on the establishment of the gut microbiota (in humans, during the early days of infancy), its influence on host development (e.g., immunity), and the mechanisms by which hosts perceive and respond to the presence of colonizing microbes. Guillemin and coworkers pursue these fundamental questions in germ-free (GF) zebrafish, an experimental system that simplifies analyses of microbial influence on host development, while closely approximating gastrointestinal tract and immune system maturation, as well as gut microbiota diversity, in mammals. This approach has demonstrated the pervasive influence of the microbiota over a variety of events in the maturation of the gastrointestinal tract, but it raises further questions regarding the potential for individual developmental variation arising from differences in microbiota from one member of a species to another. In humans, such variation could accrue among contemporaries who live in different environments or have different diets, as well as over the course of history.

Once established, the gut microbiota acts as an exquisitely tuned metabolic "organ" within the host, according to presenter Jeffrey Gordon, senior author of the second paper in this chapter. He and coworkers review current knowledge of the structure and function of the human gut microbiota, as well as recent research that reveals coevolution between humans and gut microbes to their mutual benefit. Over the course of evolution, symbiotic gut bacteria have become, in Gordon's words, "master physiological chemists," employing a broad range of strategies to manipulate host genomes.

Details of these microbial strategies are revealed in the final contribution to this chapter, in which presenter Abigail Salyers surveys the microbial activities in the human colon that are influenced by diet and that in turn affect human health. These include genetic exchanges among microbes that occur through transformation, phage transduction, and conjugation—interactions that are known to contribute to antibiotic resistance and which may also influence the evolution and virulence of pathogens. Salyers notes that several basic and longstanding questions regarding the composition, function, and evolution of the human intestinal microflora can now be investigated with the advent of molecular technology.

THE ROLE OF THE INDIGENOUS MICROBIOTA IN ZEBRAFISH GASTROINTESTINAL TRACT DEVELOPMENT

Karen Guillemin, Ph.D.
University of Oregon

Although the anatomy of the human gastrointestinal (GI) tract has been explored since at least the time of Leonardo da Vinci, who secretly produced detailed drawings of human organs at a time when such studies were considered heretical, our understanding of this organ is still largely incomplete. That is because we know so little about its cellular composition, which is dominated by microbes. The bacterial community of the GI tract contains an enormous wealth of unsequenced genomic information, and it raises important questions as to its function in the normal physiology and development of this organ.

My coworkers and I are interested in the role commensal bacteria play in animal development, a phenomenon that has gone largely unexplored by developmental biologists. We are using a model vertebrate, the zebrafish, to study GI tract development in the presence and absence of the microbiota. Here I will describe how we have used this system to explore the establishment and role of the intestinal microbiota in early development and the means by which the host perceives and responds to its microbiota.

The Zebrafish Model

Zebrafish offer a number of advantages as a model for microbiota development and establishment. The embryos develop ex utero, which facilitates our ability to create GF animals. We harvest embryos and surface-sterilize them with a bleaching procedure that has been shown not to cause developmental defects; the embryos are then grown in sterile tissue culture flasks containing sterile media. The larvae are transparent, allowing us to follow the development of internal organs and monitor the dynamics of bacteria in live animals. GI tract development and physiology in zebrafish closely resemble those of mammals. Zebrafish also possess both adaptive and innate immune systems similar to those in mammals. Finally, zebrafish are readily amenable to genetic analysis.

The zebrafish gut is simpler than the human equivalent, but it exhibits regional specialization similar to the human organ: the proximal tract is specialized for lipid absorption, while most protein absorption occurs in the distal tract. This area near the anal vent is thought to be involved in osmoregulation. Figure 1-1 shows some of the key events in gut maturation and immune system development; our focus is on zero through eight day postfertilization (dpf). The embryos hatch out of their eggshells between 2 and 3 dpf, prior to the completion of gut maturation.

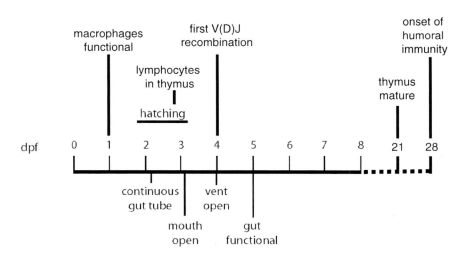

FIGURE 1-1 Important events in zebrafish development.
SOURCE: Guillemin (2005).

One of the first questions we addressed was how the gut microbiota is established. We have used scanning electron microscopy to visualize the rich microbial community on the surface of the embryonic chorion. We have also performed fluorescent in situ hybridization to look at the distribution of bacteria during development. Using a combination of three eubacterial probes that recognize sequences of 16S ribosomal RNA genes, we found that there is a dense community of microbes on the surface of the early embryo, but the interior of the embryo appears sterile. Microbes do not begin to accumulate within the embryo's internal organs, as viewed in transverse sections of the GI tract, until after the embryo hatches. In adult zebrafish, microbes are distributed throughout the lumen of the gut; the fish also appear to have immune cells that sample the microbial contents of the gut, possibly like mammalian dendritic cells. We quantified the bacterial load over the course of zebrafish development using quantitative polymerase chain reaction (PCR), producing results similar to those obtained through in situ hybridization and suggesting that the microbial load of the zebrafish GI tract, relative to its weight, is roughly comparable to that in humans.

Enumeration studies of the zebrafish microbiota reveal a preponderance of *Aeromonas* and *Pseudomonas* species, so we wanted to examine the distribution of these genera during developmental time. We hybridized the proximal and distal intestine of zebrafish at both 4 and 8 dpf with the eubacterial probes, as well as with specific probes for *Aeromonas* or *Pseudomonas*. At 4 dpf, we found a preponderance of *Pseudomonas* species in the distal intestine. By 8 dpf, these were largely replaced with *Aeromonas* species, but a large number of *Pseudomonas* species remained in the proximal intestine of these animals. Acquisition of this microbiota happens concurrently with the later events of gut maturation; a similar process of postnatal gut maturation occurs in mammals as they acquire their microflora.

Role of the Microbiota in Gut Development and Function

To examine the functional significance of the temporal relationship between microbiota establishment and gut maturation, we turned to gnotobiology, the use of GF animals (see subsequent paper by Bäckhed et al.). We raised GF zebrafish under sterile conditions, as previously described. For both GF and control fish, the egg yolk was the sole source of nutrients during these experiments. We verified the sterility of the GF zebrafish by plating fish homogenates on tryptic soy agar, by PCR with 16S panbacterial primers, and by conventional and scanning electron microscopy. To determine whether adding bacteria to GF zebrafish at a later stage of development would restore them to the same status as control animals, we raised GF animals until 5 dpf, when the conventionally-reared animals' guts become functional, then exposed the GF fish to a mixture of bacteria found in the water of their conventionally reared clutch mates.

We examined a variety of traits to compare the phenotypes of control and experimental animals, including the expression of an enzyme on the brush border of the intestinal epithelium, alkaline phosphatase. This enzyme is known to be induced during the developmental period; by staining for its activity in transverse sections of the gut, we found that by 8 dpf, alkaline phosphatase activity was considerably higher in the control zebrafish than in the GF animals. Alkaline phosphatase activity was restored to control levels in GF animals that were exposed, 5 dpf, to bacteria from their siblings.

Another marker of maturation we examined was glycan expression. The glycan landscape of the GI tract is known to be very sensitive to the presence of microbes, so we used a number of different lectins to sensitively detect the expression of a variety of sugar moieties. Using image analysis software to quantify sugar expression, we found that galactoseα1,3galactosyl (Galα1,3Gal) is down-regulated in conventionally reared animals, but persists at high levels in GF zebrafish; exposure to bacteria reduces the expression of this glycan in formerly GF fish. Experiments in GF rats have found that the number of mucus-secreting goblet cells in the GI tract is reduced in the GF animals (Ishikawa et al., 1986; Sharma and Schumacher, 1995). We found that in GF zebrafish the number of goblet cells at 8 dpf is less than in conventionally reared 8 dpf animals and similar to the number found in 5 dpf conventionally reared animals. Exposure to the microbiota again reverses this GF trait to that of a conventional animal of the same age.

We are also examining the relationship between microbiota establishment and GI tract function. For example, we have compared the ability of GF and control zebrafish to absorb proteins in their distal intestines. This trait can be evaluated by feeding the fish a high concentration of protein in the form of the enzyme horseradish peroxidase, then assaying the enzyme's activity after it is absorbed into cells. In these experiments, the GF animals—which we know to be equally proficient at swallowing as the conventionally raised controls—were found to be dramatically defective in protein absorption. This deficiency was reversed in GF animals following exposure to the microbiota. We also visualized GI motility in GF and control animals, which is possible in the transparent zebrafish. The GF animals had markedly shorter and more regular peristaltic waves along their GI tract, a trait that was once again reversed by exposure to the microbiota.

Host Perception of and Response to the Microbiota

Having accumulated evidence that the microbiota plays important roles in maturation and function of the zebrafish GI tract, we next explored how the host perceives the presence of the microbes, and attempted to identify the types of signals sent by the microbiota to its host that promote gut development. To do this, we created monocolonized animals by inoculating GF zebrafish, at 5 dpf, with pure cultures of either of two major bacterial constituents of the zebrafish GI tract: *Aeromonas sobria* and *Pseudomonas fluorescens*. We found that monoassociation with either bacterial strain was sufficient to reverse the previously discussed traits of low alkaline phosphatase activity and high Galα1,3Gal levels in GF zebrafish.

We next tested whether live bacteria were required to reverse these phenotypes or whether a heat-killed preparation of the microbiota was sufficient to signal to the host to promote gut maturation. We found that heat-killed microbiota was sufficient to induce alkaline phosphatase activity in GF animals; preliminary studies also indicate that bacterial lipopolysaccharide produces the same effect. By contrast, heat-killed bacteria failed to suppress the expression of Galα1,3Gal in GF animals. Thus, we have found evidence for two different modes of host perception for the presence of microbes: one that uses a generic signal of microbial-associated molecular patterns and another that requires active signaling from constituents of the microbiota.

Conclusion

Our findings on the role of the microbiota in the development of the GI tract in zebrafish show this to be a promising model for investigating the role of microbial communities in the developmental biology of the host. We have been able to show that the microbiota is required for gut maturation—as indicated by patterns of expression of glycans, by alkaline phosphatase activity, and by goblet cell census—and that the microbiota is important for such functions as protein absorption and GI motility.

The possibility that alkaline phosphatase enzymatic activity can be upregulated by a heat-killed bacterial preparation immediately brings to mind the toll-like receptors (TLRs) of the innate immune system, and their ability to recognize generic microbial-associated molecular patterns. Much attention has been focused on the role of TLRs in protection against infection, but it is also important to consider these molecules in the context of gut development and homeostasis. A recent publication by Rakoff-Nahoum et al. (2004) examines susceptibility to intestinal injury in animals that are deficient for TLR signaling. In this study, wild-type mice survived an intestinal injury, while animals deficient in MyD88, an adaptor molecule essential for TLR-mediated induction of inflammatory cytokines, manifested severe morbidity and mortality in response to the same insult. A similar phenotype was observed in animals in which the ligand for TLRs was depleted by an antibiotic reduction of the microbiota. This trait was reversed, and the animals' viability restored, by exposing them to lipopolysaccharide and lipoteichoic acid, two conserved molecular products of microorganisms recognized by TLRs. These results indicate that the constituents of the microbiota continually shape GI tract homeostasis.

Given such findings, it will now be important to determine the extent to which the microbiota is stereotyped during development. Most of us would agree that the human microbiota has probably changed very much since the time of Leonardo da Vinci, due to the onset of antimicrobial therapies and modern sanitation. In that regard, it may be somewhat comforting to imagine that certain aspects of the microbial-directed maturation of the GI tract require generic signals that many different possible constituents could supply. However, it is also clear that certain complex and specific signaling events influence GI tract maturation and function. The gnotobiotic zebrafish model will help elucidate the various signaling mechanisms between animals and their resident microbes.

HOST-BACTERIAL MUTUALISM IN THE HUMAN INTESTINE

*Fredrik Bäckhed, Ruth E. Ley, Justin L. Sonnenburg,
Daniel A. Peterson, Jeffrey I. Gordon*[1]
Reprinted with permission from *Science* (Bäckhed et al. 2005).
Copyright 2005 AAAS.

The distal human intestine represents an anaerobic bioreactor programmed with an enormous population of bacteria, dominated by relatively few divisions that are highly diverse at the strain/subspecies level. This microbiota and its collective genomes (microbiome) provide us with genetic and metabolic attributes we have not been required to evolve on our own, including the ability to harvest otherwise inaccessible nutrients. New studies are revealing how the gut microbiota has coevolved with us and how it manipulates and complements our biology in ways that are mutually beneficial. We are also starting to understand how certain keystone members of the microbiota operate to maintain the stability and functional adaptability of this microbial organ.

The adult human intestine is home to an almost inconceivable number of microorganisms. The size of the population—up to 100 trillion—far exceeds that of all other microbial communities associated with the body's surfaces and is ~10 times greater than the total number of our somatic and germ cells (Savage, 1977). Thus, it seems appropriate to view ourselves as a composite of many species and our genetic landscape as an amalgam of genes embedded in our *Homo sapiens* genome and in the genomes of our affiliated microbial partners (the microbiome).

Our gut microbiota can be pictured as a microbial organ placed within a host organ: It is composed of different cell lineages with a capacity to communicate with one another and the host; it consumes, stores, and redistributes energy; it mediates physiologically important chemical transformations; and it can maintain and repair itself through self replication. The gut microbiome, which may

---

[1]Materials and methods are available as supporting material on *Science* Online. We thank L. Angenent for many helpful discussions. Work cited from the authors' lab is supported by the NIH and NSF. F.B. and J.L.S. are supported by postdoctoral fellowships from the Wenner-Gren and W. M. Keck Foundations, respectively. Supporting online material: www.sciencemag.org/cgi/content/full/ 307/5717/1915/ DC1MaterialsandMethodsTablesS1toS3References.10.1126/science.1104816.

contain > 100 times the number of genes in our genome, endows us with functional features that we have not had to evolve ourselves.

Our relationship with components of this microbiota is often described as commensal (one partner benefits and the other is apparently unaffected) as opposed to mutualistic (both partners experience increased fitness). However, use of the term commensal generally reflects our lack of knowledge, or at least an agnostic (noncommittal) attitude about the contributions of most citizens of this microbial society to our own fitness or the fitness of other community members.

The guts of ruminants and termites are well-studied examples of bioreactors "programmed" with anaerobic bacteria charged with the task of breaking down ingested polysaccharides, the most abundant biological polymer on our planet, and fermenting the resulting monosaccharide soup to short-chain fatty acids. In these mutualistic relationships, the hosts gain carbon and energy, and their microbes are provided with a rich buffet of glycans and a protected anoxic environment (Brune and Friedrich, 2000). Our distal intestine is also an anaerobic bioreactor that harbors the majority of our gut microorganisms; they degrade a varied menu of otherwise indigestible polysaccharides, including plant-derived pectin, cellulose, hemicellulose, and resistant starches.

Microbiologists from Louis Pasteur and Ilya Mechnikov to present-day scientists have emphasized the importance of understanding the contributions of this microbiota to human health (and disease). Experimental and computational tools are now in hand to comprehensively characterize the nature of microbial diversity in the gut, the genomic features of its keystone members, the operating principles that underlie the nutrient foraging and sharing behaviors of these organisms, the mechanisms that ensure the adaptability and robustness of this system, and the physiological benefits we accrue from this mutualistic relationship. This review aims to illustrate these points and highlight some future challenges for the field.

Microbial Diversity in the Human Gut Bioreactor

The adult human gastrointestinal tract contains all three domains of life—bacteria, archaea, and eukarya. Bacteria living in the human gut achieve the highest cell densities recorded for any ecosystem (Whitman et al., 1998). Nonetheless, diversity at the division level (superkingdom or deep evolutionary lineage) is among the lowest (Hugenholtz et al., 1998); only 8 of the 55 known bacterial divisions have been identified to date (Figure 1-2A), and of these, 5 are rare. The divisions that dominate—the *Cytophaga-Flavobacterium-Bacteroides* (CFB) (e.g., the genus *Bacteroides*) and the Firmicutes (e.g., the genera *Clostridium* and *Eubacterium*)—each comprise ~30 percent of bacteria in feces and the mucus overlying the intestinal epithelium. Proteobacteria are common but usually not dominant (Seksik et al., 2003). In comparison, soil (the terrestrial biosphere's GI tract, where degradation of organic matter occurs) can contain 20 or more bacterial divisions (Dunbar et al., 2002).

Our knowledge of the composition of the adult gut microbiota stems from culture-based studies (Moore and Holdeman, 1974), and more recently from culture-independent molecular phylogenetic approaches based on sequencing bacterial ribosomal RNA (16S rRNA) genes. Of the > 200,000 rRNA gene sequences currently in GenBank, only 1,822 are annotated as being derived from the human gut; 1,689 represent uncultured bacteria. rRNA sequences can be clustered into relatedness groups based on their percent sequence identity. Cutoffs of 95 and 98 percent identity are used commonly to delimit genera and species, respectively. Although these values are somewhat arbitrary and the terms "*genus*" and "*species*" are not precisely defined for microbes, we use them here to frame a view of human gut microbial ecology. When the sequences (n = 495 greater than 900 base pairs) are clustered into species, and a diversity estimate model is applied, a value of ~800 species is obtained (Figure 1-3). If the analysis is adjusted to estimate strain number (unique sequence types), a value > 7,000 is obtained (Figure 1-3). Thus, the gut microbiota, which appears to be tremendously diverse at the strain and subspecies level, can be visualized as a grove of eight palm trees (divisions) with deeply divergent lineages represented by the fan(s) of closely related bacteria at the very top of each tree trunk.

Diversity present in the GI tract appears to be the result of strong host selection and coevolution. For example, members of the CFB division that are predominantly associated with mammals appear to be the most derived (i.e., farthest away from the common ancestor of the division), indicating that they underwent accelerated evolution once they adopted a mutualistic lifestyle. Moreover, a survey of GenBank reveals that several subgroups in CFB are distributed among different mammalian species (Figure 1-2B), suggesting that the CFB-mammal symbiosis is ancient and that distinct subgroups coevolved with their hosts.

The structure and composition of the gut microbiota reflect natural selection at two levels: at the microbial level, where lifestyle strategies (e.g., growth rate and substrate utilization patterns) affect the fitness of individual bacteria in a competitive ensemble, and at the host level, where suboptimal functionality of the microbial ensemble can reduce host fitness. Microbial consortia whose integrated activities result in a cost to the host will result in fewer hosts, thereby causing loss of their own habitat. Conversely, microbial consortia that promote host fitness will create more habitats. Thus, the diversity found within the human GI tract, namely, a few divisions represented by very tight clusters of related bacteria, may reflect strong host selection for specific bacteria whose emergent collective behavior is beneficial to the host. This hypothesis has two important implications: (1) A mechanism exists to promote cooperation, and (2) the structure promotes functional stability of the gut ecosystem.

To benefit the host, bacteria must be organized in a trophic structure (food web) that aids in breaking down nutrients and provides the host with energetic substrates. Cooperative behavior that imposes a cost to the individual while benefiting the community can emerge within groups of bacteria (Rainey and Rainey,

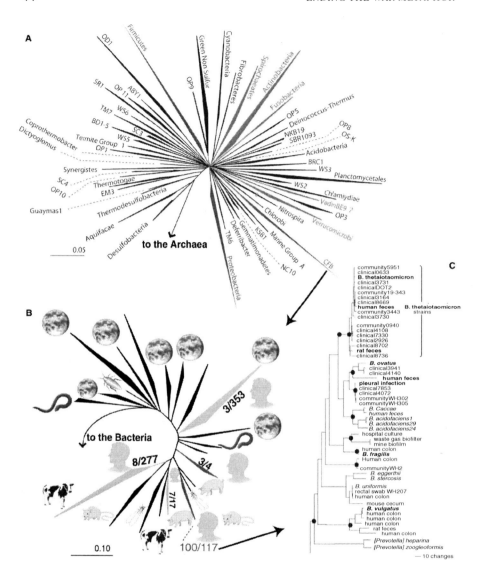

FIGURE 1-2 Representation of the diversity of bacteria in the human intestine. (A) Phylogenetic tree of the domain bacteria based on 8,903 representative 16S rRNA gene sequences. Wedges represent divisions (superkingdoms): Those numerically abundant in the human gut are red, rare divisions are green, and undetected are black (for colors please refer to the original article). Wedge length is a measure of evolutionary distance from the common ancestor. (B) Phylogenetic tree of the CFB division based on 1561 sequences from GenBank (> 900 nucleotides) and their ecological context. Wedges are major sub-

caption continues at right

2003) and can be maintained by group selection as long as consortia are isolated and new consortia form periodically (e.g., new GI tracts). Furthermore, selection must act simultaneously at multiple levels of biological organization (Travisano and Velicer, 2004). These criteria are met in the human GI tract where new acts of colonization occur at birth, with a small founding population of noncheaters from the mother, and selection occurs both at the microbial and host level.

Diversity is generally thought to be desirable for ecosystem stability (McCann, 2000). One important way diversity can confer resilience is through a wide repertoire of responses to stress (referred to as the insurance hypothesis [Yachi and Loreau, 1999]). In man-made anaerobic bioreactors used to treat wastewater (a system analogous to the gut but where no host selection occurs), rates of substrate degradation can remain constant, whereas bacterial populations fluctuate chaotically as a result of blooms of subpopulations (Fernandez et al., 2000). Functional redundancy in the microbial community ensures that key processes are unaffected by such changes in diversity (Goebel and Stackebrandt, 1994). By contrast, in the human gut, populations are remarkably stable within individuals (Zoetendal et al., 1998), implying that mechanisms exist to suppress blooms of subpopulations and/or to promote the abundance of desirable bacteria. A study of adult monozygotic twins living apart and their marital partners has emphasized the potential dominance of host genotype over diet in determining microbial composition of the gut bioreactor (Zoetendal et al., 2001). The role of the immune system in defining diversity and suppressing subpopulation blooms remains to be defined. One likely mediator of bacterial selection is secretory immunoglobulin A (Suzuki et al., 2004).

The human gut is faced with a paradox: How can functional redundancy be maintained in a system with low diversity (few divisions of bacteria), and how

groups of CFB; symbols are sources of the sequences [Earth, environmental; cow, ruminants; rodent, rat and/or mouse; person, human GI tract; others are termite, cockroach, worm (including hydrothermal), and pig]. Ratios are the number of sequences represented in the human gut relative to the total number in the subgroup: red, yellow, and black indicate majority, minority, and absence of sequences represented in human GI tract, respectively. (C) Phylogenetic (parsimony) tree of *Bacteroides*. Strains classified as *B. thetaiotaomicron* based on phenotype are in red; 16S rRNA analysis did not confirm this classification for all strains. *Bacteroides* spp. with sequenced genomes are in bold. Black circles indicate nodes with high (> 70 percent) bootstrap support. Scale bars indicate the degree of diversity (evolutionary distance) within a division or subgroup ([A] and [B]), respectively] in terms of the fraction of the 16S rRNA nucleotides that differ between member sequences; in (C), the evolutionary distance between organisms is read along branch lengths, where scale indicates number of changes in 16S rRNA nucleotide composition.
SOURCE: Bäckhed et al. (2005).

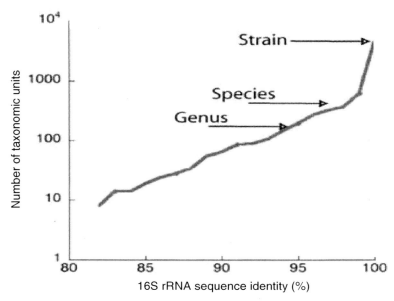

FIGURE 1-3 Taxon richness estimates for bacteria in the human GI tract. Taxon richness estimates for varying levels of 16S rRNA sequence identity, ranging from below the "genus" level (95 percent identity), to the "species" level (98 percent identity), to the strain level (unique sequences). Estimates are based on sequences available in GenBank, annotated as derived from the human GI tract, after alignment and clustering into taxonomic units ranging from 80 to 100 percent identity.
SOURCE: Bäckhed et al. (2005).

can such a system withstand selective sweeps in the form of, for example, phage attacks? The estimated 1,200 viral genotypes in human feces (Breitbart et al., 2003) suggest that a phage attack is a powerful shaper of the gut's microbial genetic landscape (Fuhrman, 1999; Winter et al., 2004). Enough diversity of genome and transcriptome must be represented at the subspecies level to lend resilience to the gut ecosystem. Ecological studies of macroecosystems have shown that less diversity is required to maintain stability if individual species themselves have a wide repertoire of responses (Yachi and Loreau, 1999). In the following section we discuss recent genome-based studies exploring how a presumed keystone bacterial species in our gut is able to adapt to (1) changing dietary conditions in ways that should stabilize the microbiota's food web, and (2) changing immune and phage selective pressures in ways that should stabilize the ecosystem.

Bacteroides thetaiotaomicron—A Highly Adaptive Glycophile

Bacteroides thetaiotaomicron is a prominent mutualist in the distal intestinal habitat of adult humans. It is a very successful glycophile whose prodigious capacity for digesting otherwise indigestible dietary polysaccharides is reflected in the fully sequenced 6.3-Mb genome of the type strain (ATCC 29148; originally isolated from the feces of a healthy adult human) (Xu et al., 2003). Its "glycobiome" contains the largest ensemble of genes involved in acquiring and metabolizing carbohydrates yet reported for a sequenced bacterium, including 163 paralogs of two outer membrane proteins (SusC and SusD) that bind and import starch (Shipman et al., 2000), 226 predicted glycoside hydrolases, and 15 polysaccharide lyases (CAZY, 2005). By contrast, our 2.85-Gb genome only contains 98 known or putative glycoside hydrolases and is deficient in the enzyme activities required for degradation of xylan-, pectin-, and arabinose-containing polysaccharides that are common components of dietary fiber (we have one predicted enzyme versus 64 in *B. thetaiotaomicron*; see Annex 1-1, Table 1-1).

The carbohydrate foraging behavior of *B. thetaiotaomicron* has been characterized during its residency in the distal intestines (ceca) of gnotobiotic mice colonized exclusively with this anaerobe (Sonnenburg et al., 2005). Scanning electron microscopy studies of the intestines of mice maintained on a standard high-polysaccharide chow diet, containing xylose, galactose, arabinose, and glucose as its principal monosaccharide components, revealed communities of bacteria assembled on small undigested or partially digested food particles, shed elements of the mucus gel layer, and exfoliated epithelial lining cells (Sonnenburg et al., 2005). Whole-genome transcriptional profiling of *B. thetaiotaomicron* (Sonnenburg et al., 2005) disclosed that this diet was associated with selective up-regulation of a subset of SusC and SusD paralogs, a subset of glycoside hydrolases (e.g., xylanases, arabinosidases, and pectate lyase), as well as genes encoding enzymes involved in delivering the products of mannose, galactose, and glucose to the glycolytic pathway and arabinose and xylose to the pentose phosphate pathway. In contrast, a simple sugar (glucose and sucrose) diet devoid of polysaccharides led to increased expression of a different subset of SusC and SusD paralogs, glycoside hydrolases involved in retrieving carbohydrates from mucus glycans, as well as enzymes that remove modifications that make these host glycans otherwise resistant to degradation (O-acetylation of sialic acids and sulfation of glycosoaminoglycans) (Sonnenburg et al., 2005).

These findings provide insights about how functional diversity and adaptability are achieved by a prominent member of the human colonic microbiota (Figure 1-4). Dining occurs on particulate nutrient scaffolds (food particles, shed mucus, and/or exfoliated epithelial cells). For a bacterium such as *B. thetaiotaomicron*, which lacks adhesive organelles, seating at the "dining table" is determined in part by the repertoire of glycan-specific outer membrane-binding proteins it produces, and this repertoire is itself shaped by the menu of available

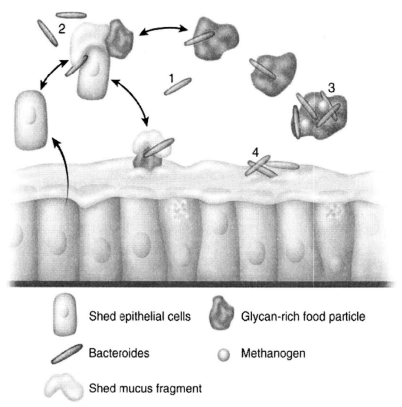

FIGURE 1-4 Lessons about adaptive foraging for glycans obtained from *B. thetaiotaomicron*. (1) *B. thetaiotaomicron* does not have adhesive organelles. Without outer membrane polysaccharide-binding protein-mediated attachment to glycan-rich nutrient platforms, it is at risk for being washed out from the intestinal bioreactor. Substrate access is limited under these conditions. (2) Small nutrient platforms are composed of undigested or partially digested food particles (e.g., dietary fiber), shed host epithelial cells, and/or mucus fragments. These platform elements may be in dynamic equilibrium with one another and with the mucus layer overlying the intestinal epithelium. Microbial fermentation of otherwise indigestible polysaccharides in these platforms is made possible by induced expression of substrate-appropriate sets of bacterial polysaccharide-binding proteins and glycoside hydrolases. (3) Mesophilic methanogens drive carbohydrate utilization by removing products of fermentation (H_2 and CO_2 are converted to methane), thereby improving the overall efficiency of energy extraction from polysaccharides. (4) When dietary polysaccharides are scarce, *B. thetaiotaomicron* turns to host mucus by deploying a different set of polysaccharide binding proteins and glycoside hydrolases. This adaptive foraging reflects the coevolved functional versatility of *B. thetaiotaomicron*'s glycobiome and the structural diversity of the host's mucus glycans.
SOURCE: Bäckhed et al. (2005).

glycans (Sonnenburg et al., 2005). Attachment to nutrient platforms helps avoid washout from the intestinal bioreactor, in much the same way as dense, well-settling, granular biofilms help oppose elimination from engineered (man-made) anaerobic upflow bioreactors (Sonnenburg et al., 2004). Attachment also presumably increases the efficiency of oligo- and monosaccharide harvest by adaptively expressed bacterial glycoside hydrolases and their subsequent distribution to other members of the microbiota whose niche overlaps that of *B. thetaiotaomicron*. In this conceptualization, microbial nutrient metabolism along the length of the intestine is a summation of myriad selfish and syntrophic relationships expressed by inhabitants of these nutrient platforms. Diversity in these microhabitats and mutualistic cooperation among their component species (including the degree to which sanctions must be applied against cheats) are reflections of a dynamic interplay between the available nutrient foundation and the degree of flexible foraging (niche breadth) expressed by microhabitat residents. *Bacteroides* spp., such as *B. thetaiotaomicron*, impart stability to the gut ecosystem by having the capacity to turn to host polysaccharides when dietary polysaccharides become scarce. The highly variable outer chain structures of mucus and epithelial cell surface glycans are influenced by host genotype and by microbial regulation of host glycosyltransferase gene expression. Coevolution of host glycan diversity and a large collection of microbial glycoside hydrolases that are regulated by nutrient availability provides insurance that the "system" (microbiota and host) can rapidly and efficiently respond to changes in the diet, and maximize energy harvest, without having to undergo substantial changes in species composition. Rather than minimizing genome size, a keystone species such as *B. thetaiotaomicron* has evolved an elaborate and sizable genome that can mobilize functionally diverse adaptive responses.

Diet-associated changes in the glycan-foraging behavior of *B. thetaiotaomicron* are also accompanied by changes in expression of its capsular polysaccharide synthesis loci, indicating that *B. thetaiotaomicron* is able to change its carbohydrate surface depending upon the nutrient (glycan) environment. This could be part of a strategy for evading an adaptive immune response. Whole-genome genotyping studies of *B. thetaiotaomicron* isolates, with the use of GeneChips designed from the sequenced genome of the type strain, disclose that their CPS loci differ, whereas their housekeeping genes are conserved (Ley and Gordon, Unpublished data). Because selective sweeps are most likely to come from the immune system and phages, both of which respond to surface structures, the associated genes are likely to be the most diverse in the genome. Accordingly, *B. thetaiotaomicron* has a remarkable apparatus for altering its genome content. The sequenced type strain contains a plasmid, 63 transposases, 43 integrases, and 4 homologs of a conjugative transposon (Xu et al., 2003). Gene transfer and mutation mechanisms endow strains of bacterial species with the (genetic) versatility necessary to withstand selective sweeps that would eradicate more clonal populations (Taddei et al., 1997).

The Gut Microbiota as a "Host" Factor That Influences Energy Storage

Comparisons of mice raised without exposure to any microorganisms, (Germ-Free), with those that have acquired a microbiota since birth, or conventionally raised (CONV-R), have led to the identification of numerous effects of indigenous microbes on host biology (see Annex 1-1, Table 1-2), including energy balance. Young adult CONV-R animals have 40 percent more total body fat than their GF counterparts fed the same polysaccharide-rich diet, even though CONV-R animals consume less chow per day (Bäckhed et al., 2004). This observation might seem paradoxical at first but can be explained by the fact that the gut microbiota allows energy to be salvaged from otherwise indigestible dietary polysaccharides (Yamanaka et al., 1977). "Conventionalization" of adult GF mice with cecal contents harvested from CONV-R donors increases body fat content to levels equivalent to those of CONV-R animals (Bäckhed et al., 2004). The increase reflects adipocyte hypertrophy rather than hyperplasia and is notable for its rapidity and sustainability (Bäckhed et al., 2004).

The mutualistic nature of the host-bacterial relationship is underscored by mechanisms that underlie this fat-storage phenotype. Colonization increases glucose uptake in the host intestine and produces substantial elevations in serum glucose and insulin (Bäckhed et al., 2004), both of which stimulate hepatic lipogenesis through their effects on two basic helix-loop-helix/leucine zipper transcription factors—ChREBP and SREBP-1c (Bäckhed et al., 2004; Towle, 2001). Short-chain fatty acids, generated by microbial fermentation, also induce lipogenesis (Rolandelli et al., 1989). Triglycerides exported by the liver into the circulation are taken up by adipocytes through a lipoprotein lipase (LPL)-mediated process. The microbiota suppresses intestinal epithelial expression of a circulating LPL inhibitor, fasting-induced adipose factor (FIAF, also known as angiopoietin-like protein-4) (Bäckhed et al., 2004). Comparisons of GF and conventionalized wild-type and FIAF –/– mice established FIAF as a physiologically important regulator of LPL activity in vivo and a key modulator of the microbiota-induced increase in fat storage (Bäckhed et al., 2004).

The caloric density of food items is portrayed as a fixed value on package labels. However, it seems reasonable to postulate that caloric value varies between individual "consumers" according to the composition and operation (e.g., transit time) of their intestinal bioreactors, and that the microbiota influences their energy balance. Relatively high-efficiency bioreactors would promote energy storage (obesity), whereas lower efficiency reactors would promote leanness (efficiency is defined in this case as the energy-harvesting and storage-promoting potential of an individual's microbiota relative to the ingested diet).

The idea that individual variations in bioreactor efficiencies may be a significant variable in the energy balance equation is supported by several observations. First, individual variations in the composition of the microbiota occur and are influenced by host genotype (Zoetendal et al., 2001). Second, small but chronic differences between energy intake and expenditure can, in principle, produce major changes in body composition [e.g., if energy balance is +12 kcal/day, 90.45 kg of fat could be gained per year if there are no compensatory responses by the host; this is the average weight increase experienced by Americans from age 25 to 55 (Flegal and Troiano, 2000)]. Third, the microbiota is a substantial consumer of energy. One group estimated that individuals on a "British Diet" must ferment 50 to 65 g of hexose sugars daily to obtain the energy required to replace the 15 to 20 g (dry weight) of bacteria they excrete per day (McNeil, 1984).

These considerations emphasize the need to assess the representation of species with large capacities for processing dietary polysaccharides, such as *Bacteroides*, in lean versus morbidly obese individuals, and in cohorts of obese individuals before, during, and after weight reduction achieved by high-polysaccharide/low-fat versus high-fat/low-polysaccharide diets, or by bariatric (gastric bypass) surgery. The results, coupled with coincident assessments of energy extraction from the diet, should provide a proof-of-concept test of whether differences in the composition of the microbiota are associated with differences in gut bioreactor efficiency (and predisposition to obesity).

Lessons that have been learned by environmental engineers who study how to optimize the efficiency of man-made anaerobic bioreactors (see Annex 1-1, Table 1-3) suggest that these enumeration studies should also include members of archaea. Thermodynamics dictates that the energy obtained from substrate conversions will be higher if low concentrations of products are maintained (Stams, 1994; Thauer et al., 1977). In the human gut, methanogenic archaea provide the last microbial link in the metabolic chain of polysaccharide processing. Bacteria degrade polysaccharides to short-chain fatty acids, carbon dioxide, and hydrogen gas. Methanogens lower the partial pressure of hydrogen by generating methane, and thereby may increase microbial fermentation rates. Defining the representation of mesophilic methanogens in the colonic microbiota of individuals, sequencing their genomes [as we are currently doing with *Methanobrevibacter smithii*, a prevalent isolate from the human colon (Miller and Wolin, 1982)], and characterizing archaeal-bacterial syntrophy in simplified gnotobiotic mouse models consuming different diets should provide a starting point for defining the role of archaea in shaping the functional diversity, stability, and beneficial contributions of our distal gut microbiota. Devising ways for manipulating archaeal populations may provide a novel way for intentionally altering our energy balance.

Looking to the Future

A comprehensive 16S rRNA sequence-based (bacterial and archaeal) enumeration of the microbiotas of selected humans, representing different ethnic groups, living in similar or distinct milieus, would provide an invaluable database for studying normal and diseased populations (Chacon et al., 2004). The concept of using the microbiota as a biomarker of impending or fully manifest diseases within or outside of the GI tract and for monitoring responses to therapeutic interventions needs to be explored.

Several groups are embarking on metagenome sequencing projects to define gene content in the human gut microbiome. If we view ourselves as being a composite of many species, this represents a logical continuation of the Human Genome Project. A complementary approach to metagenomic analysis is to determine genome-level diversity among bacterial populations belonging to a specific genus or species residing within a defined gut habitat of a single individual or a few individuals. Members of *Bacteroides* provide a natural experiment for examining the impact of habitat on genome content since they have yet to be encountered in any environment other than animal GI tracts. Figure 1-2C illustrates how a collection of just 29 isolates phenotyped as *B. thetaiotaomicron* provided a broad range of 16S rRNA sequences, including several new species. We are close to producing finished genome sequences for two prominent members of the colonic microbiota, *B. vulgatus* and *B. distasonis* (GSC, 2005). *B. fragilis*, a less prominent member, has recently been sequenced (Cerdeño-Tárraga et al., 2005; Kuwahara et al., 2004). The results will allow us to ask how evolutionary history relates to genome content and what constitutes a minimal *Bacteroides* genome.

We also need to obtain a direct view of how the metabolites originating from the microbiome influence host physiology. This will be a formidable task, requiring new techniques for measuring metabolites generated by single and defined collections of symbionts during growth under defined nutrient conditions in single-vessel chemostats, in more elaborate mechanical models of the human gut, and in vivo after colonization of specified habitats of the intestines of gnotobiotic mice. The results should help formulate and direct hypothesis-based investigations of the microbiota's "metabolome" in humans.

Databases that connect molecular data with ecosystem parameters are still rare (Galperin, 2004). A human intestinal microbiome database is needed to organize genomic, transcriptomic, and metabolomic data obtained from this complex natural microbial community, and would provide a substrate for generating testable hypotheses.

Finally, just as microbiotas have coevolved with their animal hosts, this field must coevolve with its academic hosts and their ability to devise innovative ways of assembling interactive interdisciplinary research groups necessary to advance our understanding.

ACTIVITIES OF HUMAN COLONIC MICROBES

Abigail A. Salyers
Department of Microbiology
University of Illinois

Overview of the Interaction

The microbes that inhabit our colons have a complex relationship with us

(Salyers, 1986; Salyers and Shipman, 2002). We are a food source for them, but they also contribute to our nutrition. Through their activities, they influence many aspects of human physiology. In fact, one could view the human intestine as an organ that was largely shaped by them during evolution. For example, the small intestine is designed to promote a fast flow of contents, a feature that has the effect of discouraging microbial growth by washing microbes through before they can establish themselves. The flow of contents through the colon, by contrast, is so slow that microbes can easily establish themselves and reach concentrations that are high enough to make up at least 30 percent of human colonic contents (Figure 1-5). In the colon, bacteria perform a service for us by digesting substances in the diet that the human stomach and small intestine cannot. The intestinal microbes also take an energy toll from us; they stimulate the turnover of intestinal mucosal cells. This constant sloughing of intestinal mucosal cells is a very effective defense that prevents bacteria that have attached to the mucosal cells from staying in the site long enough to invade.

In the colon, resident microbes also interact with each other genetically. Bacteria exchange genes in order to acquire new traits. One type of gene that is exchanged is antibiotic resistance genes, but many other genes are also exchanged. Diet influences this genetic interaction because it can include antibiotics or even antibiotic-resistant bacteria that can interact with the normal inhabitants of the site.

Finally, colonic bacteria modify substances such as bile acids, cholesterol, and xenobiotic compounds. The effects of these modifications on human health are still uncertain, but they surely occur.

In this chapter, we survey in detail the different types of microbial activities that are affected by the human diet and, in turn, affect human health. We also identify some basic questions, most of which were posed years ago, but are only now beginning to be addressed because modern molecular technology has made such investigations much more feasible than were previously possible.

Composition of the Intestinal Microflora

The microbial population of the human colon consists primarily of bacteria. It has been estimated that there are at least several hundred to a thousand distinct species of bacteria, although a smaller number, about 20 species, account for the majority of isolates (Bäckhed et al., 2005; Salyers, 1986). A smaller group of microbes in the colon are the methanogenic archaea. These methane-producing microbes are sufficiently active, and the methane they produce can be detected, not only in intestinal contents, but also in the breath. Most of the numerically predominant bacteria are carbohydrate fermenters. These methanogens live on byproducts of carbohydrate fermentation such as carbon dioxide and acetate.

The colonic microflora is unusual in that in contrast to most microbial populations about 50 percent of the microbes can be cultivated. More recently, molecular techniques such as 16S rRNA PCR amplification and sequencing have

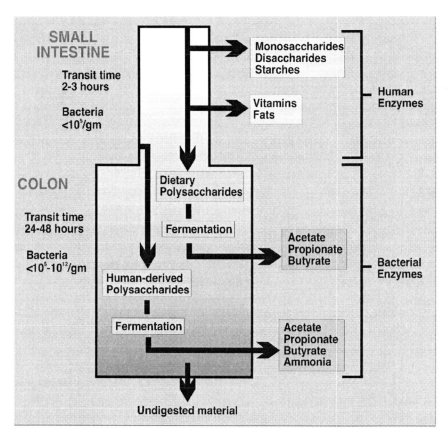

FIGURE 1-5 The flow of contents through the small intestine and colon.
SOURCE: Salyers (2005).

been applied to take a molecular census of the bacterial population (Wilson and Blitchington, 1996). Although molecular techniques have revealed some new species, there is general agreement between cultivation-based and molecular characterizations of the population. A striking feature of the colonic microflora is that the majority of colonic bacteria are gram-positive bacteria, virtually all of which are obligate anaerobes (Bäckhed et al., 2005; Salyers, 1986; Salyers and Shipman, 2002; Wilson and Blitchington, 1996). Gram-positive anaerobes account for at least 65 percent of the isolates. Gram-negative anaerobes, such as *Bacteroides* species, account for another 20 to 30 percent. Numerically minor populations, such as the enterics and the enterococci, account for less than 2 percent (Bäckhed et al., 2005).

It is important to note that numerically minor populations may still play an important role despite their relatively low numbers. Because the numerically major populations of bacteria are packed in the colon lumen, separated from the colonic mucosa by a mucin layer, any numerically minor population that succeeds in reaching the mucosa and adhering to mucosal cells could have a disproportionate effect on the colonic mucosa. Little is known about the bacteria that occupy the mucin layer, but colonic bacteria that degrade mucin have been isolated (McGarr et al., 2005).

A question that has not been answered conclusively is whether there are different populations of bacteria on the mucosal surface compared to the population in the lumen of the colon or whether there is population variation in the varying parts of the colon. It has not been easy to answer this question because mucosal samples from unmedicated healthy volunteers cannot be ethically obtained. Samples that are available tend to come from people with underlying conditions that require surgery, and these patients have invariably been treated extensively with antibiotics.

There is one older study in which samples were obtained from the intestinal tracts of sudden death victims. This was made possible by the fact that in some U.S. states, autopsy of such persons is mandated by law (Moore et al., 1978). At the time, such a study was possible only because some pathologists would provide post-autopsy samples. Such a study could probably not be done today. The results of this study supported the hypothesis that there were no distinct microbial subpopulations in different colonic locations, a conclusion that is difficult to believe in view of the fact that most environments contain niches that support distinct bacterial populations. The mouth and skin are human examples of such niche differentiation. A major limitation of this study, however, was that at least four hours elapsed between death and the availability of the specimens. During this time, extensive sloughing of the colonic mucosa would have occurred and peristalsis would have ceased. This might have eliminated, to some extent, any unique populations that exist in living humans. Because the human colon is not as accessible to sampling as other areas of the human body, mice—or some other animal such as the pig—will have to be accepted as models for colonic populations if progress in understanding niches in the colon is to be made.

As has already been mentioned, gram-positive bacteria account for at least 65 percent of colonic isolates. This is also true of other areas of the body such as the mouth, skin, and vaginal tract. The numerical predominance of gram-positive bacteria is a curious feature of the microflora of the human body because gram-positive bacteria represent only a minority of the types of bacteria found in the world at large. Gram-negative bacteria are much more diverse and much more numerous. To our knowledge, no one has yet proposed an explanation of why gram-positive bacteria should be such prominent members of the human microflora. Part of the problem with speculating about the reasons for this predominance is that virtually nothing is known about the gram-positive majority in the human colon.

Dore and coworkers (De La Cochetiere et al., 2005) were among the first to identify colonic bacteria using molecular methods. Surprisingly, most of them proved to be members of the genus *Clostridium*. Earlier cultivation-based studies had classified them in such genera as *Eubacterium, Peptostreptococcus,* and *Bifidobacterium*. This apparent difference between the results of molecular analyses and cultivation-based analyses may not be due so much to the presence of uncultivated bacteria as to the fact that much of the cultivated gram-positive bacteria may have been misclassified using phenotypic traits. It has certainly been the case that the relatively easily cultivable gram-negative colonic anaerobes have undergone many reclassifications in recent years based on 16S rRNA phylogenetic analysis. Two groups of the numerically predominant clostridia emerged, the *Clostridium leptum* group and the *Clostridium coccoides* group. Subsequent molecular studies have confirmed this identification. If you have never heard of these species, you are in good company. Virtually no studies of their metabolic characteristics have been done, and so far no genome sequences are available. These bacteria may receive more attention in the future due to interest in the possibility that the colonic microflora play a role in inflammatory bowel disease and colon cancer.

The preponderance of these previously unknown gram-positive bacteria in the normal human colon raises an interesting practical question. Should probiotics, preparations of bacteria ingested intentionally with a view of maintaining or restoring a healthy colonic microflora, include these species of gram-positive anaerobes? At present, probiotics that are available on the market consist of species of *Lactobacillus* or *Bifidobacterium* that are either not present in the human colon or are present in very low concentrations.

Given that *C. leptum, C. coccoides,* and their close relatives are normally predominant components of the colonic microflora, they are the logical species to use in probiotic products. Selling *C. leptum* or *C. coccoides* to the probiotics industry and to the regulatory agencies, however, is going to be a tough job. The genus *Clostridium* has a widely known reputation for pathogenicity, with *Clostridium botulinum* (botulism), *Clostridium perfringens* (gas gangrene), *Clostridium tetani* (tetanus), and *Clostridium difficile* (pseudomembraneous colitis) being its best known representatives. Of course, most genera that contain serious pathogens also contain a much greater number of benign species. But, at present, *Clostridium* is definitely considered a "scarce genus."

The issue of probiotic formulation is not just the concern of those who patronize health food stores and natural healers. Restoration of the colonic microflora in people who have taken antibiotics that diminish the normally predominant anaerobes or have had cancer chemotherapy, which for some reason affects the microflora in some people, is a serious medical problem that has long worried gastroenterologists.

Post-antibiotic or post-chemotherapy diarrhea is a nuisance, but the consequences of microflora changes can be much more serious. The best documented example is pseudomembraneous colitis, a condition in which depletion of the normally predominant population allows the pathogenic *Clostridium difficile*—usually a very minor component of the microflora and one that is found in only about five percent of the human population—to overgrow and produce two potent toxins (Brierley, 2005). The resulting damage to the colonic mucosa can be rapidly lethal within a few days.

The Forgotten Eukaryotes

A group of microbes in the colonic microflora that has been routinely ignored in most studies is the eukaryotic microbes (Moreels and Pelckmans, 2005). In developing countries, there is a eukaryotic component to the microflora that consists of protozoans, flatworms, and helminths. This eukaryotic component of the microflora has been a fact of human life for millions of years. Only during the last couple of centuries, and only in certain parts of the world, has the eukaryotic component of the microflora been virtually eliminated due to clean water and a high-quality food supply.

We tend to think of protozoa and helminths as pathogens, but is this picture entirely correct? In areas of the world where such eukaryotes are endemic, a majority of the population maintains them without any adverse effects. Is it possible that the abrupt (in evolutionary terms) loss of the eukaryotic component of the microflora by people who live in developed countries has had some adverse effects?

One recent, but still very speculative, answer to this question arises from the fact that helminthes—and possibly protozoa as well—stimulate the arm of the immune system that consists of eosinophils, mast cells, and other cell types that are also associated, on the negative side, with allergies and inflammatory bowel disease (Moreels and Pelckmans, 2005). The hypothesis that arises from this observation is that early stimulation of the GI immune system by eukaryotes allows this part of the immune response to develop normally. Conversely, failure to experience this type of stimulation may, in some people, predispose them to autoimmune disease such as allergies and inflammatory bowel disease.

Is there a eukaryotic component of the microflora in people from developed countries today? Although the eukaryotic intestinal pathogens are rarely seen, normal eukaryotic microflora may still exist. This population deserves investigation.

Nutritional Interactions

The colon has been called a second organ of digestion because dietary material that is not digested in the small intestine by human enzymes is fermented by the colonic microflora to produce short-chain fatty acids such as acetate, propionate, and butyrate (Bäckhed et al., 2005; Salyers, 1986; Salyers and Shipman,

2002). See Figure 1-5. These short-chain fatty acids are absorbed through the colonic mucosa and can be detected in the bloodstream. They are used by mammalian cells as sources of carbon and energy. In humans, the digestion of such materials as plant polysaccharides (dietary fiber) has been estimated to account for as much as 8 percent of the nutrition of the average person. In hard times, when only low quality, non-nutritious foods low in dietary fiber are available, the contribution to human nutrition may be higher.

There is also evidence that colonic bacteria produce vitamins (Salyers, 1986; Salyers and Shipman, 2002). The extent to which vitamin production is important to us is unknown, but it is interesting that scientists who breed and maintain populations of mice that lack any bacterial microflora (gnotobiotic or GF mice) have found it necessary to provide them with vitamin-enriched chow.

An extreme example of the importance of bacteria as sources of mammalian nutrition is the rumen of a cow. A cow relies absolutely on the bacterial population of its rumen for survival. Fermentation of plant polysaccharides by the ruminal bacteria provide the cow with almost 100 percent of the carbon and energy it needs. A cow unfortunate enough to experience an imbalance in its rumen microflora suffers from a painful and deadly condition called bloat.

Given that the residuum of the human diet that reaches the human colon is an important part of the diet of colonic microbes, a question that naturally arises is whether changes in the human diet cause changes in the microflora. Although numerous attempts have been made in the past, using cultivation-based techniques, to answer this question, the results are ambivalent (Salyers, 1986). Most studies report diet-associated changes in the microflora, but these changes are usually small and differ with the studies. No consensus emerges. It makes sense that the colonic microflora is in some sense "buffered" from changes in the human diet by the ability of colonic bacteria to utilize an amazing variety of substances and to change their activities very quickly (Salyers, 1986; Sonnenburg et al., 2005). The newly emerging molecular techniques should make such studies easier and more reliable and may perhaps reveal changes that were missed previously.

Possible Detoxifying Activities of the Human Colonic Microflora

Another interesting example of a beneficial interaction between cows and bacteria comes from scientists who were trying to solve the problem of animals in Australia and many tropical and subtropical countries that cope with toxic plants. The main toxin is mimosine, a plant compound that can kill a ruminant. Scientists observed that some small tropical ruminants ate plants that produced this compound with impunity. From the rumens of these animals, they isolated bacteria capable of detoxifying mimosine. These bacteria are now being introduced into cattle in Hawaii and Australia and they seem to confer some protection from mimosine-producing weeds (Jones and Megarrity, 1986).

The possible toxin-inactivating activities of the human colonic microflora have attracted some attention. There are a number of studies that demonstrate the ability of some colonic microbes to modify xenobiotics such as food dyes and other potential carcinogens. So far, the actual contribution of this type of activity to human health has not been demonstrated, and it is not clear that the compounds studied are the ones that may actually cause human health problems. It is an area that deserves attention because such materials in the diet spend a much longer time in the colon than in the rest of the GI tract. For this reason, toxic substances in the diet are likely to have a disproportionate effect on colonic mucosal cells or on cells they encounter if they are absorbed.

Looming behind interest in this topic is the question of whether colon cancer risk might be affected, positively or negatively, by activities of the colonic microflora. It is important to note that, although the assumption is generally made that xenobiotic-modifying activities of the colonic microbes is beneficial, scientists who are interested in bioremediation of toxic waste dumps have found many examples in which bacterial transformations of toxic waste components have produced substances that are even more toxic. More careful studies are needed of xenobiotic transformation that take a careful account of what compounds are actually likely to be found regularly in the human colon and of possible negative effects of bacterial activities.

Yet another activity of the colonic microflora that has not received much attention is recycling of human-produced substances, such as mucin and sloughed mucosal cells. These substances, mostly polysaccharides, contain—in addition to fermentable sugars—a substantial amount of nitrogen in the form of amino-sugars. Fermentation of these sugars releases not only short-chain fatty acids, but also ammonia. If the ammonia is absorbed from the colon by mucosal cells, it may contribute to the host's nitrogen balance.

Genetic Interactions Among Colonic Bacteria

Recent studies in our laboratory and other laboratories have produced evidence for an old idea called the *reservoir hypothesis*. This hypothesis, which so far has focused on antibiotic resistance genes, is illustrated in Figure 1-6. The ability of bacteria to transfer DNA to each other by a direct cell-to-cell transfer process called conjugation has been well documented in laboratory experiments. This process is of interest because it is the type of genetic exchange between bacteria that can cross species and genus barriers. Thus, one could imagine a scenario in which bacteria in the colon are not only constantly exchanging genes with each other, but also with bacteria that have been swallowed and are only transiently present in the colon (Salyers et al., 2004).

Why would such a scenario be of any interest to us, especially since most of the bacteria coexist with us without causing any problems? The reason is that a subset of these bacteria can cause infections. For example, swallowed bacteria

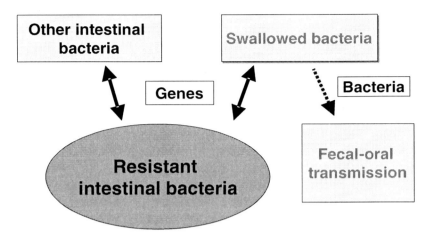

FIGURE 1-6 Flow of antibiotic resistance genes (hypothetical).
SOURCE: Salyers (2005).

include *Streptococcus pneumoniae*, the main cause of bacterial pneumonia and a major cause of infectious disease deaths in developed, as well as developing, countries. Moreover, normal colonic inhabitants such as *Bacteroides* species, *E. coli*, and *Enterococcus* species are notorious causes of potentially lethal post-surgical infections. Increasingly, these bacteria are becoming resistant to many antibiotics.

In recent years, molecular methods have been used to show how resistance gene transfers have been occurring at a surprising level in the human colon. The amount of transfer detected in the colon was surprising because in the laboratory, under supposedly optimum conditions, frequencies of transfer are relatively low. Only one in 10,000 or 100,000 possible recipients acquire transferred DNA. Yet, in the colon, some antibiotic resistance genes have obviously transferred widely within a period of a few decades (Salyers et al., 2004).

This extensive transfer has loomed large in the debate over possible adverse consequences of the use of antibiotics on the farm. The concern is that antibiotic-resistant bacteria that arise due to selection from the use of antibiotics as prophylactic treatments or as feed additives are moving through the food supply and into the human intestinal tract, where the resistance genes could be transferred to bacteria that permanently or temporarily reside in the human colon. How important this process is for the development of resistance in bacteria—that are serious causes of human infections—has not been conclusively established, but it remains a concern.

The subject of genetic interactions could be extended from concern about bacterium-to-bacterium transfer to a larger scale. Conjugation can transfer DNA, at least in the laboratory, not only from prokaryote to prokaryote but also from prokaryote to yeast. Do the bacteria that come into contact with our mucosal cells ever transfer DNA to them, and if they do, is this DNA ever fixed in the eukaryotic recipients? The latter question is important because it is unlikely that there will be much sequence homology between the bacteria and eukaryotic cell, nor are bacterial genes that encode the integrases that mediate homology-independent integration events likely to be expressed. Are there forms of illegitimate recombination that mediate integration of bacterial DNA into the genome of a eukaryotic host? Such events have been well documented in the case of the transfer of DNA from *Agrobacterium tumifaciens* to plants, but this phenomenon has not been reported for other eukaryotes. The lack of such reports may be more a reflection of lack of studies than lack of actual phenomena. Moreover, one could argue that even if such events occur in the colon, most mucosal cells are short lived and are sloughed into the lumen of the colon. There are, however, colonic stem cells whose germline is much more permanent. If the stem cells receive bacterial DNA and if it becomes fixed in their genome, such an event could have long-term effects. This is yet another area that has so far received no attention, but might be worth considering in the future.

At the very least, it is certain that transfer among bacteria in the colon involves many genes other than antibiotic resistance genes. Genes that enhance the ability of bacteria to cause disease or to survive in new niches such as the roots of plants are known to be transferred as well. The trafficking in genes among intestinal bacteria could have more global effects than just the transfer of antibiotic resistance genes.

What Needs to Be Done?

This discussion has surveyed briefly some of the issues that have been raised in connection with the normal microflora of the human colon and its possible role, if it becomes unbalanced, in human disease. A theme that has run through this article is the surprising lack of information about some very basic aspects of the human microflora. We know remarkably little about the "silent majority" of gram-positive anaerobes that are the basis of the microflora. There is little reliable information about how much person-to-person variation there is, whether nonhuman animals are good models for the human microflora or the way in which changes in diet or medical therapies affect the microflora.

One excuse given in the past for this dismal record is that cultivation-based analyses were not only time consuming and expensive, but also inherently unreliable given the variety of bacteria involved. The new molecular methods remove this technical barrier and make it possible to survey large numbers of samples cheaply and reliably. Surprisingly, there is still no microarray that represents the predominant species of colonic bacteria, although rumors have been circulating during the past several years that one laboratory or another is hard at work on developing such a microarray. At present, no such microarray is commercially available.

Moreover, having a microarray is only the first step to having a valuable screening tool. Given the large number of bacteria species in the colon and the possible presence of interfering substances in human intestinal contents or feces, it will be necessary to do a substantial amount of work on optimizing protocols for use of such a microarray in the real world. Microarrays that could detect expression of bacterial genes in the colon are also needed, but pose even more daunting challenges. This remark is not meant to make it sound as if such challenges pose a barrier that is unscalable at the present time. Microbiologists working with even more challenging environments such as soil have managed to make impressive progress in recent years. Enlisting their help makes a lot of sense.

An even bigger challenge facing us, however, is how to switch from a mind set that focuses on one microbe at a time, with disease as the end point, to a mind set that can comprehend population changes. Once again, the environmental microbiologists have been blazing this intellectual trail for the last decade and would be valuable allies in making the transition from viewing colonic bacteria one microbe at a time to viewing it as a population. Some promising work of this type is beginning to appear.

Perhaps the greatest challenge of all is educating the funding agencies. Understandably, research on human health issues has focused on disease. "Normal" is not an easily fundable research objective. This perspective needs to be changed. The irony is that the funding agencies that have supported the revolution in bacterial population studies, such as the Department of Energy and the National Science Foundation, have been discouraged from making any forays into issues traditionally associated with human or animal health. This means that the microfloras of mammalian bodies have fallen into a funding vacuum unless they can be tied to disease.

No one questions the importance of studies on inflammatory bowel disease or colon cancer, but without a normal baseline or criterion for how external factors such as diet might affect this baseline, modern studies of these diseases are likely to fall to the same fate that was previously met by the cultivation-based studies: studies whose results contradict each other because they lack any consensus as to what is normal and what amount of variation can be counted as significant. The one group that seems to have become immune to this problem is the dental microbiologists. Their example would be a good one for scientists and funding agencies interested in emulating the colonic microflora and its multifaceted interactions with the human body.

Philosophers and theologians are fond of telling us that humans are the crown of creation, but in reality we are microbial planets, the proverbial free lunch for microbes. They were here billions of years before we appeared. They made the Earth habitable for us, but it is well to remember that we were born into their world and we can only know ourselves if we understand our complex interactions with them. Disease is only a tiny part of this picture. Perhaps the time has come to remove the jeweler's eyepiece we have been using to examine a detail in the painting and take a good look at the whole picture.

ANNEX 1-1

TABLE 1-1 Comparison of the Glycoside Hydrolase and Polysaccharide Lyases in the Human, Mouse, and *B. thetaiotaomicron* Genomes

Glycoside Hydrolase (GH) or Polysaccharide Lyase (PL) Family	Known Activities	*Homo sapiens*	*Mus musculus*	*B. theta*
GH 1	beta-glucosidase (EC 3.2.1.21) beta-galactosidase (EC 3.2.1.23) beta-mannosidase (EC 3.2.1.25) beta-glucuronidase (EC 3.2.1.31) beta-D-fucosidase (EC 3.2.1.38) Phlorizin hydrolase (EC 3.2.1.62) 6-phospho-beta-galactosidase (EC 3.2.1.85) 6-phospho-beta-glucosidase (EC 3.2.1.86) strictosidine beta-glucosidase (EC 3.2.1.105) lactase (EC 3.2.1.108) prunasin beta-glucosidase (EC 3.2.1.118) oligoxyloglucan beta-glycosidase (EC 3.2.1.120) raucaffricine beta-glucosidase (EC 3.2.1.125) thioglucosidase (EC 3.2.1.147) beta-primeverosidase (EC 3.2.1.149) hydroxyisourate hydrolase (EC 3.-.-.-)	6	5	0
GH 2	beta-galactosidase (EC 3.2.1.23) beta-mannosidase (EC 3.2.1.25) beta-glucuronidase (EC 3.2.1.31)	3	2	33
GH 3	beta-glucosidase (EC 3.2.1.21) xylan 1,4-beta-xylosidase (EC 3.2.1.37) beta-N-acetylhexosaminidase (EC 3.2.1.52) glucan 1,3-beta-glucosidase (EC 3.2.1.58) glucan 1,4-beta-glucosidase (EC 3.2.1.74) exo-1,3-1,4-glucanase (EC 3.2.1.-) alpha-L-arabinofuranosidase (EC 3.2.1.55)	1	0	10
GH 5	chitosanase (EC 3.2.1.132) beta-mannosidase (EC 3.2.1.25) cellulase (EC 3.2.1.4) glucan 1,3-beta-glucosidase (EC 3.2.1.58) licheninase (EC 3.2.1.73) glucan endo-1,6-beta-glucosidase (EC 3.2.1.75)	0	0	1

continues

TABLE 1-1 Continued

Glycoside Hydrolase (GH) or Polysaccharide Lyase (PL) Family	Known Activities	Homo sapiens	Mus musculus	B. theta
	mannan endo-1,4-beta-mannosidase (EC 3.2.1.78) endo-1,4-beta-xylanase (EC 3.2.1.8) cellulose 1,4-beta-cellobiosidase (EC 3.2.1.91) endo-1,6-beta-galactanase (EC 3.2.1.-) beta-1,3-mannanase (EC 3.2.1.-)			
GH 9	endoglucanase (EC 3.2.1.4) cellobiohydrolase (EC 3.2.1.91) beta-glucosidase (EC 3.2.1.21)	1	0	0
GH 13	alpha-amylase (EC 3.2.1.1) pullulanase (EC 3.2.1.41) cyclomaltodextrin glucanotransferase (EC 2.4.1.19) cyclomaltodextrinase (EC 3.2.1.54) trehalose-6-phosphate hydrolase (EC 3.2.1.93) oligo-alpha-glucosidase (EC 3.2.1.10) maltogenic amylase (EC 3.2.1.133) neopullulanase (EC 3.2.1.135) alpha-glucosidase (EC 3.2.1.20) maltotetraose-forming alpha-amylase (EC 3.2.1.60) isoamylase (EC 3.2.1.68) glucodextranase (EC 3.2.1.70) maltohexaose-forming alpha-amylase (EC 3.2.1.98) branching enzyme (EC 2.4.1.18) trehalose synthase (EC 5.4.99.16) 4-alpha-glucanotransferase (EC 2.4.1.25) maltopentaose-forming alpha-amylase (EC 3.2.1.-) amylosucrase (EC 2.4.1.4) sucrose phosphorylase (EC 2.4.1.7) malto-oligosyltrehalose trehalohydrolase (EC 3.2.1.141) isomaltulose synthase (EC 5.4.99.11)	7	5	10
GH 16	xyloglucan:xyloglucosyl transferase (EC 2.4.1.207) keratan-sulfate endo-1,4-beta-galactosidase (EC 3.2.1.103)	0	0	3

TABLE 1-1 Continued

Glycoside Hydrolase (GH) or Polysaccharide Lyase (PL) Family	Known Activities	Homo sapiens	Mus musculus	B. theta
	glucan endo-1,3-beta-D-glucosidase (EC 3.2.1.39) endo-1,3(4)-beta-glucanase (EC 3.2.1.6) licheninase (EC 3.2.1.73) agarase (EC 3.2.1.81) kappa-carrageenase (EC 3.2.1.83)			
GH 18	chitinase (EC 3.2.1.14) endo-beta-N-acetylglucosaminidase (EC 3.2.1.96) non-catalytic proteins: xylanase inhibitors concanavalin B narbonin	8	11	7
GH 20	beta-hexosaminidase (EC 3.2.1.52) lacto-N-biosidase (EC 3.2.1.140)	2	2	15
GH 22	lysozyme type C (EC 3.2.1.17) and alpha-lactalbumins	6	7	0
GH 23	lysozyme type G (EC 3.2.1.17)	4	1	3
GH 24	lysozyme (EC 3.2.1.17)	1	0	0
GH 25	lysozyme (EC 3.2.1.17)	0	0	1
GH 27	alpha-galactosidase (EC 3.2.1.22) alpha-N-acetylgalactosaminidase (EC 3.2.1.49) isomalto-dextranase (EC 3.2.1.94)	2	2	5
GH 28	polygalacturonase (EC 3.2.1.15) exo-polygalacturonase (EC 3.2.1.67) exo-polygalacturonase (EC 3.2.1.82) rhamnogalacturonase (EC not defined)	0	0	9
GH 29	alpha-L-fucosidase (EC 3.2.1.51)	2	2	9
GH 30	glucosylceramidase (EC 3.2.1.45) beta-1,6-glucanase (EC 3.2.1.75)	2	1	2
GH 31	alpha-glucosidase (EC 3.2.1.20) glucoamylase (EC 3.2.1.3) sucrase-isomaltase (EC 3.2.1.48) (EC 3.2.1.10)	8	7	6

continues

TABLE 1-1 Continued

Glycoside Hydrolase (GH) or Polysaccharide Lyase (PL) Family	Known Activities	Homo sapiens	Mus musculus	B. theta
	alpha-xylosidase (EC 3.2.1.-) alpha-glucan lyase (EC 4.2.2.13) isomaltosyltransferase (EC 2.4.1.-)			
GH 32	invertase (EC 3.2.1.26) inulinase (EC 3.2.1.7) levanase (EC 3.2.1.65) exo-inulinase (EC 3.2.1.80) sucrose:sucrose 1-fructosyl transferase (EC 2.4.1.99) fructan fructan 1-fructosyltransferase (EC 2.4.1.100)	0	0	4
GH 33	sialidase or neuraminidase (EC 3.2.1.18) trans-sialidase (EC 2.4.1.-)	4	4	1
GH 35	beta-galactosidase (EC 3.2.1.23)	5	4	3
GH 36	alpha-galactosidase (EC 3.2.1.22) alpha-N-acetylgalactosaminidase (EC 3.2.1.49) stachyose synthase (EC 2.4.1.67) raffinose synthase (EC 2.4.1.82)	0	0	3
GH 37	trehalase (EC 3.2.1.28)	1	1	0
GH 38	alpha-mannosidase (EC 3.2.1.24) (EC 3.2.1.114)	5	5	2
GH 39	alpha-L-iduronidase (EC 3.2.1.76) beta-xylosidase (EC 3.2.1.37)	1	1	0
GH 42	beta-galactosidase (EC 3.2.1.23)	0	0	1
GH 43	beta-xylosidase (EC 3.2.1.37) alpha-L-arabinofuranosidase (EC 3.2.1.55) arabinanase (EC 3.2.1.99) xylanase (EC 3.2.1.8)	0	0	31
GH 47	alpha-mannosidase (EC 3.2.1.113)	8	8	0
GH 51	alpha-L-arabinofuranosidase (EC 3.2.1.55) endoglucanase (EC 3.2.1.4)	0	0	4
GH 53	endo-1,4-beta-galactanase (EC 3.2.1.89)	0	0	1
GH 56	hyaluronidase (EC 3.2.1.35)	6	7	0
GH 57	alpha-amylase (EC 3.2.1.1) 4-alpha-glucanotransferase (EC 2.4.1.-)	0	0	1

TABLE 1-1 Continued

Glycoside Hydrolase (GH) or Polysaccharide Lyase (PL) Family	Known Activities	Homo sapiens	Mus musculus	B. theta
	alpha-galactosidase (EC 3.2.1.22) amylopullulanase (EC 3.2.1.41)			
GH 59	galactocerebrosidase (EC 3.2.1.46)	1	1	0
GH 63	processing alpha-glucosidase (EC 3.2.1.106)	1	1	0
GH 65	trehalase (EC 3.2.1.28) maltose phosphorylase (EC 2.4.1.8) trehalose phosphorylase (EC 2.4.1.64) kojibiose phosphorylase (EC 2.4.1.-)	1	1	0
GH 66	cycloisomaltooligosaccharide glucanotransferase (EC 2.4.1.-) dextranase (EC 3.2.1.11)	0	0	1
GH 67	alpha-glucuronidase (EC 3.2.1.139)	0	0	1
GH 73	endo-beta-N-acetylglucosaminidase (EC 3.2.1.96) beta-1,4-N-acetylmuramoylhydrolase (EC 3.2.1.17)	0	0	1
GH 76	alpha-1,6-mannanase (EC 3.2.1.101)	0	0	10
GH 77	amylomaltase or 4-alpha-glucanotransferase (EC 2.4.1.25)	0	0	1
GH 78	alpha-L-rhamnosidase (EC 3.2.1.40)	0	0	6
GH 79	endo-beta-glucuronidase / heparanase (EC 3.2.1.-)	2	1	0
GH 84	N-acetyl beta-glucosaminidase (EC 3.2.1.52) hyaluronidase (EC 3.2.1.35)	1	1	1
GH 85	endo-beta-N-acetylglucosaminidase (EC 3.2.1.96)	1	1	0
GH 88	unsaturated glucuronyl hydrolases (EC 3.2.1.-)	0	0	4
GH 89	alpha-N-acetylglucosaminidase (EC 3.2.1.50)	1	1	3
GH 92	alpha-1,2-mannosidase (EC 3.2.1.-)	0	0	23
GH 93	exo-arabinanase (EC 3.2.1.55)	0	0	1
GH 95	alpha-L-fucosidase (EC 3.2.1.51)	0	0	5
GH 97	alpha-glucosidase (EC 3.2.1.20)	0	0	10

continues

TABLE 1-1 Continued

Glycoside Hydrolase (GH) or Polysaccharide Lyase (PL) Family	Known Activities	*Homo sapiens*	*Mus musculus*	*B. theta*
PL 1	pectate lyase (EC 4.2.2.2) pectin lyase (EC 4.2.2.10)	0	0	5
PL 8	hyaluronate lyase (EC 4.2.2.1) chondroitin ABC lyase (EC 4.2.2.4) chondroitin AC lyase (EC 4.2.2.5) xanthan lyase (EC 4.2.2.12)	0	0	4
PL 9	pectate lyase (EC 4.2.2.2) exopolygalacturonate lyase (EC 4.2.2.9)	0	0	2
PL 10	pectate lyase (EC 4.2.2.2)	0	0	1
PL 11	rhamnogalacturonan lyase (EC 4.2.2.-)	0	0	1
PL 12	heparin-sulfate lyase (EC 4.2.2.8)	0	0	2
PL 13	heparin lyase (EC 4.2.2.7)	0	0	1

NOTE: Based on information available at http://afmb.cnrs-mrs.fr/CAZY/.

SOURCE: Bäckhed et al. (2005).

TABLE 1-2 Effects of the Microbiota on Host Biology, Defined by Comparing Germ-Free (GF) and Conventionally-Raised (CONV-R) Rodents

Phenotype	Comments	References
Gut structure and function		
GF mice and rats have enlarged ceca	Likely a consequence of accumulation of undegraded host and dietary polysaccharides that bind water	(Gordon et al., 1966a; Wostmann and Bruckner-Kardoss, 1959)
GF mice villi are thinner	Mesenchymal core is less cellular; reduced immune population (see below)	(Banasaz et al., 2002)
GF mice have slower epithelial renewal rates	Evolutionary conserved response, also seen in germ-free zebrafish; mechanisms to be defined (e.g., what is contribution of undeveloped mucosal immune system). Epithelial regeneration markedly reduced in GF mice with dextran sodium sulfate-induced colitis: effect requires Myd88-dependent signaling through mesenchymal cells and recruitment of pericryptal macrophages.	(Banasaz et al., 2002; Pull et al., 2005; Rawls et al., 2004; Savage et al., 1981)
GF mice have slower gut motility	Migrating motor complexes move more slowly with more restricted spatial distribution; detailed comparisons of the enteric nervous system in GF versus CONV-R animals are needed; potential implications concerning the pathogenesis of irritable bowel syndrome in humans	(Abrams and Bishop, 1967)
GF rats have reduced bile acid deconjugation	Impaired excretion of bile acids	(Gustafsson et al., 1966)
GF rats produce more bile acids	This effect, together with deconjugation defect, results in increased bile acid pools; impact on cholesterol homeostasis	(Wostmann, 1973)
GF rats have fewer enteroendocrine cells	There are multiple subpopulations on enteroendocrine cells, defined by their peptide hormone products. The effects of microbiota on these subpopulations has not been well-defined.	(Uribe et al., 1994)
GF rats have mesenteric microvaculture that is hyporesponsive to norepinephrine and pitressin	Kallikrein-like molecules produced by GF cecum may contribute to phenotype	(Baez and Gordon, 1971; Gordon, 1964)

continues

TABLE 1-2 Continued

Phenotype	Comments	References
GF mice have reduced capillary network complexity in their villus mesenchymal cores	Potential influence on nutrient absorption and mucosal barrier functions	(Stappenbeck et al., 2002)
Cardiac function		
GF mice and rats have lower cardiac weight	Detailed morphometric studies lacking, mechanism not described	(Bruckner-Kardoss and Wostmann, 1974; Gordon et al., 1966a, 1966b; Wostmann et al., 1982)
GF rats have lower cardiac output	Physiological mechanisms, myocardial energetics not defined	(Gordon et al., 1963; Wostmann et al., 1968)
Endocrine system		
GF mice are more insulin sensitive than CONV-R animals	Could reflect, at least in part, reduced fat stores; other similarities to mice that are subjected to chronic caloric restriction need to be delineated	(Bäckhed et al., 2004)
GF mice have lower circulating levels of leptin and adiponectin	Associated with reduced fat stores	(Bäckhed et al., 2004; Bäckhed and Gordon, unpublished observation)
Nutrition/metabolism		
GF mice are vulnerable to vitamin deficiencies	The gut microbiota produces vitamin K, B_6, B_{12}, biotin, folic acid, and pantothenate	(Gustafsson et al., 1962; Sumi et al., 1977; Wostmann et al., 1963)
GF rats do not extract as much energy from their diet	See text for details	(Wostmann et al., 1983; Yamanaka et al., 1977)

TABLE 1-2 Continued

Phenotype	Comments	References
GF mice and rats have lower metabolism (VO_2)	Hexose monophosphate shunt and TCA cycle activity reduced. Mechanisms remain ill-defined; possible role for leptin	Bruckner-Kardoss and Wostmann, 1978; Levenson et al., 1969; Wostmann et al., 1982, 1968
GF mice absorb more cholesterol	GF mice have large bile acid pools	(Gustaffsson et al., 1975)

Immune system development

Phenotype	Comments	References
B-cells and immunoglobulin secretion	GF mice have 40–1000 fold less serum IgM/IgG and intestinal IgA	(Horsfall et al., 1978)
Natural immunoglobulin	GF mice have normal levels of natural Ig and B1 B-cells. However the majority of IgA that reacts with components of the microbiota originates from B2 B-cells. While class switching can occur in a T-cell independent pathway, most reactive antibodies are generated in a classical T-cell dependent manner.	(Bos et al., 2001; Macpherson and Uhr, 2004; Ochsenbein et al., 1999; Thurnheer et al., 2003)
Anti-'commnesal' IgA	The segmented filamentous bacteria (SBF; *Clostridia*) are stronger inducers of intestinal IgA than other bacteria (including Bacteroidetes). Interestingly, SBF found to be enriched in the intestines of mice lacking secretory IgA.	(Fagarasan et al., 2002; Suzuki et al., 2004)
Intraepithelial lymphocytes	Both $\gamma\delta$ and $\alpha\beta$ T-cells are significantly decreased in the intraepithelial lymphocyte population of GF mice: $\gamma\delta > \alpha\beta$	(Bandeira et al., 1990)
Cytotoxic T lymphocytes	Size and composition of CD8 repertoire to non-gut related antigen is unaffected by presence of absence of the microbiota.	(Bousso et al., 2000)
T-cells ($\alpha\beta$)	General T-cell function and number is not reduced in GF rats	(Nielsen, 1972)
T-cells ($\gamma\delta$)	Decreased number of mesenteric lymph node $\gamma\delta$ T-cells in GF mice	(Yoshikai et al., 1988)
Mucosal-associated invariant T-cells	Invariant $V\alpha 19$-$J\alpha 33$ TCR+ cells located in lamina propria, fail to develop in GF mice	(Treiner et al., 2003)
CD4+CD25+ T-cells	Levels and function are the same in GF and CONV-R mice	(Gad et al., 2004)

continues

TABLE 1-2 Continued

Phenotype	Comments	References
Modulation of Immunity and Disease		
GF mice are resistant to developing inflammatory bowel disease	GF mice with aberrations in T-cell development and function (IL2–/–, IL10–/–, TCRα–/–) do not develop spontaneous colitis, unlike their CONV-R counterparts	(Dianda et al., 1997; (Mizoguchi et al., 2000; Sadlack et al., 1993; Sellon et al., 1998)
GF rodents have reduced susceptibility to arthritis	CONV-R β2-microglobulin-HLA-B27 transgenic rats develop spontaneous colitis and arthritis; B10.BR mice develop enthesopathy; GF counterparts do not	(Rath et al., 1996; Rehakova et al., 2000)
GF NOD mice have higher rate of autoimmune diabetes	No primary papers; phenotype mentioned in reviews	(Bach, 1994a,1994b; Wicker et al., 1987)
Xenobiotic metabolism		
The gut microbiota metabolizes dietary oxalates	50 percent of GF rats have kidney stones versus 0 percent for CONV-R. Oxalate-degrading *Oxalobacter formigenes* reduces kidney stone formation in a rat model; currently in clinical trials.	(Allison et al., 1985; (Gustaffson and Norman, 1962; Sidhu et al., 2001)
The gut microbiota is required for nitroreduction of xenobiotics	See http://umbbd.ahc.umn.edu/ for a database of microbial biocatalytic/biodegradation reactions involving xenobiotics and various chemical compound classes. Consider microbiota when defining factors that influence bioavailability of orally administered drugs.	(Larsen et al., 1998)
General health and disease		
GF rats live longer than their CONV-R counterparts	Mechanism to be determined; possible similarities to insulin-sensitive, calorie-restricted animals	(Gordon et al., 1966b; Pollard and Wostmann, 1985)
Removing the microbiota decreases incidence of intestinal neoplasia in some mouse models	GF *IL-10–/–* mice and *Tgfβ-1–/–*, *Rag2–/–*; *Tcrb–/–*, *p53–/–*; and *Gpx1–/–*,*Gpx2–/–* compound homozygous knockout mice have reduced inflammation and tumor formation. Microbial communities associated with pre-neoplastic and neoplastic lesions in mouse models and humans have yet to be enumerated.	(Balish and Warner, 2002; Chu et al., 2004; Engle et al., 2002; Kado et al., 2001)
GF mice are more radioresistant	Mechanism to be defined; potential implications for ameliorating GI syndrome in patients receiving radiotherapy for abdominal/pelvic malignancies	(Matsuzawa, 1965)

SOURCE: Bäckhed et al. (2005).

TABLE 1-3 Six Ways Environmental Engineers Improve Bioreactor Efficiency

Approach	Method	Reference
Engineering	Altering reactor configuration: e.g., changing to a plug-flow reactor with higher substrate levels at the entrance to the reactor increases conversion rates according to Monod kinetics and promotes staging of the reactor by compartmentalization. This results in differing local environmental conditions that are optimal for sequential functional subpopulations.	(Angenent et al., 2002; Rittmann and McCarty, 2001)
Engineering	Removal of product. Even if the product is not inhibiting, thermodynamics dictate that the energy for the conversion will be higher if the concentration of products are maintained at a very low level.	(Stams, 1994; Thauer et al., 1977)
Operational	Elongation of the sludge retention time (mean residence time) by adding an attachment matrix to the reactor.	(Zaiat et al., 2001)
Microbial Ecology	Selection of a different community: e.g., sulfate reducers (SRBs) are not wanted in anaerobic methanogenic bioreactors because they produce a toxic product—H_2S. Preventing SRBs improves reactor efficiency.	(Elferink et al., 1994)
Microbial Ecology	Bioaugmentation: addition of a functional microbe that can remove a specific substrate at higher rates.	(Abeysinghe et al., 2002; Patureau et al., 2001)
Microbial Ecology	Bacteriophage addition: bacteriophage modulate bacterial population dynamics in bioreactors and, therefore, can be used to optimize reactor efficiency (e.g., as a biocontrol agent to prevent foam formation by microbes).	(Hantula et al., 1991; Lu et al., 2003; Thomas et al., 2002)

SOURCE: Bäckhed et al. (2005).

REFERENCES

Abeysinghe DH, De Silva DG, Stahl DA, Rittmann BE. 2002. The effectiveness of bioaugmentation in nitrifying systems stressed by a washout condition and cold temperature. *Water and Environmental Research* 74(2):187–199.

Abrams GD, Bishop JE. 1967. Effect of the normal microbial flora on gastrointestinal motility. *Proceedings for the Society of Experimental Biology and Medicine* 26(1):301–304.

Allison MJ, Dawson KA, Mayberry WR, Foss JG. 1985. Oxalobacter formigenes gen. nov., sp. nov.: Oxalate-degrading anaerobes that inhabit the gastrointestinal tract. *Archives of Microbiology* 141(1):1–7.

Angenent LT, Zheng D, Sung S, Raskin L. 2002. Microbial community structure and activity in a compartmentalized, anaerobic bioreactor. *Water and Environmental Research* 74(5):450–461.

Bach JF. 1994a. Insulin-dependent diabetes mellitus as an autoimmune disease. *Endocrine Reviews* 15(4):516–542.

Bach JF. 1994b. Predictive medicine in autoimmune diseases: From the identification of genetic predisposition and environmental influence to precocious immunotherapy. *Clinical Immunology and Immunopathology* 72(2):156–161.

Bäckhed F, Gordon JI. Unpublished observation as cited in Bäckhed F, Ley RE, Sonnenburg JL, Peterson DA, Gordon JI. 2005. Host-bacterial mutualism in the human intestine. *Science* 307(5717):1915–1920.

Bäckhed F, Ding H, Wang T, Hooper LV, Koh GY, Nagy A, Semenkovich CF, Gordon JI. 2004. The gut microbiota as an environmental factor that regulates fat storage. *Proceedings of the National Academy of Science USA* 101(44):15718–15723.

Bäckhed F, Ley RE, Sonnenburg JL, Peterson DA, Gordon JI. 2005. Host-bacterial mutualism in the human intestine. *Science* 307(5717):1915–1920.

Baez S, Gordon HA. 1971. Tone and reactivity of vascular smooth muscle in germfree rat mesentery. *Journal of Experimental Medicine* 134(4):846–856.

Balish E, Warner T. 2002. *Enterococcus faecalis* induces inflammatory bowel disease in interleukin-10 knockout mice. *American Journal of Pathology* 160(6):2253–2257.

Banasaz M, Norin E, Holma R, Midtvedt T. 2002. Increased enterocyte production in gnotobiotic rats mono-associated with *Lactobacillus rhamnosus* GG. *Applied Environmental Microbiology* 68(6):3031–3034.

Bandeira A, Mota-Santos T, Itohara S, Degermann S, Heusser C, Tonegawa S, Coutinho A. 1990. Localization of gamma/delta T cells to the intestinal epithelium is independent of normal microbial colonization. *Journal of Experimental Medicine* 172(1):239–244.

Bos NA, Jiang HQ, Cebra JJ. 2001. T cell control of the gut IgA response against commensal bacteria. *Gut* 48(6):762–764.

Bousso P, Lemaitre F, Laouini D, Kanellopoulos J, Kourilsky P. 2000. The peripheral CD8 T cell repertoire is largely independent of the presence of intestinal flora. *International Immunology* 12(4):425–430.

Breitbart M, Hewson I, Felts B, Mahaffy JM, Nulton J, Salamon P, Rohwer F. 2003. Metagenomic analyses of an uncultured viral community from human feces. *Journal of Bacteriology* 185(20):6220–6223.

Brierley R. 2005. *Clostridium difficile*—a new threat to public health? *Lancet Infectious Diseases* 5(9):535.

Bruckner-Kardoss E, Wostmann BS. 1974. Blood volume of adult germfree and conventional rats. *Laboratory Animal Science* 24(4):633–635.

Bruckner-Kardoss E, Wostmann BS. 1978. Oxygen consumption of germfree and conventional mice. *Laboratory Animal Science* 28(3):282–286.

Brune A, Friedrich M. 2000. Microecology of the termite gut: structure and function on a microscale. *Current Opinion in Microbiology* 3(3):263–269.

CAZY (Carbohydrate-Active Enzymes). 2005. Homepage. [Online]. Available: http://afmb.cnrs-mrs.fr/CAZY [accessed December 20, 2005].

Cerdeõno-Tárraga AM, Patrick S, Crossman LC, Blakely G, Abratt V, Lennard N, Poxton I, Duerden B, Harris B, Quail MA, Barron A, Clark L, Corton C, Doggett J, Holden MTG, Larke N, Line A, Lord A, Norbertczak H, Ormond D. 2005. Extensive DNA inversions in the *B. fragilis* genome control variable gene expression. *Science* 307(5714):1463–1465.

Chacon O, Bermudez LE, Barletta RG. 2004. Johne's disease, inflammatory bowel disease, and *Mycobacterium paratuberculosis*. *Annual Review of Microbiology* 58:329–363.

Chu FF, Esworthy RS, Chu PG, Longmate JA, Huycke MM, Wilczynski S, Doroshow JH. 2004. Bacteria-induced intestinal cancer in mice with disrupted Gpx1 and Gpx2 genes. *Cancer Research* 64(3):962–968.

De La Cochetiere MF, Durand T, Lepage P, Bourreille A, Galmiche JP, Dore J. 2005. Resilience of the dominant human fecal microbiota upon short-course antibiotic challenge. *Journal of Clinical Microbiology* 43(11):5588–5592.

Dianda L, Hanby AM, Wright NA, Sebesteny A, Hayday AC, Owen MJ. 1997. T cell receptor-alpha beta-deficient mice fail to develop colitis in the absence of a microbial environment. *American Journal of Pathology* 150(1):91–97.

Dunbar J, Barns SM, Ticknor LO, Kuske CR. 2002. Empirical and theoretical bacterial diversity in four Arizona soils. *Applied Environmental Microbiology* 68(6):3035–3045.

Elferink O, Visser A, Stams A. 1994. Sulfate reduction in methanogenic bioreactors. *FEMS Microbiology Review* 15(2–3):119.

Engle SJ, Ormsby I, Pawlowski S, Boivin GP, Croft J, Balish E, Doetschman T. 2002. Elimination of colon cancer in germ-free transforming growth factor beta 1-deficient mice. *Cancer Research* 162(22):6362–6366.

Fagarasan S, Muramatsu M, Suzuki K, Nagaoka H, Hiai H, Honjo T. 2002. Critical roles of activation-induced cytidine deaminase in the homeostasis of gut flora. *Science* 298(5597):1424–1427.

Fernandez AS, Hashsham SA, Dollhopf SL, Raskin L, Glagoleva O, Dazzo FB. Hickey RF, Criddle CS, Tiedje JM. 2000. Flexible community structure correlates with stable community function in methanogenic bioreactor communities perturbed by glucose. *Applied Environmental Microbiology* 66(9):4058–4067.

Flegal KM, Troiano RP. 2000. Changes in the distribution of body mass index of adults and children in the US population. *International Journal of Obesity-Related Metabolic Disorders* 24(7): 807–818.

Fuhrman JA. 1999. Marine viruses and their biogeochemical and ecological effects. *Nature* 399(6736): 541–548.

Gad M, Pedersen AE, Kristensen NN, Claesson MH. 2004. Demonstration of strong enterobacterial reactivity of CD4+CD25– T cells from conventional and germ-free mice which is counter-regulated by CD4+CD25+ T cells. *European Journal of Immunology* 34(3):695–704.

Galperin MY. 2004. The Molecular Biology Database Collection: 2004 update. *Nucleic Acids Research* 32(Database issue):D3–D22.

Genome Sequencing Center (GSC). 2005. Comparative microbial genome analysis of the human-Bacteroides symbiosis. [Online]. Available: http://genomeold.wustl.edu/projects/bacterial/cmpr_microbial/index.php?cmpr_microbial01 [accessed: December 21, 2005].

Goebel BM, Stackebrandt E. 1994. Cultural and phylogenetic analysis of mixed microbial populations found in natural and commercial bioleaching environments. *Applied Environmental Microbiology* 60(5):1614–1621.

Gordon HA. 1965. A bioactive substance in the caecum of germ-free animals: Demonstration of a bioactive substance in caecal contents of germ-free animals. *Nature* 205(4971):571.

Gordon HA, Wostmann BS, Bruckner-Kardoss E. 1963. Effects of microbial flora on cardiac output and other elements of blood circulation. *Proceedings of the Society of Experimental Biology and Medicine* 114:301–304.

Gordon HA, Bruckner-Kardoss E, Wostmann BS. 1966a. *Acta Anatomica* 64:367.

Gordon HA, Bruckner-Kardoss E, Wostmann BS. 1966b. Aging in germ-free mice: Life tables and lesions observed at natural death. *Journal of Gerontology* 21(3):380–387.

Guillemin K. 2005 (March 17). *Session I: Host-Pathogen Interactions: Defining the Concepts of Pathogenicity, Virulence, Colonization, Commensalism, and Symbiosis.* C Presentation at the Forum on Microbial Threats Workshop Ending the War Metaphor: The Changing Agenda for Unraveling the Host-Microbe Relationship. Washington, D.C., Institute of Medicine, Forum on Microbial Threats.

Gustafsson BE, Norman A. 1962. Urinary calculi in germfree rats. *Journal of Experimental Medicine* 116:273–284.

Gustafsson BE, Daft FS, McDaniel DE, Smith JC, Fitzgerald RJ. 1962. Effects of vitamin K-active compounds and intestinal microorganisms in vitamin K-deficient germfree rats. *Journal of Nutrition* 78:461–468.

Gustafsson BE, Midtvedt T, Norman A. 1966. Isolated fecal microorganisms capable of 7-alpha-dehydroxylating bile acids. *Journal of Experimental Medicine* 123(2):413–432.

Gustafsson BE, Einarsson K, Gustafsson J. 1975. Influence of cholesterol feeding on liver microsomal metabolism of steroids and bile acids in conventional and germ-free rats. *Journal of Biological Chemistry* 250(21):8496–8502.

Hantula J, Kurki A, Vuoriranta P, Bamford DH. 1991. Ecology of bacteriophages infecting activated sludge bacteria. *Applied Environmental Microbiology* 57(8):2147–2151.

Horsfall DJ, Cooper JM, Rowley D. 1978. Changes in the immunoglobulin levels of the mouse gut and serum during conventionalisation and following administration of *Salmonella typhimurium*. *Austrian Journal of Experimental Biology and Medical Science* 56(6):727–735.

Hugenholtz P, Goebel BM, Pace NR. 1998. Impact of culture-independent studies on the emerging phylogenetic view of bacterial diversity. *Journal of Bacteriology* 180(18):4765–4774.

Ishikawa K, Satoh Y, Tanaka H, Ono K. 1986. Influence of conventionalization on small-intestinal mucosa of germ-free Wistar rats: Quantitative light microscopic observations. *Acta Anaomicat (Basel)* 127:296–302.

Jones RJ, Megarrity RG. 1986. Successful transfer of DHP-degrading bacteria from Hawaiian goats to Australian ruminants to overcome the toxicity of Leucaena. *Australian Veterinary Journal* 63(8):259–262.

Kado S, Uchida K, Funabashi H, Iwata S, Nagata Y, Ando M, Onoue M, Matsuoka Y, Ohwaki M, Morotomi M. 2001. Intestinal microflora are necessary for development of spontaneous adenocarcinoma of the large intestine in T-cell receptor beta chain and p53 double-knockout mice. *Cancer Research* 61(6):2395–2398.

Kuwahara T, Yamashita A, Hirakawa H, Nakayama H, Toh H, Okada N, Kuhara S, Hattori M, Hayashi T, Ohnishi Y. 2004. Genomic analysis of *Bacteroides fragilis* reveals extensive DNA inversions regulating cell surface adaptation. *Proceedings of the National Academy of Science USA* 101(41):14919–14924.

Larsen GL, Huwe JK, Bakke JE. 1998. Intermediary metabolism of pentachloronitrobenzene in the control and germ-free rat and rat with cannulated bile ducts. *Xenobiotica* 28(10):973–984.

Levenson SM, Doft F, Lev M, Kan D. 1969. Influence of microorganisms on oxygen consumption, carbon dioxide production and colonic temperature of rats. *Journal of Nutrition* 97(4):542–552.

Ley RE, Gordon JI. Unpublished data as cited in Bäckhed F, Ley RE, Sonnenburg JL, Peterson DA, Gordon JI. 2005. Host-bacterial mutualism in the human intestine. *Science* 307(5717):1915–1920.

Lu Z, Breidt F, Plengvidhya V, Fleming HP. 2003. Bacteriophage ecology in commercial sauerkraut fermentations. *Applied Environmental Microbiology* 69(6):3192–3202.

Macpherson AJ, Uhr T. 2004. Induction of protective IgA by intestinal dendritic cells carrying commensal bacteria. *Science* 303(5664):1662–1665.

Matsuzawa T. 1965. Survival time in germfree mice after lethal whole body x-irradiation. *Tohoku Journal of Experimental Medicine* 85:257–263.

McCann KS. 2000. The diversity-stability debate. *Nature* 405(6783):228–233.

McGarr SE, Ridlon JM, Hylemon PB. 2005. Diet, anaerobic bacterial metabolism and colon cancer: A review of the literature. *Journal of Clinical Gastroenterology* 39(2):98–109.

McNeil NI. 1984. The contribution of the large intestine to energy supplies in man. *American Journal of Clinical Nutrition* 39(2):338–342.

Miller TL, Wolin MJ. 1982. Enumeration of *Methanobrevibacter smithii* in human feces. *Archives of Microbiology* 131(1):14–18.

Mizoguchi A, Mizoguchi E, Saubermann LJ, Higaki K, Blumberg RS, Bhan AK. 2000. Limited CD4 T-cell diversity associated with colitis in T-cell receptor alpha mutant mice requires a T helper 2 environment. *Gastroenterology* 119(4):983–995.

Moore WE, Holdeman LV. 1974. Human fecal flora: the normal flora of 20 Japanese-Hawaiians. *Applied Microbiology* 27(5):961–979.

Moore WE, Cato EP, Holdeman LV. 1978. Some current concepts in intestinal bacteriology. *American Journal of Clinical Nutrition* 31(10 Suppl):S33–S42.

Moreels TG, Pelckmans PA. 2005. Gastrointestinal parasites: potential therapy for refractory inflammatory bowel diseases. *Inflammatory Bowel Disease* 11(2):178–184.

Nielsen HE. 1972. Reactivity of lymphocytes from germfree rats in mixed leukocyte culture and in graft-versus-host reaction. *Journal of Experimental Medicine* 136(3):417–425.

Ochsenbein AF, Fehr T, Lutz C, Suter M, Brombacher F, Hengartner H, Zinkernagel RM. 1999. Control of early viral and bacterial distribution and disease by natural antibodies. *Science* 286(5447):2156–2159.

Patureau D, Helloin E, Rustrian E, Bouchez T, Delgenes JP, Moletta R. 2001. Combined phosphate and nitrogen removal in a sequencing batch reactor using the aerobic den trifier, *Microvirgula aerodenitrificans*. *Water Research* 35(1):189–197.

Pollard M, Wostmann BS. 1985. Increased life span among germfree rats. *Progress in Clinical Biology Research* 181:75–76.

Pull SL, Doherty JM, Mills JC, Gordon JI, Stappenbeck TS. 2005. Activated macrophages are an adaptive element of the colonic epithelial progenitor niche necessary for regenerative responses to injury. *Proceedings of the National Academy of Science USA* 102(1):99–104.

Rainey PB, Rainey K. 2003. Evolution of cooperation and conflict in experimental bacterial populations. *Nature* 425(6953):72–74.

Rakoff-Nahoum S, Paglino J, Eslami-Varzaneh F, Edberg S, Medzhitov R. 2004. Recognition of commensal microflora by toll-like receptors is required for intestinal homeostasis. *Cell* 118(2):229–241.

Rath HC, Herfarth HH, Ikeda JS, Grenther WB, Hamm TE Jr, Balish E, Taurog JD, Hammer RE, Wilson KH, Sartor RB. 1996. Normal luminal bacteria, especially Bacteroides species, mediate chronic colitis, gastritis, and arthritis in HLA-B27/human beta2 microglobulin transgenic rats. *Journal of Clinical Investigation* 98(4):945–53.

Rawls JF, Samuel BS, Gordon JI. 2004. Gnotobiotic zebrafish reveal evolutionarily conserved responses to the gut microbiota. *Proceedings of the National Academy of Science USA* 101(13):4596–4601.

Rehakova Z, Capkova J, Stepankova R, Sinkora J, Louzecka A, Ivanyi P, Weinreich S. 2000. Germfree mice do not develop ankylosing enthesopathy, a spontaneous joint disease. *Human Immunology* 61(6):555–558.

Rittmann BE, McCarty PL. 2001. *Environmental Biotechnology: Principles and Applications.* Boston: McGraw Hill International.

Rolandelli RH, Koruda MJ, Settle RG, Leskiw MJ, Stein TP, Rombeau JL. 1989. The effect of pectin on hepatic lipogenesis in the enterally-fed rat. *Journal of Nutrition* 119(1):89–93.

Sadlack B, Merz H, Schorle H, Schimpl A, Feller AC, Horak I. 1993. Ulcerative colitis-like disease in mice with a disrupted interleukin-2 gene. *Cell* 75(2):253–261.

Salyers AA. 1986. Diet and the colonic environment: Measuring the response of human colonic bacteria to changes in the host's diet. In: Vahouny G, Kritchevsky D, eds. *Dietary Fiber: Basic and Clinical Aspects.* New York: Plenum Press. Pp. 119–130.

Salyers AA. 2005 (March 16). Session I: Host-Pathogen Interactions: Defining the Concepts of Pathogenicity, Virulence, Colonization, Commensalism, and Symbiosis. Presentation at the Forum on Microbial Threats Workshop Ending the War Metaphor: The Changing Agenda for Unraveling the Host-Microbe Relationship, Washington, D.C., Institute of Medicine, Forum on Microbial Threats.

Salyers AA, Shipman JA. 2002. Getting in touch with your prokaryotic self: Mammal-microbe interactions. In: Staley JT, Reysenbach AL, eds. *Biodiversity of Microbial Life: Foundation of Earth's Biosphere.* New York: Wiley-Liss, Inc. Pp. 315–341.

Salyers AA, Shoemaker NB, Bonheyo GT. 2002. The ecology of antibiotic resistance genes. In: *Bacterial Resistance to Antimicrobials.* New York: Marcel Dekker. Pp. 1–17.

Salyers AA, Gupta A, Wang Y. 2004. Human intestinal bacteria as reservoirs for antibiotic resistance genes. *Trends in Microbiology* 12(9):412–416.

Savage DC. 1977. Microbial ecology of the gastrointestinal tract. *Annual Review of Microbiology* 31:107–133.

Savage DC, Siegel JE, Snellen JE, Whitt DD. 1981. Transit time of epithelial cells in the small intestines of germfree mice and ex-germfree mice associated with indigenous microorganisms. *Applied Environmental Microbiology* 42(6):996–1001.

Seksik P, Rigottier-Gois L, Gramet G, Sutren M, Pochart P, Marteau P, Jian R, Dore J. 2003. Alterations of the dominant faecal bacterial groups in patients with Crohn's disease of the colon. *Gut* 52(2):237–242.

Sellon RK, Tonkonogy S, Schultz M, Dieleman LA, Grenther W, Balish E, Rennick DM, Sartor RB. 1998. Resident enteric bacteria are necessary for development of spontaneous colitis and immune system activation in interleukin-10-deficient mice. *Infection and Immunity* 66(11):5224–5231.

Sharma R., Schumacher U. 1995. Morphometric analysis of intestinal mucins under different dietary conditions and gut flora in rats. *Digestive Diseases and Sciences* 40:2532–2539.

Shipman JA, Berleman JE, Salyers AA. 2000. Characterization of four outer membrane proteins involved in binding starch to the cell surface of Bacteroides thetaiotaomicron. *Journal of Bacteriology* 182(19):5365–5372.

Sidhu H, Allison MJ, Chow JM, Clark A, Peck AB. 2001. Rapid reversal of hyperoxaluria in a rat model after probiotic administration of Oxalobacter formigenes. *Journal of Urology* 166(4):1487–1491.

Sonnenburg JL, Angenent LT, Gordon JI. 2004. Getting a grip on things: How do communities of bacterial symbionts become established in our intestine? *Nature of Immunology* 5(6):569–573.

Sonnenburg JL, Xu J, Leip DD, Chen CH, Westover BP, Weatherford J, Buhler JD, Gordon JI. 2005. Glycan foraging in vivo by an intestine-adapted bacterial symbiont. *Science* 307(5717):1955–1959.

Stams AJ. 1994. Metabolic interactions between anaerobic bacteria in methanogenic environments. *Antonie Van Leeuwenhoek* 66(1–3):271–294.

Stappenbeck TS, Hooper LV, Gordon JI. 2002. Developmental regulation of intestinal angiogenesis by indigenous microbes via Paneth cells. *Proceedings of the National Academy of Science USA* 99(24):15451–15455.

Sumi Y, Miyakawa M, Kanzaki M, Kotake Y. 1977. Vitamin B-6 deficiency in germfree rats. *Journal of Nutrition* 107(9):1707–1714.

Suzuki K, Meek B, Doi Y, Muramatsu M, Chiba T, Honjo T, Fagarasan S. 2004. Aberrant expansion of segmented filamentous bacteria in IgA-deficient gut. *Proceedings of the National Academy of Science USA* 101(7):1981–1986.

Taddei F, Matic I, Godelle B, Radman M. 1997. To be a mutator, or how pathogenic and commensal bacteria can evolve rapidly. *Trends in Microbiology* 5(11):427–428.

Thauer RK, Jungermann K, Decker K. 1977. Energy conservation in chemotrophic anaerobic bacteria. *Bacteriological Reviews* 41(1):100–180.

Thomas JA, Soddell JA, Kurtboke DI. 2002. Fighting foam with phages? *Water Science and Technology* 46(1–2):511–518.

Thurnheer MC, Zuercher AW, Cebra JJ, Bos NA. 2003. B1 cells contribute to serum IgM, but not to intestinal IgA, production in gnotobiotic Ig allotype chimeric mice. *Journal of Immunology* 170(9):4564–4571.

Towle HC. 2001. Glucose and cAMP: adversaries in the regulation of hepatic gene expression. *Proceedings of the National Academy of Science USA* 98(24):13476–13478.

Travisano M, Velicer GJ. 2004. Strategies of microbial cheater control. *Trends in Microbiology* 12(2):72–78.

Treiner E, Duban L, Bahram S, Radosavljevic M, Wanner V, Tilloy F, Affaticat P, Gilfillan S, Lantz O. 2003. Selection of evolutionarily conserved mucosal-associated invariant T cells by MR1. *Nature* 422(6928):164–169.
Uribe A, Alam M, Johansson O, Midtvedt T, Theodorsson E. 1994. Microflora modulates endocrine cells in the gastrointestinal mucosa of the rat. *Gastroenterology* 107(5):1259–1269.
Whitman WB, Coleman DC, Wiebe WJ. 1998. Prokaryotes: The unseen majority. *Proceedings of the National Academy of Science USA* 95(12):6578–6583.
Wicker LS, Miller BJ, Coker LZ, McNally SE, Scott S, Mullen Y, Appel MC. 1987. Genetic control of diabetes and insulitis in the nonobese diabetic (NOD) mouse. *Journal of Experimental Medicine* 165(6):1639–1654.
Wilson K, Blitchington R. 1996. Human colonic biota studied by ribosomal DNA sequence analysis. *Applied Environmental Microbiology* 62(7):2273–2278.
Winter C, Smit A, Herndl GJ, Weinbauer MG. 2004. Impact of virioplankton on archaeal and bacterial community richness as assessed in seawater batch cultures. *Applied Environmental Microbiology* 70(2):804–813.
Wostmann B. 1973. Intestinal bile acids and cholesterol absorption in the germfree rat. *Journal of Nutrition* 103(7):982–990.
Wostmann B, Bruckner-Kardoss E. 1959. Development of cecal distention in germ-free baby rats. *American Journal of Physiology* 197:1345–1346.
Wostmann BS, Knight PL, Keeley LL, Kan DF. 1963. Metabolism and function of thiamine and naphthoquinones in germfree and conventional rats. *Federation Proceedings* 22:120–124.
Wostmann BS, Bruckner-Kardoss E, Knight PL. 1968. Cecal enlargement, cardiac output, and O2 consumption in germfree rats. *Proceedings of the Society of Experimental Biology and Medicine* 128(1):137–141.
Wostmann BS, Bruckner-Kardoss E, Pleasants JR. 1982. Oxygen consumption and thyroid hormones in germfree mice fed glucose-amino acid liquid diet. *Journal of Nutrition* 112(3):552–559.
Wostmann BS, Larkin C, Moriarty A, Bruckner-Kardoss E. 1983. Dietary intake, energy metabolism, and excretory losses of adult male germfree Wistar rats. *Laboratory Animal Science* 33(1):46–50.
Xu J, Bjursell MK, Himrod J, Deng S, Carmichael LK, Chiang HC, Hooper LV. Gordon JI. 2003. A genomic view of the human-bacteroides thetaiotaomicron symbiosis. *Science* 299(5615):2074.
Yachi S, Loreau M. 1999. Biodiversity and ecosystem productivity in a fluctuating environment: The insurance hypothesis. *Proceeding of the National Academy of Science USA* 96(4):1463–1468.
Yamanaka M, Nomura T, Kametaka M. 1977. Influence of intestinal microbes on heat production in germ-free, gnotobiotic and conventional mice. *Journal of Nutritional Science and Vitaminology (Tokyo)* 23(3):221–226.
Yoshikai Y, Matsuzaki G, Kishihara K, Nomoto K, Yokokura T, Nomoto K. 1988. Age-associated increase in the expression of T-cell antigen receptor gamma-chain gene in conventional and germfree mice. *Infection and Immunity* 56(8):2069–2074.
Zaiat M, Rodrigues JA, Ratusznei SM, de Camargo EF, Borzani W. 2001. Anaerobic sequencing batch reactors for wastewater treatment: A developing technology. *Applied Microbiology and Biotechnology* 55(1):29–35. Review.
Zoetendal EG, Akkermans AD, De Vos WM. 1998. Temperature gradient gel electrophoresis analysis of 16S rRNA from human fecal samples reveals stable and host-specific communities of active bacteria. *Applied Environmental Microbiology* 64(10):3854–3859.
Zoetendal EG, Akkermans AD, Vliet WMA, Arjan J, de Visser GM, de Vos WM. 2001. The host genotype affects the bacterial community in the human gastro-intestinal tract. *Microbial Ecology in Health and Disease* 13(3):129–134.

2

Beyond the Gut: Insights from Other Host-Microbe Systems

OVERVIEW

Equally compelling but less studied than the host-microbe environment of the human gut, microbial communities in plants, insects, and the soil are also likely to yield important scientific and medical insights. The two papers in this chapter offer intriguing perspectives on nonhuman host-microbe systems, beginning with a description of the microbial communities that exist on and inside plants and how these microbial communities contribute to protecting their hosts from infectious disease. The first paper is also coauthored by workshop presenter Jo Handelsman.

Contending that the advancement of infectious disease research lies in understanding the nature of cooperation within microbial communities and its contribution to host health, the authors lead a guided tour of insights, derived from studies of plant pathology, that raise the possibility of harnessing the natural microbial communities of humans for disease prevention. She notes that many microbiological milestones—among them the germ theory of disease and the discovery and characterization of viruses—were first achieved by plant biologists, but were not recognized at the time by their peers in other disciplines. Thus, while it is not surprising that studies of plants and their associated microbial communities have added considerably to knowledge of host-microbe relationships, these findings have not been widely appreciated, nor have they been well integrated with current understanding of the human gut microbiota.

Handelsman and coworkers have demonstrated that intermicrobe communications that lead to disease could be disrupted, and that beneficial lines of communication could be protected against pathogenic saboteurs. For example, they observed that plant diseases can be suppressed by treatments that modify the microbial community of the root to make it more like the community in the soil, a conclusion which they have dubbed the "camouflage hypothesis." By analogy, the human intestinal microflora may influence the success of pathogens by either presenting a barrier to invasion that is predicated on the composition of the entire community, or conversely by potentiating activity, facilitating infection, or aggravating disease symptoms.

The second contribution to this chapter, by plant biologist Brian Staskewicz, describes similarities among the strategies used by plant and animal pathogens and compares the defenses mounted against them by their disparate hosts. The complexity of disease resistance in plants is illustrated through Staskewicz's description of his laboratory's efforts to describe the function and regulation of a key disease resistance protein in the plant *Arabidopsis thaliana*, in response to the pathogenic bacterium, *Pseudomonas syringae*.

Conserved cellular defense responses in plants resemble certain innate immune responses to pathogens in vertebrates and insects, suggesting that these defense pathways may be inherited from a common ancestor. The preponderance of conserved motifs and, presumably, mechanisms among plant and animal proteins involved with innate immunity has encouraged communication and even collaboration among the scientists who study these systems in widely different species—an unfortunately rare occurrence that may yield significant insights on the structure, function, and evolution of innate immunity.

IT TAKES A VILLAGE: ROLE OF INDIGENOUS MICROBIAL COMMUNITIES IN INFECTIOUS DISEASE

Christina Matta and Jo Handelsman[1]

Summary

The microbial communities that reside on and inside plants and animals are a key to host health. In addition to contributing to digestion and nutrition, they present a formidable barrier to pathogens, which may invade the community or arise from it. The future of infectious disease research needs to focus on ways to enlist the natural community in prevention of disease rather than solely on the traditional warfare model, which requires direct killing of the pathogen with a chemical agent. The future of this field will depend on insights into the nature of cooperation within communities and the features that make them resistant to invasion. In these areas, the field of plant pathology, or infectious disease of plants, has much to offer. Plant pathologists have long recognized the role of the micro-

---

[1] C. Matta is from the Department of History of Science and J. Handelsman is from the Department of Plant Pathology, both of the University of Wisconsin, Madison, WI.

bial community in host health. But biomedical research in the late 20th and early 21st century has tended to ignore recent developments in plant pathology that may enrich medical understanding of human disease. Examination of 19th and early 20th century microbiology illustrates the power of communication between scientists who study plant and human diseases. In fact, the development of the germ theory and experimental evidence for it were predicated on an intimate discussion among scientists who studied plants and humans. For both the plant sciences and biomedicine to benefit from each other's expertise, we need to rebuild the ties and foster collaboration between plant pathology and human infectious disease.

Crossing the Disciplinary Divide: Microbiology in Historical Perspective

The role plant sciences have played in shaping the content and methods of modern bacteriology has been overshadowed by the popular appeal of medical breakthroughs. Indeed, to the lay public, the very terms *microbiology* and *bacteriology*, are almost synonymous with contagious disease of humans. Likewise, medical microbiologists have tended to overlook their discipline's debts to botany, plant pathology, soil science, and the agricultural sciences. Historically, however, medical and nonmedical microbiology were enmeshed in an intricate, subtle relationship based upon shared methodologies that were equally applicable in both medical and nonmedical contexts. In many instances, breakthroughs heralded as triumphs of medical research echoed knowledge or practices that had been standard or assumed in the plant sciences for years or decades. The relevance of plant research to microbiology more broadly—something that biologists of all specialties actively recognized and drew upon even into the mid-20th century—has largely faded from view.

Cohn, Koch, and the Germ Theory

Plant pathology has historically offered novel approaches for investigating disease causality and pathogenesis that have proven crucial to the understanding of human and animal infectious disease. From Mathieu du Tillet's extensive epidemiological studies of wheat smut in 1755, to de Bary's thorough demonstration in 1863 that *Phytophthora infestans* was without a doubt the cause of late blight of potato, to USDA plant pathologist Erwin Frink Smith's insistence that crown gall of tomatoes could provide a model for understanding tumor growth in human cancers, plant scientists have repeatedly anticipated medical methods and discoveries (Campbell et al., 1999).

Even Robert Koch, who is generally credited as the architect of the germ theory (Brock, 1988), worked within an intricate web of knowledge derived by botanists, bacteriologists, and mycologists. In the 19th century, changes in academic botany in Europe led to the inclusion of bacteria with other microscopic organisms such as algae and fungi—organisms traditionally considered plants. It is no surprise, then, that the most prominent of the early bacteriologists was a botanist: Ferdinand Cohn, professor of botany at the University of Breslau (now Wroclaw, Poland). (Figure 2-1) As early as 1872, Cohn had presented strong evidence that bacteria cause disease when he published his observations of bacteria in diseased organisms and the loss of disease-causing ability when an infectious fluid was filtered. Moreover, Cohn's taxonomic and morphological study of bacteria provided the observations necessary to quell continuing debates about pleomorphism, a doctrine that posited that all bacteria were a single species and that the shape of a bacterium was either determined by the organism's stage in its life cycle or by environmental conditions (or some combination of both). If the doctrine of pleomorphism were correct, specific causality of disease would not be possible; if distinct bacterial species did not exist, then it would be impossible to identify a particular set of disease symptoms with one particular organism. Cohn amassed enough morphological, developmental, and physiological data on various species of bacteria to create a taxonomic system with four "tribes" of bacteria, which contained genera that were differentiated based upon both physiological and morphological criteria (Cohn, 1872).

Without Cohn's careful observations and focused arguments against pleomorphism, the germ theory of the 1870s and 1880s could not have become the basis for our current understanding—that contagious diseases are each caused by a unique microorganism. It was, in fact, Cohn to whom a then-unknown physician named Robert Koch turned for an expert opinion on his demonstration of the life cycle of *Bacillus anthracis*.

Some microbiologists have argued that Cohn's claims about monomorphism

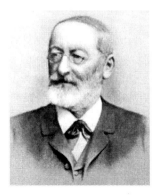 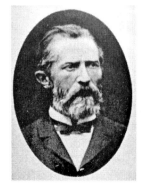 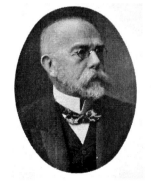

FIGURE 2-1 Left to right: Ferdinand Julius Cohn (1828–1898), Heinrich Anton de Bary (1832–1888), and Robert Koch (1843–1910).
SOURCE: Handelsman (2005).

could not have been confirmed until after Koch published his pure culture techniques (Brock, 1961), but this assessment overlooks a very important detail: that pure culture techniques had been standard practice in mycology at least since the late 1860s when mycologist Oskar Brefeld proposed a set of techniques for cultivating fungi on sterile media and in pure culture. It was these methods that botanist and developmental mycologist Anton de Bary, for example, used in his studies of plant pathogens such as *Phytophthora infestans* and *Puccinia graminis*. Furthermore, botanist Joseph Schroeter (one of Cohn's students) had begun experimenting with obtaining pure cultures of pigmented bacteria as early as 1870. By the time Koch published his methods for studying pathogenic organisms in culture in 1881, then, methods for isolating individual organisms and reintroducing them to host tissue were widespread in mycology and already under development in bacteriology.

A Mosaic from Tobacco to Polio

By far the most notable example of research in plant science that profoundly influenced the development of medical science is tobacco mosaic virus (TMV). In 1892, Russian botanist Dmitri Ivanowski published his observations that filtering sap from tobacco plants infected with tobacco mosaic disease did not prevent the sap from infecting other plants, even when he used the filtration techniques developed by Charles Chamberlain that were so effective in removing pathogenic bacteria from media (Ivanowski, 1892). Six years later, the Dutch soil microbiologist and plant pathologist Martinus W. Beijerinck attributed the symptoms to an unfilterable, noncellular, infectious particle that he termed a *virus* (Beijerinck, 1898). In 1901, U.S. Army physician Walter Reed echoed this conclusion when he pronounced yellow fever as nonbacterial, arguing instead that it was caused by a filterable agent.

The exact particle involved in TMV remained unidentified until 1935, when biochemist Wendell Stanley purified the virus and isolated its crystalline form. Stanley's work provided the first physical evidence of a material infectious agent, and as a result, TMV became an experimental model for early research in virology. Both plant scientists and medical microbiologists recognized that the results of research on TMV and the methods used therein could be applied to other viral diseases. Stanley himself used techniques he had developed for working with TMV in his research on influenza. More important, however, Stanley regarded TMV as a means of unlocking the secrets of poliovirus. In the late 1940s and early 1950s, his laboratory used TMV as a standard against which to compare the viral structures, mutations and corollary amino acid changes, and host-viral interactions of the three types of poliovirus then recognized (Creager, 2002). The methods of crystallization and purification that Stanley had pioneered using a plant virus were crucial to understanding the polio epidemic of the mid-20th century.

Communication Breakdown Between Independent Universes

Since the 1950s, communication between the plant sciences (and related fields such as soil microbiology) and biomedicine has disintegrated, even when the questions that engage practitioners in both areas are the same. The breakdown of this interdisciplinary exchange has led biomedical scientists to overlook recent breakthroughs in the plant sciences that might advance their own scientific progress.

Trapping Promoters on Two Continents

In 1988, for example, Michael Daniels' group at the John Innes Institute published their elegant method for isolating promoters from the plant pathogen *Xanthomonas campestris*, which involved cloning fragments of the *X. campestris* genome upstream of a promoterless tetracycline resistance determinant (Osbourn et al., 1987). He inoculated the clone library into plants that were grown in a solution containing tetracycline, ensuring that only those clones that carried a promoter that was induced inside the plant would survive. Daniels' paper predated the introduction of IVET, or *in vivo* expression technology, into the microbiological literature by six years, but the methods were essentially the same, except that the host was a plant rather than an animal (Figure 2-2). In the first IVET paper, the Mekalanos group at Harvard cloned fragments of the *Salmonella typhimurium* genome upstream of a promoterless *purA* gene in a purine auxotroph and injected the resulting library into mice, which provide a sufficiently purine-limited environment that selects for prototrophic strains (Mahan et al., 1993); therefore, the bacterium would only survive if the DNA upstream of the *purA* gene carried a promoter that was active inside the animal. The surviving clones could then be retrieved from the spleens of infected mice, and the promoters and genes they regulate could be identified in *S. typhimurium*, from which they arose. This powerful strategy has been applied to many host-microbe relationships and has provided sweeping insights into mutualistic and pathogenic relationships, yet despite Daniels' priority of publication, his paper is only rarely cited in papers about IVET or promoter trapping (Brown and Allen, 2004).

Protection, Probiotics, and Biocontrol

Probiotics, or consumable preparations of live bacterial cultures, have become fashionable in health food stores, in food animal production facilities, and research laboratories as a means of preventing or curing numerous ailments in animals and humans. Explanations for the benefits of such preparations have, at their core, two proposed mechanisms: first, that the probiotic strains outcompete detrimental bacteria at the site of pathogen infection, thus preventing the onset of disease symptoms. The second mechanism claims that probiotics induce a systemic response in the host that enhances resistance to infection. Yet neither of

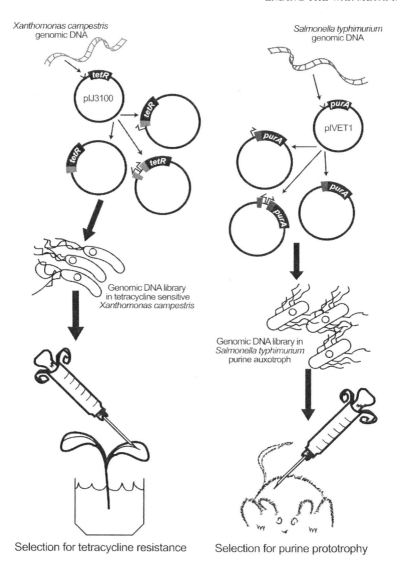

FIGURE 2-2 Schematic depiction of the first strategies to select in vivo for promoters that are induced by plant (left panel) or animal (right panel) hosts (Mahan et al., 1993; Osbourn et al., 1987). The strategies both use a chemical condition in the host (tetracycline or low availability of purines) to select for clones that carry host-inducible promoters. The scheme on the right is a simplified version of that published by Mahan et al. (1993); it does not show, for example, the integration of the vector into the chromosome, which was an aspect of the original strategy that differentiated it from the Osbourn et al. method (1987).
SOURCE: Handelsman (2005). Figure 2-2 was created with the help of Jo Handelsman's graduate student, Zakee Sabree.

these mechanisms is new to probiotics; they are both established mechanisms that govern the successful biological control (or biocontrol) of plant disease. Biocontrol agents, in the form of microbial inoculants applied to seed, soil, or leaves, have been used to enhance plant health and agricultural yield since the early 20th century. These agents typically work by suppressing a disease—some biocontrol strains colonize plant surfaces and exclude pathogens by competitive or antagonistic strategies such as occupying desirable niches or reducing pathogen populations through secretion of antibiotics. Others incite systemic acquired resistance, an induced response that makes the entire plant less susceptible to infection. Although both past and present work on biological control provides rich data that could inform the much younger field of probiotics, the potential for integration of these fields has not been recognized in current literature on probiotics.

Because of the breakdown in communication, therefore, knowledge developed within the plant sciences community has not been adopted by the biomedical community as successfully as in the 19th and early 20th centuries. Given the frequency with which conceptual change in the plant and agricultural sciences has enriched—and, often, preceded—similar developments in biomedicine, overlooking recent breakthroughs in the former can only be detrimental to the future growth of biomedicine. Of special importance at present is the seminal work in plant pathology and microbial ecology that considers the role of microbial communities in infectious disease.

Role of Communities in Infectious Disease

Pathogens live in a microbiological stew. When between hosts, they must survive in the environment among competitors who garner their scarce resources. When they contact a host, pathogens often must breach a protective microbiological barrier to reach the host tissue and induce disease. Pathogens frequently constitute part of this protective barrier, making a switch from commensal to pathogen whose triggers and governors are poorly understood.

The study of pathogenesis has traditionally ignored the microbial context of disease. It is time to examine the role of the microbial communities that live on and in host plants and animals to identify factors that reduce the effectiveness of host-associated communities as barriers and that incite commensals in these communities to turn on their host and cause disease. Plant disease, more often than human disease, has been studied in a microbial context, so there is much to learn from plant pathology that may affect our understanding of pathogenesis in humans.

Suppressive Soils, Biocontrol, and Latent Pathogens

The study of plant pathogens has typically included attention to microbial communities, in part because some attempts to assign responsibility for an effect to a single species have been dismal failures, indicating that mechanisms of disease suppression include coordination of responses in a community. Suppressive soils are an excellent case in point. It has long been observed that after growing a crop at the same site for many consecutive years, the frequency of certain diseases decreases. The soil becomes "suppressive" to that disease. Although the effect is demonstrably of biotic origin, disappearing upon biocidal treatment and spreading to other soils when a small soil inoculum is transferred to a new site, attempts to isolate a single organism responsible for the suppressiveness have been unsuccessful (Baker and Cook, 1974). Analysis of microbial communities in suppressive soils indicates that they differ from nonsuppressive soils in composition and structure, and certain disease-suppressive microorganisms have been isolated, but the exact complement of organisms required for suppressiveness has not been identified in most cases.

We found that introduction of *Bacillus cereus*, a biocontrol agent that suppresses root diseases of alfalfa and soybean plants caused by oomycete pathogens, altered the structure of the community associated with soybean roots, which is known as the rhizosphere community (Gilbert et al., 1993). Whether this community change is required for disease suppression, or just associated with it, remains unknown, but some features of the community change are noteworthy. First, *B. cereus* induces a dramatic increase in the proportion of the community that is represented by *Cytophaga johnsoniae*, a member of the *Cytophaga/Flavobacterium* group of the Bacteroidetes phylum (Gilbert et al., 1993). When *B. cereus* is isolated from field-grown roots, it frequently carries along with it "hitchhikers," what are difficult to separate from it initially. Interestingly, these coisolates are most often members of the *Cytophaga/Flavobacterium* group, and *B. cereus* provides a growth benefit for them under some conditions (Dunn et al., 2003).

In addition to the increase in representation of the *Cytophaga/Flavobacterium* group, *B. cereus* induces a global change in composition of the rhizosphere community that causes it to resemble the community in raw soil more than a typical rhizosphere. This finding led us to suggest the "camouflage hypothesis," which posits that microbial communities can prevent detection of a root by pathogens by altering the chemical composition of root exudates, making the root resemble soil, thereby "camouflaging" the root to resemble its surroundings (Gilbert et al., 1994). Many results reported in the first half of the 20th century are consistent with the camouflage hypothesis. For instance, biocontrol agents, plant disease resistance genes, and certain cultural practices have all been shown to be associated with reduction of disease as well as a change in the rhizosphere community that makes it resemble the soil more than the typical rhizosphere (Gilbert et al., 1993, 1996). As the study of plant disease became more reductionist in the latter half of the 20th century, attention to microbial communities decreased and a causal relationship between the composition of the rhizosphere community and disease suppression was not established. The camouflage hypothesis is attractive because a broad-based mechanism of disease suppression that is founded upon the contributions of many organisms that comprise a community might be more robust to the evolution of pathogens than are disease resistance genes and synthetic pesticides.

The camouflage hypothesis might have parallels in human infectious disease. The gut community, for example, may govern pathogen success by presenting a barrier to invasion that is predicated on the composition of the entire community, not one species. Alternatively, members of the natural community may potentiate the activity of the pathogen, facilitating infection or aggravating disease symptoms.

Future Focus

Understanding both plant and human infectious disease will be enhanced by understanding the communities in which the pathogens must function. The following key questions about community-pathogen interactions are especially crucial to constructing a comprehensive understanding of disease.

Community Robustness

To induce disease, many pathogens must colonize their hosts. If the tissue they infect carries a normal microflora, then the pathogen must invade the community on the host to cause disease. Little is understood about the nature of community robustness (resistance to and recovery from change) or the basis for pathogen invasiveness of communities. Identifying the components of community structure (species richness, functional redundancy, abundance of certain members) that contribute to robustness and the genes that make pathogens invasive will advance the understanding of the role of communities in disease (Handelsman et al., 2005).

Commensal-Pathogen Switch

Many pathogens reside peacefully in the communities that colonize infection sites on healthy host tissue and are triggered by certain cues to incite disease. Perturbation of the community, changes in host resistance, or convergence of physical or chemical features of the environment (such as availability of certain dietary components) to stimulate pathogen population or alter gene expression in the pathogen may be responsible for the switch from commensal to pathogen. An understanding of community structure and function that accounts for the effects of such changes will provide the basis for building quantitative models that predict disease events.

Microbial Cooperation

Little is known about polymicrobial diseases, but there is no doubt that in both plants and animals, certain diseases require the presence of two or more species. For example, a particular sequence of invasion events is required for biofilm formation on teeth. Certain bacteria require the prior establishment of other species in order to colonize (Kolenbrander et al., 2002). Although *Streptococcus mutans* is directly responsible for tooth decay, other members of the community are required for its establishment. In plant disease, similar synergies are abundant. Verticillium wilt disease of potatoes, for example, is substantially intensified on potato plants when their roots are infected by the root lesion nematode *Pratylenchus penetrans* (MacGuidwin and Rouse, 1990).

Mathematical Models

Predictive models that integrate biological and physical characteristics of the community are needed to generate principles of microbial ecology. Models that predict invasion events in many different communities will reveal the variables that govern robustness, invasion, and microbial cooperation, thereby forming the basis for predicting outcomes in new experimental or biological landscapes. Modeling has traditionally provided the basis for establishing broad principles in areas of biology as diverse as enzyme kinetics and macroecology (Anderson and May, 1986; Berg, 1983; Levin et al., 1989; Michaelis and Menten, 1913). Similarly, it is such models that will furnish microbial ecology with the power to revolutionize approaches to avoiding, preventing, treating, and curing infectious disease of plants and animals.

Conclusion

Much is made these days of interdisciplinary science that spans many fields, often uniting the biological and physical or mathematical sciences. These efforts have yielded extraordinary collaborations and insights into the natural world. But collaborations among closely related fields also remain powerful. The history of communication and collaboration between plant pathologists and medical microbiologists is a testament to this power. Such interactions contributed to the development of pure culture techniques, establishment of the germ theory of disease, and understanding of viral structure and function among many other great discoveries that punctuate the early history of microbiology. The more recent division between the fields has led to embarrassing ignorance at its best and wasteful delays in progress at its worst.

As one final case in point, consider the career of Selman Waksman. Waksman was trained as a soil microbiologist and considered himself an agricultural scientist throughout his career. Yet, through his discovery of streptomycin, produced by actinomycetes from soil, he made one of the most significant advances in medicine in the 20th century, for which he was awarded the 1952 Nobel Prize in Medicine. Waksman expressed great satisfaction in the fact that the National Academy of Sciences created divisions for both of his two great loves, agriculture and microbiology, during his lifetime (Waksman, 1958).

Waksman's discovery came toward the end of the Second World War—the first war in which there were fewer deaths from infection than from battle itself— because of the availability of antibiotics. Similarly, in the 21st century, we now face medical challenges of daunting proportions. An impending flu pandemic, the spread of antibiotic resistance among bacterial pathogens, and the recognition of the role of bacteria in far more conditions than we ever anticipated all present us with an opportunity. Plant pathology has addressed the role of microbial communities in plant disease, host genes that mediate resistance to disease, and environmental factors in development of disease epidemics. And as the United States confronts the potential for human epidemics derived from natural events or bioterrorism, we need to be equally cognizant of the vulnerability of our food supply to pathogens and microbial toxins. Perhaps the urgency of preparing for dire events will encourage the cooperation between these two fields that have so much to share.

THE MOLECULAR BASIS OF BACTERIAL INNATE IMMUNITY IN *ARABIDOPSIS THALIANA*

Brian Staskawicz
University of California, Berkeley

As Jo Handelsman has described in her contribution to this workshop (see the previous paper), plant disease epidemics have changed the course of human history on many occasions. One such epidemic, a rust that wiped out coffee plantations in British colonies, turned the country into a nation of tea drinkers. Today, the interactions of plants and infectious diseases—the major interest of my laboratory—are studied in model systems such as *Arabidopsis thaliana*, a plant that researchers have developed as a sort of "fruit fly" for plant genetics. Figure 2-3 depicts *Arabidopsis*, as well as rice, the plant that feeds most of the world, and the various classes of pathogens known to infect these plants, and indeed, all other higher eukaryotes.

Arabidopsis is a member of the Brassica family, which also includes such familiar vegetables as broccoli and cauliflower. There are many advantages to using *Arabidopsis* as a model system for studying plant-pathogen interactions. The plant completes a life cycle, from seed to seed, within seven weeks, and its entire genome has been sequenced. It is easily transformed (to produce a transgene) with *Agrobacterium tumefaciens*, known as nature's genetic engineer due to its facility for introducing DNA into plant (and yeast) cells. *Arabidopsis* transformation is performed by soaking the plant, while in flower, in a beaker contain-

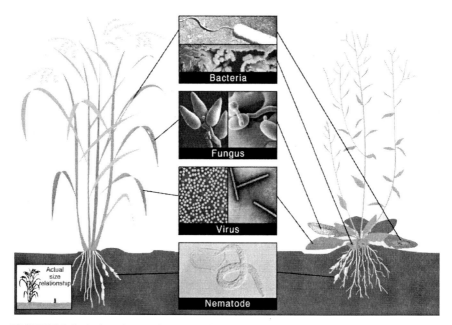

FIGURE 2-3 A rice plant (left) and *Arabidopsis thaliana* (right), a model plant for host-pathogen interactions. The establishment of numerous pathosystems in the genetically tractable plant species *A. thaliana* leads to rapid identification of components of host resistance and defense signaling pathways. Within each group, related bacterial, fungal, viral, and nematode pathogens cause diseases in both rice and *Arabidopsis*. Scanning electron micrographs (center panels) and disease reaction phenotypes of representative phytopathogens of *Oryza* and *Arabidopsis* are shown. The rice bacterial pathogen *X. oryzae pv. oryzae* causes chlorotic water-soaked stripes on rice leaves and lesions on *Arabidopsis* leaves. The bacterial pathogen *P. syringae* induces small water-soaked chlorotic lesions on *Arabidopsis*. The fungus *Erysiphe cihoracearum* causes powdery mildew disease on *Arabidopsis*. The most important fungal pathogen of rice is *Magnoportha grisea*, which produces gray necrotic lesions on all parts of the shoot. Tobacco mosaic virus infects and spreads throughout the *Arabidopsis* plant with few detectable symptoms. The spherical form of rice tungro virus causes yellow discoloration of the leaves. The plant parasitic nematode infects and causes disease in both rice and *Arabidopsis*.
SOURCE: Baker et al. (1997).

ing genetically engineered *Agrobacterium* in a liquid medium. Seeds from transformed plants are harvested and screened, with a typical transformant yield of 0.5 percent.

Thanks to the ease of conducting genetic research on *Arabidopsis*, a large international community of scientists works with this organism. An additional tool at our disposal is a comprehensive collection of transposon mutants in

Arabidopsis, created through random insertion of *Agrobacterium* transfer DNA (T-DNA) throughout the genome. The ends of the inserted transgenes have been sequenced and catalogued, so researchers who wish to examine a specific knock-out mutant can simply order seed and grow it.

Breeding for Pathogen Resistance

One of the major techniques for controlling plant disease is through classical plant breeding. The science of plant breeding is considered to have begun in 1906 in England, when the first (intentional) genetic cross was performed in wheat. The basis of plant breeding for disease resistance is to identify pathogen-resistant germplasm at the geographical origin of the plant species, where the plant and its pathogen coevolved. Researchers have discovered many wild species of agronomically important plants that can be genetically crossed with their cultivated relatives. This repertoire of diversity is the source of all disease resistance genes in a particular plant species.

To introduce resistance genes into cultivated plants, breeders create interspecific hybrids by taking pollen from a wild species and crossing it into the agronomic species. This is followed by selection for resistance and many rounds of backcrossing to produce a stable, resistant cultivar—a process that can take as long as 10 years. Most resistance traits that have been incorporated through plant breeding are single dominant genes because plant breeders like to look at single traits, and they find them in the first generation; however, there are many instances of multiple and recessive genes controlling resistance. Because of the ease of manipulation of single-gene traits, a century of plant breeding for disease resistance has produced agronomic fields that are genetically uniform. The human equivalent of this situation would occur if every one of us had exactly the same genetic resistance to flu virus, and the virus mutated to avoid our defenses: it would kill us all. Plant breeding establishes a huge selection pressure for pathogens to mutate, and they do. Then the breeding cycle begins all over again, with continued natural genetic variation occurring in both host resistance (R) genes and genes for pathogen effector proteins.

A Model System of Plant Innate Immunity

Immunity to pathogens, while strategically similar among plants and animals, manifests itself in different ways in each kingdom. In keeping with their lack of mobility, plants have very sophisticated ways of dealing with both biotic and abiotic stress. The plant's innate immune system employs hundreds of germline encoded pathogen receptors, most of which recognize type III effector proteins of bacterial pathogens. Plants have no system for adaptive immunity comparable to that in animals.

We study plant immunity through a discipline we call functional pathogenomics, in which we examine both the host (*Arabidopsis*) and the pathogen (*Pseudomonas syringae*). *Arabidopsis* can be manipulated in much the same way as a microbe: everything you can do with yeast or with *Pseudomonas*, you can do with *Arabidopsis*, with the exception of gene replacement. *Arabidopsis* has 125 megabases of DNA and about 25,000 genes, but many of these genes are regulated as families and are therefore redundant, as is typical of plants. For example, a particular protein might be encoded by a family of genes, each of which functions only in the leaves, or in the roots, or in the stem. This redundancy complicates genetic forward screens and makes it difficult to reveal recessive mutations, but it also means that the *Arabidopsis* genome is far simpler than 25,000 genes might suggest.

The pathogen in our study system, *P. syringae*, is a gram-negative bacterium. It is a facultative parasite that lives on the leaf surface, and has been found to obtain populations of 10^5 colony-forming units per centimeter squared on the leaf surface without causing disease. Under appropriate environmental conditions, *P. syringae* enters the leaf through the stomates (openings in the epidermis where gas exchange occurs) or through wounds. It multiplies in the intercellular spaces and remains outside plant cells. Another interesting trait of *P. syringae* is its capacity to produce ice nucleation proteins; by ordering water molecules, these proteins can induce premature freezing, which kills the host plant. The advantage of this trait for the bacterium appears to be in promoting dissemination: bacteria on the leaf surface become incorporated into water droplets that return to the atmosphere and, eventually, rain down on other plants.

P. syringae has an inner and an outer membrane; the plant cell has a very complex plant cell wall, a plasma membrane, and various membrane-bound organelles within its cytoplasm. The bacterium delivers as many as 40 different effector proteins through the plant cell wall in order to suppress or modify the host plant's immune response and thereby permit colonization, much as effector proteins from animal pathogens do. A type III secretion system, essentially a molecular syringe, injects the bacterial effector proteins into the plant cell. All 40 or so effector proteins have different (and some have multiple) targets within the plant cell that are either destroyed or altered in some fashion.

In response to such invasions, plants have evolved resistance proteins to deal with specific bacterial effector proteins. Plant resistance proteins have long been hypothesized to recognize—directly or indirectly—specific bacterial effector proteins. This notion, known as the gene-for-gene hypothesis, was first proposed in the 1940s by the plant pathologist H. H. Flor (Loegering and Ellingboe, 1987; Staskawicz, 2001). This concept is the essence of innate immunity in plants. However, until a decade or so ago, all that was known about plant *R* genes is that they typically segregated as a single trait. It was expected that *R* genes would encode receptors that served as ligands for the bacterial effector proteins, and that effector protein binding would cause the resistance protein to trigger a signal cascade leading to the disease resistance phenotype.

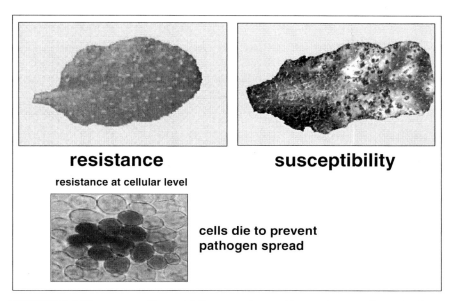

FIGURE 2-4 Phenotypes of bacterial disease resistance. Leaves from two isogenic plants that differ only as follows: the plant on the left has a single dominant disease resistance gene (*RPS2*); the plant on the right has a recessive (inactive) allele (*rps2*) of the same gene. Following inoculation of both plants with *P. syringae*, the plant on the left expresses resistance to the pathogen. At the microscopic level, it can be seen that infected cells in the resistant plant are undergoing programmed cell death, in a localized hypersensitive reaction.
SOURCE: Staskawicz (2005).

In 1994, our lab and several others cloned some disease resistance genes, and we have since found that in only a couple of cases, the ligand-receptor model does not apply. However, a key finding from these studies is that resistance genes confer upon plant cells the ability to undergo programmed cell death upon recognizing a pathogen. By committing suicide, infected cells prevent the pathogen from spreading through the plant. This phenomenon, known as the hypersensitive reaction, is depicted in Figure 2-4.

Structural Comparisons of Disease Resistance Proteins

There are two main classes of *Arabidopsis* disease resistance proteins: the cytosolic "nucleotide-binding site plus leucine-rich repeat" (NBS-LRR) type, of which there are several subtypes, and the membrane-bound "leucine-rich repeat transmembrane kinase" (LRR-TM kinase) type. Figure 2-5 shows the distribution of the 150 disease resistance gene loci among the five *Arabidopsis* chromo-

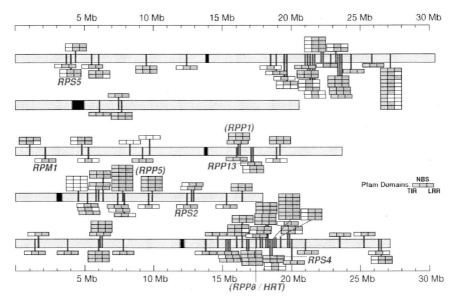

FIGURE 2-5 *Arabidopsis* disease resistance genes.
SOURCE: Michelmore (2001).

somes. The clustering of the *R* genes is thought to promote allelic diversity, and perhaps recombination as well (through unequal crossing over or possibly through gene conversion). After all, the 150 *R* genes in *Arabidopsis* not only encode the capacity for resistance to bacteria, but also resistance to viruses, fungi, nematodes, and insects. There must be some mechanism(s) that enable the plant to deal with the diversity of pathogen effector genes that it encounters.

Figure 2-6 shows similar motifs that occur in animal innate immune receptors and plant disease resistance proteins. For example, the *Arabidopsis* flagellin sensitivity 2 (FLS2) protein and the mammalian toll-like receptor 5 (TLR5) proteins both contain leucine-rich repeats and transmembrane domains; however, in the analogous cytoplasmic location to the FLS2 protein kinase domain, TLR5 has the toll interleukin 1 receptor. Both FLS2 and TLR5 interact with the bacterial protein, flagellin. The pervasive similarities in plant and animal innate immune receptor structure have become a focus for interaction among plant and animal molecular biologists studying these systems, as the entire community attempts to learn how these molecules actually function.

Disease Resistance at the Molecular Level

To illustrate the intricacy of disease resistance protein function and the methods we have used to elucidate how plant and pathogen components of disease

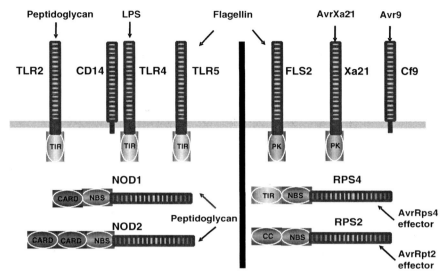

FIGURE 2-6 Representative protein motifs found in immune receptors of plants and animals. Schematic diagram of several proteins present in plants (left) and animals (right) that initiate signal transduction cascades after pathogen infection.
SOURCE: Staskawicz (2005).

resistance work together, I will describe research in my laboratory on a particular *Arabidopsis* disease resistance protein, RPS2 (*R*esistance to *P. syringae* 2). This protein recognizes a *P. syringae* effector protein called AvrRpt2. As shown in Figure 2-6, RPS2 is a membrane-associated NBS-LRR-type protein, with a coiled-coil "leucine zipper" nucleotide binding site at its N-terminus. As shown in Figure 2-7, RPS2 forms a complex with another *Arabidopsis* protein called RIN4 (for *R*PM1-*i*nteracting *p*rotein 4; RPM1 is also a disease resistance protein, *R*esistance to *P. syringae* pv *maculicola* 1).

It turns out that this system is under negative regulation, which appears to be a common theme of signal transduction networks in plants. In this case, the negative regulator RIN4 renders RPS2 inactive. This was shown to be the case by overexpressing RPS2 relative to RIN4, either transgenically or transiently, which produces a constitutive defense response: cell death. On the other hand, if RIN4 is overexpressed relative to RPS2, disease resistance is inhibited, so these plants are more susceptible to *P. syringae*. Homozygous *rin4* mutants were found to be lethal in the presence of the RPS2 gene; this makes sense, because a constitutively activated defense response would result in whole-plant suicide by the hypersensitive response.

Recent work in my laboratory shows how these proteins function in the presence of AvrRpt2, the *P. syringae* effector protein (Axtell and Staskawicz, 2003;

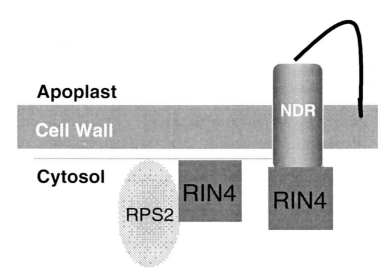

FIGURE 2-7 Model for RPS2-mediated innate immunity. RIN4 complexes with disease resistance proteins. RPS2 forms a complex with RIN4, a negative regulator of RPS2 activity (see Figure 2-8). RIN4 also forms a complex with and negatively regulates NDR1, a glycosylphatidylinositol membrane-anchored protein that is presumed to be involved in disease resistance downstream of the RPS2-RIN4 interaction.
SOURCE: Staskawicz (2005).

Axtell et al., 2003; Belkhadir et al., 2004). The bacterium delivers an inactive form of AvrRpt to the plant cell via a type III secretion system. The effector protein becomes active following processing by a plant protein factor (cyclophilin), after which 71 N-terminal amino acids are cleaved to produce the mature, 184-residue effector protein. After cloning and sequencing AvrRpt2, we analyzed its predicted secondary structure and found it had functional resemblance to the cysteine protease, staphopain.

We also isolated the plant protein factor that enables the processing of AvrRpt2 into its active form, and learned that it was common to all eukaryotes. This was significant because it meant that we could develop an assay for AvrRpt2 processing in yeast, which is even easier to manipulate than *Arabidopsis*. We took a biochemical approach, using the pure recombinant full-length AvrRpt2 protein and assaying chromatographic (hydrophobic interaction ion exchange gel filtration) fractions from yeast in order to isolate the eukaryotic proteins that processed the bacterial effector protein. Analysis of the active fraction by tandem mass spectrometry identified the eukaryotic processing factor as cyclophilin, a peptidyl-prolyl isomerase (PPIase) that is thought to act as a molecular chaperone or folding catalyst. Cyclophilin has been widely studied in association with protein folding, signal transduction, protein trafficking and assembly, and cell cycle variation; it is required for assembly of the HIV-1 virion. Clearly, it is an important constituent of eukaryotic cells.

Next we used cyclophilin cDNA from yeast to find the orthologous gene in *Arabidopsis*. Pure recombinant protein from the *Arabidopsis* gene was then successfully tested in place of the yeast fraction in the processing assay. It worked as predicted, and we also found that cyclosporin A, which is known to bind specifically to cyclophilin, inhibited effector processing, while rapamycin, which inhibits another class of PPIases, did not.

The actual cleavage of AvrRpt2 occurs through autocatalysis, following processing (presumably refolding) by cyclophilin. Two regions encoding a 7-amino acid sequence of the autocatalytic cleavage site in AvrRpt2 occur in the negative regulator of disease resistance, RIN4. This suggests that RIN4 is inactivated when cleaved byAvrRpt2, which in turn permits activation of RPS2-mediated disease resistance. These findings are summarized in Figure 2-8. Researchers in my lab and others are now trying to determine the molecular basis of RPS2 activation.

A bioinformatics prediction has found putative AvrRpt2 cleavage sequences in approximately 20 proteins in the *Arabidopsis* genome, all of which are thus potential targets of that effector protein. By extension, it seems likely that among the 40 effector proteins produced by *P. syringae*, there are others that have multiple targets within the plant cell.

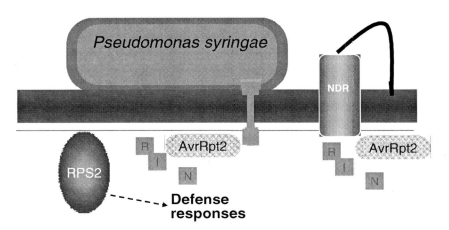

FIGURE 2-8 Model of RPS2-mediated immunity in *Arabidopsis*. In the presence of *P. syringae* effector protein AvrRpt2, RIN4 is eliminated and RPS2 disease resistance is activated.
SOURCE: Staskawicz (2005).

REFERENCES

Anderson RM, May RM. 1986. *The Dynamics of Human Host-Parasite Systems.* Princeton, NJ: Princeton University Press.
Axtell MJ, Staskawicz BJ. 2003. Initiation of RPS2-specified disease resistance in Arabidopsis is coupled to the AvrRpt2-directed elimination of RIN4. *Cell* 112(3):369–377.
Axtell MJ, Chisholm ST, Dahlbeck D, Staskawicz BJ. 2003. Genetic and molecular evidence that the Pseudomonas syringae type III effector protein AvrRpt2 is a cysteine protease. *Molecular Microbiology* 49(6):1537–1546.
Baker KF, Cook RJ. 1974. *Biological Control of Plant Pathogens.* San Francisco, CA: W.H. Freeman.
Baker B, Zambryski P, Staskawicz B, Dinesh-Kumar SP. 1997. Signaling in plant-microbe interactions. *Science* 276(5313):726–733.
Beijerinck MW. 1898. Ueber ein contagium vivum fluidum als ursache der fleckenkrankheit der tabaksblätter. *Verhandelingen der Koninklyke Akademie van Wettenschappen te Amsterdam* 65:3–21.
Belkhadir Y, Nimchuk Z, Hubert DA, Mackey D, Dangl JL. 2004. *Plant Cell* 16(10):2822–2835.
Berg HC. 1983. *Random Walks in Biology.* Princeton, NJ: Princeton University Press.
Brock T. 1961. *Milestones in Microbiology.* Englewood Cliffs, NJ: Prentice-Hall.
Brock T. 1988. *Robert Koch: A Life in Medicine and Bacteriology.* Berlin, Germany: Springer-Verlag.
Brown DG, Allen C. 2004. *Ralstonia solanacearum* genes induced during growth in tomato: An inside view of bacterial wilt. *Molecular Microbiology* 53:1641–1660.
Campbell CL, Peterson PD, Griffith CS. 1999. *The Formative Years of Plant Pathology in the United States.* St. Paul, MN: APS Press.
Cohn F. 1872. Untersuchungen über Bacterien. *Beiträge zur Biologie der Pflanzen.* 1:127–224.
Creager ANH. 2002. *The Life of a Virus: Tobacco Mosaic Virus as an Experimental Model, 1930–1965.* Chicago, IL: University of Chicago Press.
Dunn AK, Klimowicz AK, Handelsman J. 2003. Use of a promoter trap to identify *Bacillus cereus* genes regulated by tomato seed exudate and a rhizosphere resident, *Pseudomonas aureofaciens. Applied Environmental Microbiology* 69(2):1197–1205.
Gilbert GS, Parke JL, Clayton MK, Handelsman J. 1993. Effects of an introduced bacterium on bacterial communities on roots. *Ecology* 74:840–854.
Gilbert GS, Handelsman J, Parke JL. 1994. Root camouflage and disease control. *Phytopathology* 84:222–225.
Gilbert GS, Clayton MK, Handelsman J, Parke JL. 1996. Use of cluster and discriminant analyses to compare rhizosphere bacterial communities following biological perturbation. *Microbial Ecology* 32:123–147.
Handelsman J. 2005 (March 17). *Session IV: Novel Approaches for Mitigating the Development of Resistance.* Presentation at the Forum on Microbial Threats Workshop Ending the War Metaphor: The Changing Agenda for Unraveling the Host-Microbe Relationship, Washington, D.C., Institute of Medicine, Forum on Microbial Threats.
Handelsman J, Robinson CJ, Raffa KF. 2005. Microbial communities in lepidopteran guts: From models to metagenomics. In: McFall-Ngai M, Henderson B, Ruby EG, eds. *The Influence of Cooperative Bacteria on Animal Host Biology.* New York: Cambridge University Press. Pp. 143–168.
Ivanowski D. 1892. Ueber die mosaikkrankheit der tabakspflanze. *St. Petersburg Academy of Imperial Sciences Bulletin Series 4* 35:67–70.
Kolenbrander PE, Andersen RN, Blehert DS, Egland PG, Foster JS, Palmer RJ Jr. 2002. Communication among oral bacteria. *Microbiolgy and Molecular Biology Reviews* 66:486–505.
Levin SA, Hallam TG, Gross LJ. 1989. *Applied Mathematical Ecology.* New York: Springer-Verlag New York, Incorporated.
Loegering WQ, Ellingboe AH. 1987. H.H. Flor: Pioneer in Phytopathology. *Annual Review of Phytopathology* 25:59–66.

MacGuidwin AE, Rouse DI. 1990. Role of *Pratylenchus penetrans* in the potato early dying disease of Russet Burbank Potato. *Phytopathology* 80:1077–1082.

Mahan MJ, Slauch JM, Mekalanos JJ. 1993. Selection of bacterial virulence genes that are specifically induced in host tissues. *Science* 259(5095):686–688.

Michaelis L, Menten M. 1913. Die kinetik der invertinwirkung. *Biochemistry Zeitung* 49:333–369.

Michelmore R. 2001. *Physical location of Arabidopsis sequences related to NBS-encoding plant R-genes.* [Online]. Available: http://niblrrs.ucdavis.edu/At_RGenes/RGenes_Phylogeny/At_RGenes_on_Chromosomes.html [accessed April 28, 2006].

Osbourn AE, Barber CE, Daniels MJ. 1987. Identification of plant-induced genes of the bacterial pathogen *Xanthomonas campestris* pathovar campestris using a promoter-probe plasmid. *European Molecular Biology Organization Journal* 6(1):23–28.

Staskawicz B. 2001. Genetics of plant-pathogen interactions specifying plant disease resistance. *Plant Physiology* 125(1):73–76.

Staskawicz BJ. 2005 (March 16). *Session I: Host-Pathogen Interactions: Defining the Concepts of Pathogenicity, Virulence, Colonization, Commensalism, and Symbiosis.* Presentation at the Forum on Microbial Threats Workshop Ending the War Metaphor: The Changing Agenda for Unraveling the Host-Microbe Relationship, Washington, D.C., Institute of Medicine, Forum on Microbial Threats.

Waksman SA. 1958. *My Life with the Microbes.* London, UK: Scientific Book Club.

3

The Ecology of Pathogenesis

OVERVIEW

Over the course of the last century, the identification of increasing numbers of microbial pathogens and the characterization of the diseases they cause has begun to reveal the extraordinary complexity and individuality of host-pathogen relationships. The vast majority of microbes does not produce overt illness in their hosts, but instead act as persistent colonists. Genetic changes in either host or microbe may disrupt this equilibrium and shift the relationship toward pathogenesis, resulting in illness and possibly death for the host. These considerations are reflected in the contributed papers collected in this chapter, which explore how pathogens coexist within host-microbial communities, placing infectious disease within an ecological and evolutionary context.

In this relatively recent, dynamic model of pathogenesis, it has become exceedingly difficult to identify what makes a microbe a pathogen. This challenge is taken up at the beginning of the chapter by Stanley Falkow, who describes the variety of circumstances that lead to pathogenesis. Recognizing that a considerable amount of infectious disease is caused by "accidents" of transmission, susceptibility, and host response to microbes, Falkow illustrates how primary pathogens pursue an adaptive strategy that produces disease in normal hosts. This perspective informs an ecological model of pathogenicity as a product of ongoing evolution between pathogen and host.

The chapter continues with a detailed exploration of a single human pathogen, the bacterium *Helicobacter pylori*, which is strongly associated with increased risk for peptic ulcer disease and gastric cancer. Martin Blaser considers this example of amphibiosis—a term coined decades ago by microbial ecologist

Theodore Rosebury to describe a relationship between two life forms that is either symbiotic or parasitic, depending on the context—as representative of most relationships between humans and their indigenous organisms. The intricate signaling that occurs between humans and *H. pylori* has provided important insight on the effects of indigenous microbes on normal human physiology, as well as on disease. It also raises questions about the consequences of the disappearance of *H. pylori* (and other less-detectable indigenous bacteria) from the human gastrointestinal tract, a trend apparently underway in the industrialized world.

In contrast to the sole human-microbe interaction known to produce peptic ulcers, a broad range of normal luminal bacteria can induce and perpetuate intestinal inflammation (and possibly extraintestinal inflammatory conditions such as arthritis) in genetically susceptible hosts. Balfour Sartor's contribution to this chapter describes bacterial factors and genetically programmed host responses that influence whether the host's response to commensal bacteria is one of coexistence or of aggressive defense via inflammation, as occurs in idiopathic inflammatory bowel disease (IBD), Crohn's disease, and ulcerative colitis. Greater understanding of the mechanisms of induction and perpetuation of intestinal inflammation may indicate how these responses could be inhibited in order to restore mucosal homeostasis, and how therapies for these conditions might be tailored to individual patients.

The chapter concludes with further reflections on the human microbiome by Maria Dominguez-Bello, who notes two promising areas for continued research on host-microbe ecology. The first is the rumen, which she portrays as a model system of host-microbe mutualism and the subject of seminal studies on digestive processes in humans and other animals. The second research area—which follows from Blaser's aforementioned observation that modern life is changing the human microbiota—is the comparative study of indigenous microbes in human populations outside the industrialized world. To this end, Dominguez-Bello describes her own work among indigenous Venezuelan Amerindian tribes that examines the association between microbiome diversity and human health.

THE ZEN OF PATHOGENICITY

Stanley Falkow
Stanford University

The following remarks are meant to present a human's idea of the microbe's "point-of-view" and the various ways that a microorganism might cause disease. In so doing, I will offer a view of host-pathogen relationships that is in keeping with the goal of this workshop of replacing the war metaphor. As a first example of the intricacies of such relationships, consider a host macrophage engulfing the plague bacillus (*Yersinia pestis*), as shown in Figure 3-1. To many, this apparently defensive moment represents the essence of the host-parasite relationship.

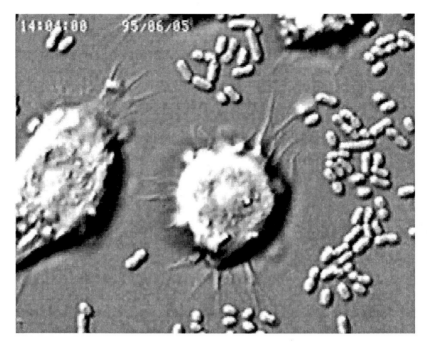

FIGURE 3-1 Host macrophage engulfing the plague bacillus (*Yersinia pestis*).
SOURCE: Falkow (2005).

In the end, the ingested bacteria are killed, but so is the host cell. There are more bacteria than host cells, and often the microbe has the last laugh.

The impact of microbes on humans extends to our culture (Cockburn, 1971; McNeill, 1976). Figure 3-2 shows variations in the human population over several centuries and notes the factors driving these changes, which are dominated by disease and war. The graph reveals an interesting trend: peaks of human population, followed by die-offs due to infectious diseases, followed by renaissance periods of peak human productivity in the resulting population valleys. If this pattern continues to hold, then we are approaching a time of epidemics, of which HIV/AIDS may be considered a harbinger.

Throughout most of our history, people have lived in small groups. Most known epidemic infections of humans require populations of 50,000 to 100,000 to spread; therefore, the diseases that are strictly adapted to our species are relatively recent in the evolutionary sense. The development of pathogens specific to humans was further encouraged by the crowding, defective hygiene, and poor nutrition associated with the transition to living in larger communities. In addition, the domestication of animals has permitted the evolution of infectious diseases such as measles (from canine distemper and rinderpest), diphtheria (from

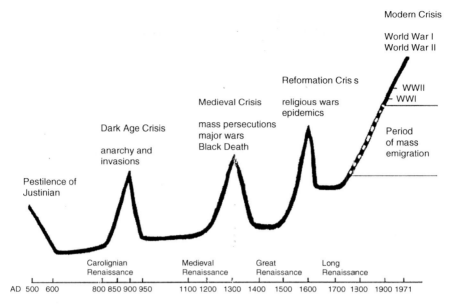

FIGURE 3-2 Infectious diseases were, and still are, the most common cause of death worldwide.
SOURCE: Falkow (2005).

cows), and influenza (from birds). Humans over time have become the preferred hosts of several species of bacteria, viruses and, in many parts of the world, worms. We really are a fertile landscape of opportunity for microbes.

What Is a Pathogen?

Once it was understood that microbes caused disease, the term *pathogen* was coined to describe *any* disease-causing organism, and this is the term still employed in medicine. Although this definition is certainly practical, it may not be entirely accurate from a biological—that is, the microbe's—standpoint. As I see it, humans play host to the following categories of microbes:

- **Transients:** Microbes that we ingest and with which we come in contact, but which do not persist on us. They are just "passing through."
- **Commensals:** (*to eat from the same table*): The hundreds of microbial species growing within each of us. Many of them are with us from the moment of birth, when we are first colonized by microbes, and remain with us to the grave. Some commensal species play essential roles in the development of our gas-

trointestinal tract and immune system. Their last role is to participate in our decomposition (think of it as recycling) after we die.

- **Pathogens:** I use the term *primary pathogen* (which is not a universally accepted term) to describe microbes that cause disease in apparently normal human hosts. By contrast, *opportunistic pathogens* cause disease only in compromised human hosts. Commensals can be opportunists, and an opportunist in one host can be a primary pathogen in another host.

Differentiating between pathogens and commensals is important to devising new ways to thwart off attacks by pathogens. However, this is not an easy distinction to make because of the considerable similarities between the colonization strategies used by both pathogens and commensals. Successful microbes of both classes must find ways to enter their hosts (us), locate a niche to colonize, interact intimately with the host, replicate, persist (although this may not be necessary for pathogens), disseminate to new hosts, and, ultimately, evolve.

I believe that the major difference between pathogens and commensals is that pathogens have the inherent ability to cross anatomic and biochemical barriers in the host that serve to limit colonization by commensals. Most pathogens establish themselves in niches devoid of other microorganisms. For example, *E. coli* that cause diarrheal disease and urinary tract infections do not occupy the same niche as the commensal strains of *E. coli* in the colon. Instead, enterohemorrhagic *E. coli* specifically colonize a special niche within the colon near the lymphatic centers, while the urinary tract pathogens leave the colon altogether for another mucosal surface. Pathogens have the inherent ability to colonize these host-protected niches, and the invasive properties pathogens use to get there are essential to their survival in nature and are often host specific. This adaptive strategy, or lifestyle, is specific to primary microbial pathogens and absent from opportunists.

A considerable amount of human infectious disease is not caused by primary pathogens. Some infectious diseases—such as Lyme disease, rabies, and botulism—occur in humans through *accidents of transmissibility*, when we are infected by microbes that are specific to other host species. Most potential bioterrorism agents fit this general description. In these cases, disease is a disadvantage to both the host and the microbe, because the host often dies before the microbe can be transmitted to another host. Other human infections are *accidents of susceptibility*, which result from noninherent defects in host immunity. These defects could be either mechanical or biochemical, but in either case allow commensals that were previously held in place by normal host defense mechanisms to cross the barriers that contain them. Finally, there are human diseases that represent *accidents of host response*, or heritable defects in host immunity like that seen in cystic fibrosis.

Although we can get disease from a variety of microorganisms, I would argue that only some of them are primary pathogens. This subset of disease-causing microorganisms has evolved specifically to cross host barriers in order to survive, and in crossing host barriers they often cause injury. The virulence factors that allow pathogens to pursue this strategy are equivalent to the fur, claws, and fangs of higher animals: adaptations to an organism's environment that favor survival. Pathogenicity in this instance reflects the ongoing evolution between a parasite and host, and disease is the product of a microbial adaptive strategy for survival. Moreover, what we recognize clinically as disease is very often our human response to microbial invasion. In some cases, disease is a host-microbe experiment gone wrong, and when that happens, the host is as likely to be "at fault" in causing disease as the microbe.

Host Defenses

Animals have evolved both innate and adaptive immune mechanisms to avoid microbial intrusion or traumatic insult. The main function of the innate immune system is to keep commensal or transient organisms in their place—that is, to limit their ability to colonize host tissues beyond the mucosal surface. Immune signal cascades mediated by toll-like receptors (TLRs), which specifically recognize molecules characteristic of prokaryotes and other kinds of parasites, alert the host to microbial intrusion. The features recognized by TLRs are not unique to pathogens, but they set off an elaborate cascade that can summon cells with antibacterial characteristics, such as the macrophages that are recruited to ingest the *Yersinia* in Figure 3-1. Invading microbes without specific mechanisms to avoid the innate immune system are destroyed. Pathogens must possess inherent ways to avoid or subvert these innate host defense mechanisms.

Adaptive immunity, or the ability to produce antibodies that can neutralize microbes, occurs in higher animals. The capacity of humans to make antibody is of course critical to the effectiveness of vaccines. If we know how to stimulate production of antibody against a particular antigen, it is relatively easy to develop a vaccine against an organism that invades the bloodstream. However, it is much more difficult to make vaccines directed against microbes that inhabit the mucosal surfaces (e.g., the gut). Thus, the development of mucosal vaccines has been a great challenge, particularly when one considers the huge differences in individual susceptibility to infection between, for example, a normal neonate and one that has a low birth weight, is preterm, or is otherwise physically compromised. Some pathogens have devised ways to get around the adaptive immune system by constantly changing their surface or by camouflaging their appearance.

Steps to Successful Pathogenesis

The following section describes the challenges faced by pathogens, and the various mechanisms they have evolved to address them.

Entry

There are 9 natural portals of microbial entry in humans (10, if the umbilicus is included); along with injured tissues, these are the typical routes of entry for pathogens. The skin and the mucosal surfaces present formidable physical barriers to microbes: tight cell junctions; the mucus "stream" that flows through the gut, capturing organisms washing them out of the body; and antimicrobial substances. All of these obstacles, along with competition from commensals, stand in the way of the microbe.

Colonization

Following entry, the microbe must find a niche to inhabit. This process is often called colonization, and the microbe usually achieves it by attaching itself to a unique host cellular target, or by adapting to host physiology. Bacteria have hairlike structures called pili that have evolved to recognize and adhere to a specific receptor on the surface of the host cell. The various forms of pili have been studied extensively in the uropathogenic strains of *E. coli*. Genomic analysis of *Salmonella* reveals at least eight different kinds of pili that the bacterium uses to find targets for attachment in different contexts, both inside and outside the host's body.

Microbes are very simple creatures, but they can perform the tasks of recognition at their surfaces through either proteins or proteinaceous appendages. The bacterial strain that causes salmonellosis, for example, recognizes specific kinds of cells in the terminal ileum.[1] Protein-based adherence mechanisms are also found in viruses; herpesviruses, for example, have proteins on their surfaces that recognize specific receptors on host cells.

Persistence

Many common pathogens are organisms such as *Pneumococcus*, group A *Streptococcus*, *Meningococcus*, and *Hemophilus influenzae* that all humans carry at some point in their lives. These microbes occasionally cause clinically apparent disease, because they have an adaptive strategy of persistence achieved through mechanisms that avoid, circumvent, or subvert host defense mechanisms. One of the common mechanisms bacteria use is encapsulation, as occurs in *Streptococcus pneumoniae* (the most common cause of bacterial pneumonia) and *Ba-*

---

[1]Such specificity might seem to suggest that one could make a vaccine based on a single kind of pilus. This might work in some cases, but more often than not this strategy would be foiled by the redundant recognition and adherence mechanisms present in most species of bacteria. Moreover, bacterial adherence is often an interactive, multicellular phenomenon, as when the presence of a device such as a prosthetic valve or indwelling catheter supports communities of microorganisms as biofilms.

cillus anthracis (anthrax). The capsule, made of carbohydrate or protein, surrounds the microorganism and interferes with phagocytosis, much as the slimy coating on a wet bar of soap makes it hard to grab. Without a capsule, *S. pneumoniae* is essentially avirulent; it can live in the human host, but it is very unlikely to cause disease.

Another means to persistence is to breach the tight junctions between epithelial cells or to get inside the cells themselves. *Salmonella* and *Shigella* can stimulate human epithelial cells and cause them to extend cytoplasmic ruffles that act to trap the bacteria and literally pull them into the cell. Other bacteria harness the cytoskeleton; the organism that causes enterohemorrhagic *E. coli* reorganizes the cytoskeletal actin of its host cell in the colon epithelium into a sort of pedestal. The bacterium sticks avidly to this pedestal, where it is bathed with host cell nutrients that the microbe uses for growth. The attached bacteria replicate to form microcolonies on the surface of the host cell.

Yet, other pathogens persist in their hosts by circumventing the intracellular trafficking that allows host phagocytes to take up commensal bacteria or other kinds of particles, put them into vacuoles, and digest them. In some cases, the digested products trigger the production of antibodies by the host's immune system. Some pathogenic bacteria divert normal trafficking by phagocytes; others (e.g., *Yersinia*) kill the phagocyte quickly after they attach or have been ingested.

Enzymes and toxins allow pathogenic bacteria to spread through local tissues and perturb host immune function. Group A *Streptococci* secrete substances that disintegrate the molecular "cement" between cells—hyaluronic acid—so that the bacteria slip easily along the tissue plane. Other secreted streptococcal toxins kill host cells. The released host cell contents form a viscous mass that might impair the ability of bacteria to spread through the tissues, but the bacteria make a DNase that dissolves this barrier. Thus, the microbe releases a series of substances exquisitely timed to permit the microbe to spread, replicate, and persist in an environment that is normally lethal for other microorganisms.

Replication

What do microbes gain from host-pathogen relationships? Replication. The successful microbe is one that can replicate sufficiently to be transmitted to a new susceptible host. What does the host gain from its associations with microbes? Usually immunity sufficient to clear the immediate threat and, in the best of circumstances, forevermore.

Some pathogens persistently colonize their hosts and continuously transmit small numbers of their kind into the host's environment. Under these conditions, disease represents an option, not a goal, for a pathogen. It is merely one means to the end of replication, not a necessary outcome of colonization. When an organism causes disease, it is but a byproduct of its survival strategy. And, disease is often as much a factor of the state of the host defenses as it is of the microbes' need to breach host barriers.

For example, while many people become ill in influenza outbreaks, even more people escape disease. In seeking to understand host-pathogen relationships, disease can distract us from understanding the actual mechanisms that underlie these associations. However, we must understand how pathogens operate in order to devise new ways to protect ourselves from their ill effects.

Dissemination

Bacteria need an exit strategy from their hosts. Microbes are conveyed between humans in a variety of ways: through respiratory droplets or saliva, fecal-oral transmission, and even in our lovemaking. Zoonotic infections, which rarely spread person-to-person, are transmitted through animal bites, feces, and insect vectors (ticks, fleas, etc.).

Even organisms such as *Salmonella typhi*, *Mycobacterium tuberculosis*, and *Helicobacter pylori*, which cause lifelong infections, must eventually find new hosts. The ease and the frequency with which a pathogen leaves its host may influence its virulence.

The Roles and Origin of Bacterial Toxins

A particularly fascinating aspect of bacterial evolution is the existence of toxins. *Vibrio cholerae*, for example, produces an extraordinarily powerful and well-known toxin that causes patients with cholera to pass copious amounts of watery stools. These patients survive only if the number of liters of fluid they lose can be balanced with the same volume of fluid going in. Humans do not carry the cholera bacterium; its reservoir is probably in marine estuaries.

Toxins appear to perform a variety of functions for bacteria, including nutrient acquisition, the breakdown of anatomic barriers, facilitation of exit and transmission, and the modulation of immune function. It seems unlikely that the original purpose of toxins was to poison mammals. Thus, if we can put aside our desire to avoid cholera or botulism or other toxic bacterial infections, and instead consider what advantages toxins confer upon bacteria, we may come up with a better way to neutralize toxin-producing pathogens.

I suspect that bacterial toxins first evolved in compost heaps when bacteria came in contact with predatory amoeba and especially with nematodes. Pound for pound, nematodes eat more bacteria than any other organism. To avoid becoming prey, bacteria harmed their predators. Thus, the toxins that bacteria initially evolved to avoid phagocytosis by amoebae became—after millions of years of evolution—the same molecules that stop the human phagocyte from engulfing bacteria.

Finally, it has been said of bacterial toxins that we incriminate the microbe for the sins of the viruses (Hayes, 1968). Many toxins are encoded by accessory genetic elements, and the advantage they confer upon the organism that possesses them is unknown. We might be able to get answers to such questions by comparing bacteria such as *Bacillus anthracis*, which carries a DNA insert known as a pathogenicity island (further discussed below), and its close relative *Bacillus cereus*, which does not carry a pathogenicity island. Such studies could also provide new insights on protecting ourselves from anthrax.

Corollaries of Pathogenicity

A better understanding of the previously described steps that pathogens must take in order to live successfully in their hosts could result in the search for new ways to protect humans from infectious diseases. Such efforts should also address the following "corollaries" of pathogen behavior, as revealed through microbiological research.

Bacteria Have Keen Senses

Pathogens and other bacterial specialists (almost all bacteria are specialists) use elaborate regulatory mechanisms based on environmental and biochemical cues. Bacteria have extremely sensitive chemical sensory systems that measure environmental variables such as oxygen and carbon dioxide concentration and pH. Significant changes in these measures signal the microbe to alter the products it makes to suit its environment. Such adjustments allow simple organisms to survive transitions.

When a bacterium in a bit of feces on the ground moves into a human's mouth, it undergoes an enormous change in pH and comes in contact with lysozyme and a variety of other antibacterial chemicals. Then the ingested bacterium is plunged into the acid vat of the stomach and quickly passes into the small bowel, where it is bathed in bile and an impressive array of digestive enzymes, all along being propelled by the forces of peristalsis. The bacterium takes all of this in stride and responds to each change in environment by rapid changes in its own structure and metabolism. These constantly changing environmental cues permit many microbes to anticipate when they will reach their optimal niche. Thus, *Salmonella* uses changes in pH, the viscosity of intestinal mucus, and the concentration of oxygen adjacent to host epithelial cells to determine when it will encounter its target cell in the terminal ileum. The bacterium quickly readies itself for infection during its transition through the gut. Clearly, it can respond far faster to us than we can to it.

Pathogens Are Opportunists

As Walt Kelly's comic strip hero, Pogo, said, "We have met the enemy, and he is us." Pathogens can respond to a host's biological and social behavior (Falkow, 1998). Many pathogens that coexist uneventfully with other hosts cause disease when they encounter humans; for example, the Lyme bacterium (*Borrelia burgdorferi*) persists in mice, deer, and ticks, and only causes disease when it colonizes humans or dogs. These hosts represent new "opportunities" for such microbes, and unfortunately may result in new diseases for hosts that (unlike mice, deer, and ticks) have not evolved a relationship with a given pathogen.

Similar scenarios involving human behavior underlie several recent infectious crises, including Legionnaire's disease and toxic shock syndrome. The increasing presence of aerosols in our environment—created by taking showers rather than sitting demurely in a bathtub, by air conditioning, by misting of produce in supermarkets—has provided new opportunities for organisms to spread in a "modern" world. The bacterium *Legionella*, for example, lives primarily in amoebae in an aquatic environment. When amoebae are dispersed in aerosols that are inhaled by humans, they—along with their bacterial hitchhikers—are taken up by macrophages in the lung. Once inside a human cell, the bacterium replicates and causes a clinical pneumonia we call Legionnaire's disease. Likewise, the response of American industry to women's demand for more absorbent tampons, which gave them greater freedom during menstruation, resulted in a product that unexpectedly encouraged growth of certain staphylococci that typically exist in small numbers in women's genital tracts. The regrettable result was the emergence of a new disease entity: toxic shock syndrome.

Bacteria Evolve Rapidly

The previous 20 years of research on bacteria reveal that they become pathogenic through a horizontal exchange of genetic information. In some ways microbial genomes comprise a genetic information network, operating much like the Internet. Mobile genetic elements such as plasmids, phages, and transposons are constantly streaming among microorganisms as they contact each other or enter into new environments. This elementary form of gene transfer enables microbes—often quite diverse ones—to share information with one another (Dobrindt et al., 2004).

For example, as described by Martin Blaser and colleagues (see paper in this chapter), there are two types of *H. pylori*: one that is associated with gastritis, and another that is associated with peptic ulcer and gastric cancer. The difference between the two types is that the more pathogenic type contains an insertion of DNA that is called a pathogenicity island. This extra DNA encodes a protein that leads to cancer and ulcers in some human hosts, although exactly how it does that remains to be determined. It is known that such islands of genes often allow bacteria to synthesize surface proteins that function much like a hypodermic needle (type III secretion). This structure makes contact with host cells and permits the bacteria to deliver other proteins, called effectors, directly into the host cell. The injected effector proteins have the ability to change or capture or manipulate normal host functions to the microbe's favor. This apparently ancient and relatively common pathogenic mechanism is present in plant pathogens as well as in those infecting animals and humans, but this remarkable microbial attribute has only been revealed and appreciated within the past decade or so.

In the larger context of host-microbe interactions, the exchange of genetic information in packets of DNA—transferred by direct contact, or through bacterial viruses, or even through the uptake of naked DNA—has enabled bacteria to experiment with their environment. In some cases, these experiments have led microbes to develop survival mechanisms that we see as pathogenicity and disease. However, it is also clear from genomics and other research that this genetic process has produced a variety of nonpathogenic microbial adaptations; for example, nitrogen fixation benefits microbes as well as crop plants (and therefore, also humans).

Conclusion

We have tried to control infectious disease with antibiotics and vaccines. Every time we attempt to control microbes by killing them, it provides them with a strong genetic selection for resistant organisms. There has been a continuous dialog over the past 50 years in regard to the problem of antimicrobial resistance. If we are going to address the problem of antibiotic resistance, I believe we will need to take a new, more sensible approach to the problem. Moreover, we will need to address the fact that pathogenicity in all microbes—not just bacteria—can occur in big genetic jumps, rather than through slow, adaptive evolution; HIV is a case in point. We also must reflect upon the lesson of bacterial genomics: many pathogens adapted to humans are relatively recent in evolution. We have to understand that the host-pathogen interaction is a dynamic process, and there are likely to be surprises in our future.

The mapping of the human genome and of bacterial genomes provides the means to better understand host-microbe relationships. In the context of infectious diseases, it is likely to be just as important to learn about the host as the microbe. For example, a single gene makes a dramatic difference in the susceptibility of mice to *Salmonella*; those that have the gene are resistant, and those that do not have it die upon infection (Govoni and Gros, 1998). Also, recent findings associate different human lymphocyte antigen (HLA) types in humans with susceptibility or resistance to infectious diseases (Segal and Hill, 2003). In the future, I expect that it will be possible to quickly genotype patients with infectious disease and understand how to moderate and mitigate therapy according to an individual's genetically determined risk. This ability should also lead to new ideas for therapies for infectious diseases.

I will conclude with a story about my experience researching plague many years ago. One summer, the fleas we used to study *Yersinia* were not doing well. When we inspected the fleas under the microscope, we discovered that they had mites. Then we examined the mites and found that they themselves had little mites, upon which there were microbes (see Figure 3-3).

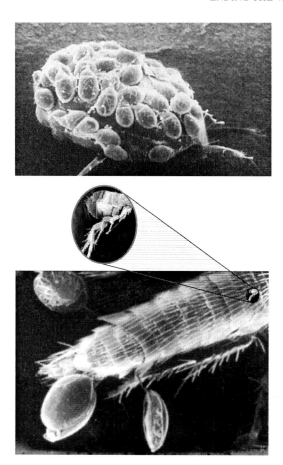

FIGURE 3-3 Illustration of the old rhyme (based on a poem by Jonathan Swift, author of *Gulliver's Travels*[2]), "Big fleas have little fleas upon their backs to bite them, and little fleas have lesser fleas and, so on, *ad infinitum*." We need to keep that idea in mind today, along with the fact that, in the end, microbes always have the last laugh.
SOURCE: Falkow (2005).

---

[2]Swift actually wrote,
"So, naturalists observe, a flea
Has smaller fleas that on him prey;
And these have smaller still to bite 'em;
And so proceed ad infinitum."
Swift J. 1733. *Poetry, a Rhapsody*. [Online]. Available: http://www.online-literature.com/quotes/quotation_search.php?author=Jonathan%20Swiftl.

Acknowledgments

I wish to thank Alison Mack and Eileen Choffnes, who made a rambling talk into prose. Many of the ideas presented here were previously published in several review articles that contain references to the following primary literature:

Falkow S. 1997. What is a pathogen? *American Society for Microbiology News* 63:359–365.
Falkow S. 1998. The microbe's view of infection. *Annals of Internal Medicine* 129(3):247–248.
Finlay BB, Falkow S. 1997. Common themes in microbial pathogenicity revisited. *Microbiology and Molecular Review* 61(2):136–139.
Monack DM, Mueller A, Falkow S. 1994. Persistent bacterial infections: The interface of the pathogen and the host immune system. *Nature Reviews Microbiology* 2(9):747–765.

PATHOGENICITY AND SYMBIOSIS: HUMAN GASTRIC COLONIZATION BY *HELICOBACTER PYLORI* AS A MODEL SYSTEM OF AMPHIBIOSIS

Martin J. Blaser[3]

Amphibiosis, a term coined by the microbial ecologist Theodore Rosebury about 50 years ago (Rosebury, 1962), is the biological condition in which the relationship between two life forms is either symbiotic or parasitic, depending on the context. This is a more precise term than commensalism and describes a more complex relationship than symbiosis. It is my hypothesis that amphibiosis best describes most relationships between humans and their indigenous organisms. A second hypothesis is that human gastric colonization by *Helicobacter pylori* is a model system for amphibiosis.

H. pylori as a Model of Our Indigenous Biota

H. pylori are curved gram-negative bacteria that live in the mucous layer of the human stomach (Blaser and Atherton, 2004). Most individuals acquire *H. pylori* early in life. It does not invade the gastric tissue, but lives in the mucous layer, persisting for the lifetime of the host in most cases (Hazell et al., 1986). Its very persistence is one of the hallmarks of amphibiosis. Although these organisms were first seen in the human stomach about 100 years ago, they were not isolated in pure culture by Warren and Marshall until in 1982 (Warren and Marshall, 1983). However, there is now extensive evidence that *H. pylori* has long been part of the human biosphere. From the population biology studies examining more than 300 *H. pylori* isolates from around the world (Falush et al., 2003), modern *H. pylori* populations are not clearly delineated (Figure 3-4A). *H. pylori* are naturally competent for transformation (Israel et al., 2000), and populations of organisms show evidence for extensive recombination (Suerbaum

---

[3] New York University School of Medicine, New York; VA Medical Center, New York.

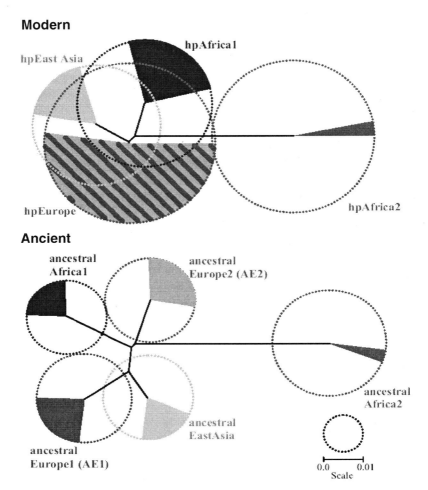

FIGURE 3-4 Modern and ancient *H. pylori* populations, determined by applying the STRUCTURE algorithm to sequences in eight conserved *H. pylori* genes in > 300 contemporary isolates (Falush et al., 2003).
SOURCE: Blaser (2005).

et al., 1998). Using an algorithm to assign ancestry to each nucleotide, Falush et al. showed that all or essentially all modern *H. pylori* populations derive from five ancestral populations. It is likely two were originally African populations and two were strongly associated with Eurasia and one with East Asia (Figure 3-4B). Relating such data to known human migrations (Ghose et al., 2002), it has become clear that *H. pylori* has been present in human populations for at least

60,000 years. Indirect evidence also suggests that an ancestral *H. pylori* strain has been present in humans, and our predecessors, for millions of years (Blaser, 1998).

These studies, suggesting that we have shared much history, are consistent with a different model of human identity; the human body is home to more microbial cells than human cells (Savage, 1977) (Figure 3-5A). Further, since our indigenous and transient microbes are varied, they have been considered by Lederberg as our "microbiome" (Lederberg, 2000). I propose an integration of the human 46 chromosome genome and the extremely large microbiome to produce a *metabolome* (Figure 3-5B). In this conception, we, along with our major constituents, have been selected for coexistence, and our metabolic circuitry is comingled and synergistic. This idea can help us understand both normal physiology and disease, and our relationship with *H. pylori* provides an important probe (and test) of the underlying biology.

Whether the normal biota are useful or harmful has been debated for more than a century (Mackowiak, 1982). Pasteur, the "father" of microbiology, considered that the normal biota (flora) are essential to life. Metchnikoff, one of the founders of immunology, believed that normal flora are antagonistic and compete with the host. There is evidence that supports both view points (Mackowiak, 1982); in its aggregate, this is amphibiosis.

Signaling

In the relationship between host and colonizing microbes, an important interface is the signaling between host and microbe. A prototypic microbe on a mucosal surface, subject to being washed away by flow, is multiplying, producing metabolites and toxins, and possibly directly adhering to the epithelium (Blaser, 1997). Each of these activities may be considered as signals to the host. The host produces a physical and chemical milieu, its own metabolites, and defense molecules that also may be considered as signals to the microbes.

Signaling between microbe and host may be unlinked. This signaling pattern would be a mirror of warfare, with an arms race between microbe and host. Acute infection by a pathogen best fits this paradigm. The alternative model is that there is a linkage between microbial and host signals that have coevolved due to selective pressure on both host and microbe to coexist. This is the model that may be most appropriate for the indigenous biota, and the cross-signaling must be dynamic, reflecting variations induced by microbial diversity, host development and aging, and other environmental cofactors.

Our interactions with *H. pylori* illustrate several aspects of these issues (Figure 3-6). *H. pylori* colonization is mostly acquired early in life (Oliveira et al., 1994; Pérez-Pérez et al., 2003), with an early population bloom leading to the gradual development of immunity. The host recognizes and responds to the organism, causing the microbial population to diminish in number, and then ensues stable equilibrium lasting decades in which effective *H. pylori* multiplication and

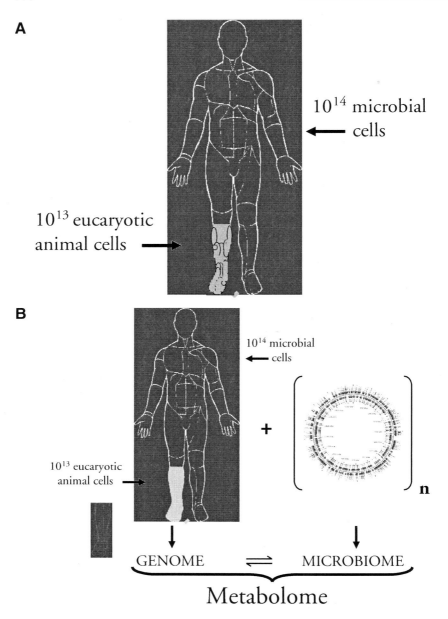

FIGURE 3-5 Who are we? A: Microbial cells outnumber all host cells in the human body. B: An integrated view of host-microbial interactions in the human body, constituting the *metabolome*. In this model, our indigenous microbes are as much a part of human physiology as is a recognized human organ, such as the liver.
SOURCE: Blaser (2005).

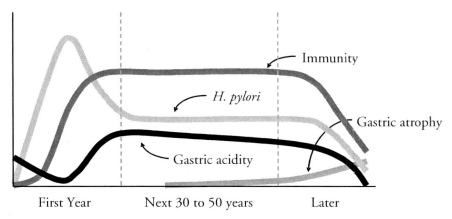

FIGURE 3-6 Schematic of the natural history of *H. pylori* populations and host characteristics in colonized individuals over their lifetime. This model is divided into an initial (transient) period, a long equilibrium, and a late decline. Host recognition and response (immunity) limits *H. pylori* populations, but the ongoing interaction progressively damages gastric tissues, leading to localized and then generalized gastric atrophy. As this continues, gastric acidity is reduced, *H. pylori* populations decline, and as they decline, host responses diminish. In this formulation, *H. pylori* may be a model for other persistent colonizers that both elicit host responses and induce tissue injury.
SOURCE: Blaser (2005).

host effector mechanisms are balanced. It is a stalemate, but with effects on gastric physiology (Calam, 1995; Moss and Calam, 1993). Over decades, the consequence of this slow inflammatory interaction is the gradual development of gastric atrophy (Kuipers et al., 1995a; Kuipers et al., 1995b). As atrophy increases, *H. pylori* populations fall, sometimes to zero, and the immune response subsequently falls as well (Karnes et al., 1991) (Figure 3-6).

Thus, there is an initial transient state, a long period of equilibrium, and then a late transitional state. A model for persistence includes both adherent and mucosal (free-living) *H. pylori* populations, nutrients derived from the host permeating the mucous layer, and a number of *H. pylori*-produced effectors that induce the flow of nutrients to feed the organism and allow them to multiply (Kirschner and Blaser, 1995). The essential feature of the model is a negative-feedback loop; this is the only way persistence can be modeled within appropriate parameters (Blaser and Kirschner, 1999; Kirschner and Blaser, 1995). The model is robust, encompassing a wide range of host, microbial, and interactive variation, but in the absence of feedback, no equilibrium can be achieved; microbial populations (MP) go to infinity or to zero. This linked signaling between coevolved species could represent a model for other persistent indigenous organisms as well.

A more specific version of the model is that *H. pylori*, the coevolved microbe living in the gastric lumen (Figure 3-7), is subject to a variety of stresses,

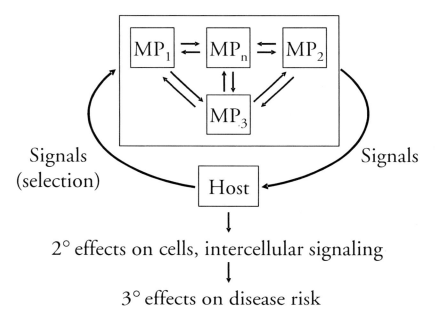

FIGURE 3-7 Equilibrium relationships between coevolved persistent microbes and their hosts. The colonizing microbe is considered as a group of highly related MP that differ in their expression of "contingency" genes, living in equilibrium with one another, with the exact relationships determined by the relative fitness of the MPs in relation to the (selecting) host signals. *H. pylori* serves as the model organism, and there are primary, secondary, and tertiary consequences of the relationship.
SOURCE: Blaser (2005).

including pH, nutrient limitation, and peristalsis. Organisms have been selected that signal specific host cells to produce effectors that abrogate the stress. Such a model represents an equilibrium relationship, but since both hosts and their *H. pylori* populations are unique (El-Omar et al., 2000; Israel et al., 2000; Kuipers et al., 2000; Machado et al., 2003), the exact relationships form unique equilibria, and in changing contexts, they form dynamic unique equilibria. My hypothesis is that this primary equilibrium affects secondary events (Blaser, 1992), including epithelial cell cycle, inflammatory responses, and neuroendocrine pathways (Blaser and Atherton, 2004), and that these in turn affect risk of disease (Figure 3-7).

The Disappearance of *H. pylori*

In developing countries, *H. pylori* is most often acquired in childhood; by the time adulthood is reached, virtually everyone is colonized by the organism

(Oliveira et al., 1994; Pérez-Pérez et al., 2003) (Figure 3-8), often with multiple strains (Ghose et al., 2005). In contrast, in developed countries such as the United States, *H. pylori* prevalence is much lower, reflecting a birth cohort phenomenon (Parsonnet, 1995; Rehnberg-Laiho et al., 2001). When current U.S. adults were children, there was much more *H. pylori* in circulation than now exists for our children. Since all developed countries were formerly developing countries, over time, the incidence of acquisition has gradually fallen (Parsonnet, 1995; Rehnberg-Laiho et al., 2001), and continues to fall (Pérez-Pérez, 2002). In fact, *H. pylori* is disappearing in developed countries. This seems puzzling. How can an organism that probably has been with humans for tens of thousands of years, if not longer, now be disappearing? In turn, this phenomenon raises two questions: why is *H. pylori* disappearing, and what are the consequences of its disappearance?

Why is *H. pylori* disappearing? Important factors probably include its less efficient transmission, based on cleaner water and smaller family size (Goodman and Correa, 2000; Klein et al., 1991). The transmission of microbes is a function of the population structure of human communities; one of the large demographic changes associated with recent socioeconomic development is that families are becoming smaller. Older siblings play an important role in *H. pylori* transmission (Goodman and Correa, 2000; Goodman et al., 1996), and there are now fewer children per family. Host survival advantage also may have been removed. If *H. pylori* protected against lethal diarrheal disease (Rothenbacher, 2000), and

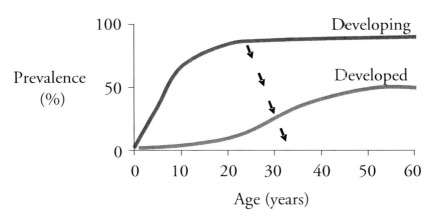

FIGURE 3-8 Prevalence of *H. pylori* in human populations in developing and developed countries. Because all developed countries were formerly developing countries, the prevalence of colonization should have shifted downward (↓) over the course of development, and much evidence supports this hypothesis. As socioeconomic development is proceeding, *H. pylori* is disappearing, especially from children.
SOURCE: Blaser (2005).

such illnesses are themselves diminished due to improved hygiene, then any positive selection for the presence of *H. pylori* may be removed. As overall *H. pylori* populations fall, there also is diminished ability for gene exchange, making the colonizers of an individual host less robust. Furthermore, we are more than 60 years into the antibiotic era. A course of amoxicillin may eliminate *H. pylori* 10–20 percent of the time (Rauws et al., 1988). This is insufficient for planned therapy to eradicate *H. pylori*, but if all the antibiotics that are given in childhood are summated, there is enormous pressure, not only on the development of resistance, but on the presence of *H. pylori* in individual hosts.

Consequences of *H. pylori* Disappearance

Regardless of why *H. pylori* is disappearing, probably for the first time in human history there are large numbers of adults who do not have the organism; thus, through clinical and epidemiologic comparisons, we can examine the consequences of colonization vis a vis its lack.

For persons colonized with *H. pylori*, within the gastric mucosa the lamina propria contains numerous lymphocytes and macrophages. Pathologists call this "chronic gastritis" (Harford et al., 2000; Tham et al., 2001). An alternative nomenclature is that these cells represent the "physiologic response to an indigenous organism." This phenomenon may be considered an analogy to the lamina propria in the colon. We consider the colon to be normally colonized by bacteria and the colonic lamina propria is replete with inflammatory/immunologic (defense) cells. A germ-free colon shows few or no such cells in the lamina propria, but when the colon is "conventionalized," there is infiltration of the lamina propria with host phagocytic and immunologic cells. Regardless of what we call the phenomenon, it is clear that the cells in the lamina propria reflect the presence of microbes in the mucous layer, clearly in the colon, and now apparently in the stomach as well (Blaser, 1990).

Why is that important? In 1975, Peleyo Correa developed a model of the pathway for the most important type of gastric carcinogenesis, involving adenocarcinoma of the stomach (Correa et al., 1975). In his model, there is a progression over decades, from normal gastric mucosa to chronic gastritis, atrophic gastritis, metaplasia, dysplasia, and then to cancer (Correa et al., 1975). A long series of investigations supports Correa's hypothesis, but it was not known what caused the initial transition from normal gastric mucosa, to chronic gastritis. As indicated above, there is overwhelming evidence that the acquisition of *H. pylori* is the main cause for this transition (Blaser, 1990). Therefore, it was a reasonable hypothesis that the presence of *H. pylori* could be a risk factor for development of gastric cancer.

On the basis of both epidemiologic and animal challenge studies, it is now clear that colonization by *H. pylori* is an important risk factor for gastric cancer (IARC, 1994; Peek and Blaser, 2002). Thus, one of the biological costs of

Helicobacter pylori gastric colonization is that some hosts will develop gastric cancer. In certain ethnic groups, such gastric cancers might affect up to 5 percent of the population, mostly at older ages, in their 60s, 70s, and beyond, in a log-linear relationship with age. Clearly, as with other "environmental" carcinogens (e.g., tobacco smoke), the cost of carrying *H. pylori* is not absolute; not everyone gets gastric cancer. It is a risk relationship, with the greatest impact late in life.

In parallel studies, gastric colonization with *H. pylori* tripled or quadrupled the risk of peptic ulcer disease (Nomura et al., 1994; Nomura et al., 2002a). There are many data from retrospective (treatment) studies that indicate the same kind of relationship (Hentschel et al., 1993). The magnitude of the risk relationship between *H. pylori* and gastric cancer is greater than the relationship with ulcer disease.

Differences Among *H. pylori* Strains

H. pylori strains can be divided by the presence or absence of the *cag* island. First discovered based on the presence of the gene, *cagA* (Covacci et al., 1993; Cover et al., 1990; Crabtree et al., 1991; Tummuru et al., 1993), a marker for the presence of the rest of the island, this is a region of about 40 kilobases on the *H. pylori* chromosome (Tummuru et al., 1995; Censini et al., 1996; Akopyants et al., 1998). The *cag* island is flanked by direct DNA repeats, and includes multiple direct DNA repeats (Aras et al., 2003a; Tomb et al., 1997); it is a metastable genetic element subject to partial or total deletion events (Censini et al., 1996), but through recombination the island also can be restored to a negative strain (Kersulyte et al., 1999). The *cag* island contains type IV secretion system (TFSS) genes that translocate the CagA protein from *Helicobacter* cells into gastric epithelial cells (Hatakeyama, 2004; Odenbreit et al., 2000). There are sites on the CagA protein that undergo tyrosine phosphorylation by host cel. Src-like kinases, and then this phosphoprotein interacts with several cellular signal transduction pathways (Amieva et al., 2003; Higashi et al., 2001; Naumann et al., 1999). I had previously postulated that there might be strong signals from *H. pylori* cells to the host (Blaser, 1992), and that these signals provide the substrate for the feedback relationship (Blaser and Kirschner, 1999; Kirschner and Blaser, 1995). In fact, the injection of the CagA protein is a very strong signal that *H. pylori* provides to host cells; recent data indicate that much of the interaction between *H. pylori* and host cells involves *cag* island genes (Segal et al., 1999; Viala et al., 2004).

Because we can differentiate between two groups of helicobacters, *cag* positive and *cag* negative, it is next reasonable to ask whether there is differential risk of disease in persons carrying one or the other strain. Studies now have shown 50 to 300 percent increases in risk of gastric cancer in persons with *cag*-positive strains compared to those with *cag*-negative strains (Blaser et al., 1995a; Nomura et al., 2002b; Parsonnet et al., 1997). How do *cag*-positive strains increase risk? There have been well over 100 studies that show effects of *cag*-

positivity on proinflammatory cytokines, tissue infiltration with inflammatory cells, epithelial cell cycle events, and intracellular signaling pathways (Blaser and Atherton, 2004; Hatakeyama, 2004; Peek and Blaser, 2002).

One of the hypotheses of how *H. pylori* colonization leads to gastric cancer risk is that the organism induces a variety of host responses that are affected by strain, host, or cofactor differences; there is evidence that each of these factors affects cancer risk (Blaser et al., 1995b; El-Omar et al., 2000; Machado et al., 2003). For example, host characteristics affect risk; particular proinflammatory genotypes drive the interactions toward atrophic gastritis, leading to effects on cell cycle and mutation leading to adenocarcinoma (El-Omar et al., 2000; Machado et al., 2003). Although this conception is the major thrust of current investigation, there is an alternative hypothesis (Figure 3-9). Atrophic gastritis, per se, alters the gastric environment, allowing for changes in gastric microecology. The development of atrophic gastritis can permit new organisms to colonize the stomach; it may be that these microecologic changes are driving toward adenocarcinoma. Thus, whether the *H. pylori*-induced increases in cancer risk are due to direct effects on the tissue or indirect, due to replacement of the biota, are two testable hypotheses.

Since *H. pylori* is a risk factor for gastric cancer (IARC, 1994; Peek and Blaser, 2002), and *H. pylori* is disappearing, gastric cancer should be disappearing. In fact, in virtually every developed country studied, 20th century gastric cancer rates are declining (Howson et al., 1986); it now is clear that the disappearance of *H. pylori* is responsible for at least a part, if not the major part, of this phenomenon. This provides a strong justification for medical attempts to make all humans *Helicobacter* free.

Esophageal Diseases

However, new cancers continue to arise. Adenocarcinoma of the esophagus has dramatically increased in the United States since at least 1970 (Devessa et al., 1998); there has been a six-fold rise over the past 25 years (Pohl and Gilbert, 2005). The evidence is clear that this is not due to a surveillance artifact. In fact, adenocarcinoma of the esophagus is the most rapidly increasing cancer in the United States, and there are data from England, Scandinavia, and Australia that confirm the rapid rise in the incidence of this tumor, and of the closely related, if not identical, adenocarcinoma of the gastric cardia. It is likely that these gastroesophageal (GE) junction tumors represent a single disease.

Why are these cancers rising at the same time that gastric cancer is falling? It is clear that the pathway for the development of these cancers relates to a condition called gastroesophageal reflux disease (GERD) (Lagergren et al., 1999), which can then lead to a metaplastic process called Barrett's esophagus, which can lead to dysplasia and adenocarcinoma; this process may take 20 to 40 years.

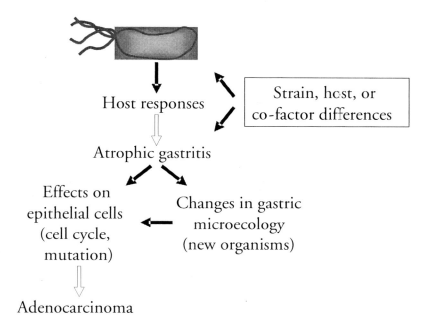

FIGURE 3-9 Potential pathways by which *H. pylori* colonization increases risk of gastric cancer. The mainstream of current research suggests that the interaction of *H. pylori* and host cells per se, as affected by strain, host, and environmental differences, leads to atrophic gastritis, and then to cancer. An alternative model is that the critical dimension of the *H. pylori*-host interactions is that they lead to the development of atrophic gastritis, and that with atrophic gastritis, there is expansion of other MPs, or replacement by microbes that cannot survive well in the normal high-acid *H. pylori*-rich stomach. It may be these other microbes that, through greater tissue injury and a more enhanced proinflammatory interaction, provide the direct oncogenic signals.
SOURCE: Blaser (2005).

Reflux esophagitis was first described in the medical literature in the 1930s, and Barrett's esophagus was first described by Dr. Norman Barrett, a surgeon, in 1950.

Are these diseases related to the disappearance of *H. pylori*? In a series of clinical and epidemiologic studies, we and others asked two questions: what is the state of the esophagus, and how does that relate to the presence of *H. pylori*? A number of studies now have shown that people who have esophageal disease are less often colonized with *H. pylori* than those with a normal esophagus (Chow et al., 1998; Loffeld et al., 2000; Vaezi et al., 2000; Vicari et al., 1998). Because we showed that *cagA*-positive strains are more interactive than *cagA*-negative strains, we particularly looked at *cagA* status. In a study of Dutch patients, we asked who carries a *cag*-positive strain. The results showed that for persons with a normal esophagus, it was 33 percent, for hiatal hernia, 14 percent; esophagitis,

16 percent; and Barrett's, 6 percent (Loffeld et al., 2000). In these cross-sectional studies, as the groups are moving nosologically from normal esophagus toward malignancy, *cag*-positive strains were becoming less prevalent. Consequently, we performed studies to examine directly whether there is a relationship between the presence of *Helicobacter*, especially *cag*-positive strains, and cancers of the GE junction. In a study of 130 cancer cases, and 220 controls, compared to the reference *Helicobacter*-negative group, the odds ratio for *cag*-negative strains was 1.1, but the odds ratio was 0.4 for *cag*-positive strains (Chow et al., 1998). Thus, an inverse association was observed for the presence of *cag*-positive strains and adenocarcinoma of the esophagus, the disease that is rising so rapidly. There have been several independent confirmations of these phenomena, concerning GERD, Barrett's, and adenocarcinoma (de Martel, 2005; Queiroz et al., 2004; Warburton-Timmsa et al., 2001; Ye et al., 2004).

A study from Sweden by Ye and colleagues showed an odds ratio of 0.2 for *cag*-positive strains (Ye et al., 2004). Recently de Martel and colleagues examined the Kaiser cohort of 130,000 people. For *H. pylori* positive persons, the odds ratio associated with developing esophageal adenocarcinoma was 0.37 (de Martel, 2005). Again, there was an inverse relationship between esophageal adenocarcinoma and *H. pylori* in this prospective study, although they did not show any differential effect for *cagA*. There now have been several epidemiologic studies showing that the presence of *Helicobacter* has an inverse association with adenocarcinomas involving the GE junction and its precursor lesions (Chow et al., 1998; de Martel, 2005; Peek et al., 1999; Ye et al., 2004); one study that did not show a significant association may have had technical artifacts (Wu et al., 2003).

H. pylori Strain Type and Risk of Disease by Location

The data suggest that in relation to diseases of the lower stomach and esophagus, such as ulcer disease and gastric cancer, carrying a *cag*-positive strain increases risk of disease (Blaser, 1999). Carrying a *cag*-negative strain enhances risk but to a much lower extent (Parsonnet et al., 1997). However, considering diseases of the upper stomach and esophagus, such as GERD, Barrett's, and adenocarcinoma, having a *cag*-positive strain appears to be protective, and *cag*-negative strains are relatively neutral (Chow et al., 1998; Loffeld et al., 2000; Queiroz et al., 2004; Vaezi et al., 2000; Vicari et al., 1998; Warburton-Timmsa et al., 2001; Ye et al., 2004). As such, most of the disease relationship concerns *cag*-positive strains, which is not surprising, since they are the more interactive with the host (Amieva et al., 2003; Hatakeyama, 2004; Higashi et al., 2001; Naumann et al., 1999; Odenbreit et al., 2000; Segal et al., 1999).

Although the mechanisms involved may be complex, Yamaji and colleagues studied more than 6,000 patients who underwent endoscopy in Japan (Yamaji et al., 2001). The investigators categorized the subjects by both *Helicobacter* and pepsinogen status to create a scale ranging from a relatively normal stomach to

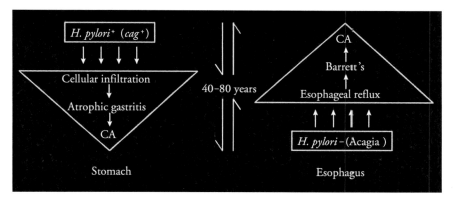

FIGURE 3-10 Proposed reciprocal relationship between adenocarcinomas of the stomach and esophagus. *H. pylori* colonization initiates a multidecade sequence of events leading to atrophic gastritis and ultimately to gastric cancer. Conversely, the absence of *H. pylori*, especially of *cag*-positive strains (a phenomenon that I have termed *acagia*), predisposes to GERD and sequelae, increasing risk of esophageal adenocarcinoma, a process that also requires multiple decades.
SOURCE: Blaser (2005).

atrophy. For individuals in categories progressively related to atrophy, gastric cancer prevalence went up, and GERD went down. Conversely, moving from atrophy to normal on the scale was associated with increased reflux and decreased gastric cancer prevalence.

As such, I propose that there is a reciprocal relationship between adenocarcinomas of the stomach and the esophagus (Figure 3-10). The data suggest that over several decades persons who have *H. pylori*, especially *cag*-positive strains, have increased risk of cellular infiltration of their stomach, and atrophic gastritis, leading to gastric cancer. In contrast, persons who are not colonized with *H. pylori*, especially not having *cag*-positive strains (a condition I have called *acagia* in 1998) (Wu et al., 2003), have increased risk for GERD, Barrett's, and esophageal cancer.

H. pylori Protection Against Esophageal Disease

How might *H. pylori* protect against esophageal disease? There could be direct or indirect effects on the esophagus, and the work of Yamaji (Yamaji et al., 2001) and others cited above (Kuipers et al., 1995a, 1995b) suggest there may be indirect effects operating through gastric physiology.

We also are interested in direct effects of *H. pylori* (or its absence) on the esophagus, involving either esophageal tissue or the esophageal biota.

Dr. Zhiheng Pei found that bacteria can be visualized in the distal esophagus in biopsies that he examined histopathologically (Yamaji et al., 2001). Consequently, studies were performed on four healthy persons to examine 16S ribosomal RNA (rRNA) clones from their esophageal biopsies (Pei et al., 2004). In these subjects, 95 species-level operational taxonomic units (SLOTU) were identified; diversity estimations predicted about 130 different SLOTU in the healthy esophagus. The 95 SLOTU belonged to 6 phyla and 41 genera; 59 SLOTU were homologous with culture-defined species, 34 were 16S clones, and 2 were not homologous with any known clones. Fourteen SLOTU were shared by all 4 individuals, accounting for 64 percent of the clones. These preliminary observations provide evidence that there is a conserved esophageal biota, and there are host-specific organisms. Ongoing studies support these observations and suggest that differences exist in the esophageal biota present in individuals with normal esophagus and with GERD (Lu et al., 2005; Pei et al., 2005).

H. pylori, Gastric Hormones, and Metabolic Effects of Colonization

The stomach may be considered an endocrine organ, since it produces the hormones gastrin and somatostatin (Calam, 1995; Moss and Calam, 1993; Moss et al., 1992). Several years ago, investigators found that the stomach produces leptin (Sobhani et al., 2002). Leptin is a hormone, first described in adipose tissue, involved in energy homeostasis; among its many effects, leptin signals the hypothalamus that appetite is sated (Matson et al., 2000). It is not surprising that the stomach was found to produce leptin since it is an organ involved in eating. Several years ago, investigators found that the stomach produces another hormone related to metabolism, called ghrelin (Lee et al., 2002). In many ways, ghrelin is a physiologic antagonist of leptin, because one activity of ghrelin is to signal the hypothalamus to eat (Horvath et al., 2001).

Recently, several investigators have examined the relationship of *H. pylori* status and gastric hormonal expression. Azuma and colleagues explored gastric leptin levels prior to and after treatment to eradicate *H. pylori* in 40 subjects; in 33, the organism was successfully removed, and in 7, treatment was unsuccessful). For pretreatment, gastric leptin RNA levels were about the same in the two groups. For those in whom treatment was not successful (i.e., *H. pylori* remained), the posttreatment leptin levels did not substantially change. However, when *H. pylori* was removed (treatment success), leptin expression diminished significantly. Interestingly, about 20 percent of the successfully treated subjects gained substantial weight during the six months subsequent to treatment (Azuma et al., 2001).

Nishi and colleagues examined plasma ghrelin levels by whether subjects were *H. pylori*-positive or not; those who were *H. pylori*-negative had significantly higher ghrelin levels than those who were positive (Isomoto et al., 2004).

Nwokolu studied the effect of *H. pylori* eradication on gastric physiology in 10 subjects (Nwokolo et al., 2003). After *H. pylori* eradication, ghrelin levels rose, leptin declined, gastrin declined, and gastric acidity rose (Nwokolo et al., 2003). The gastrin and acidity results confirmed prior studies and directly illustrate the effects of *H. pylori* on local (gastric) physiology. In total, the above studies provide evidence that in the hormonally active stomach, *H. pylori* colonization has an effect on local hormone production, which has both local and systemic effects. This is an important confirmation of the metabolome concept.

Variation in *H. pylori* Genotypes Within an Individual Host

There now is extensive evidence that *H. pylori* populations within a host are changing over the course of colonization (Israel et al., 2001; Kuipers et al., 2000). There is competition between strains as well as recombination (Falush et al., 2001; Kersulyte et al., 1999). However even for a single strain, variation is ongoing. For example, even in a population of *cag*-positive strains, there will be strains in which all or part of the *cag* island is deleted, so that the *H. pylori* population of an individual's stomach is heterogeneous with regard to *cagA* presence (Occhialini et al., 2001; Wirth et al., 1999).

The 3' region of *cagA* is highly polymorphic due to repetitive DNA (Azuma et al., 2002; Yamaoka et al., 1998). In a single individual, biopsies from the antrum and the corpus may show size differences in this region because of the direct DNA repeats (Aras et al., 2003b). Translation of these regions shows heterogeneity in the presence of the tyrosine phosphorylation domain (Aras et al., 2003b). *H. pylori* has evolved into a system using deletion and recombination, based on repetitive DNA motifs, so that cells can change phenotype (Aras et al., 2001, 2002, 2003a). In the important *cag* signaling moiety, this variation is biologically relevant; in any individual with a *cag*-positive strain, there can be variants that produce and inject the protein-containing phosphorylation sites, as well as variants without the sites or that are unable to inject or do not have the island. Each of these organisms signals the host differently; the *cag* island is a model for other loci in the genome.

Conclusions

I have presented a model in which *H. pylori* evolves within a single host (Figure 3-11). The population of strains is undergoing genetic change through a variety of mechanisms, including point mutation and intragenomic and intergenomic recombination. There is much evidence to suggest that *H. pylori* becomes a quasispecies, similar to HIV or hepatitis C (Kuipers et al., 2000). Two strains can recombine into a broader quasispecies that is being selected for fitness in a microniche. The microniches are in communication with one another, and the

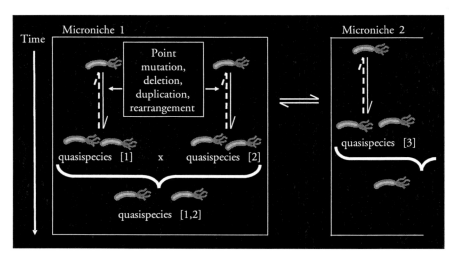

FIGURE 3-11 Schematic of *H. pylori* variation in a single host. The genomes of *H. pylori* cells are highly plastic, subject to point mutation and intra- and intergenomic variation. A model is proposed in which related microbial individuals, a quasispecies, compete with one another in a microniche. Multiple quasispecies may compete or recombine. Local selection determines the population structure in that niche, and by competing and cooperating, populations from adjacent niches influence the overall *H. pylori* composition.
SOURCE: Blaser (2005).

sum of the microniches determines the macroniche. The presence of microniches permits multiple independent strains to colonize one individual's stomach (Blaser and Kirschner, 1999).

In conclusion, there is increasing evidence that *H. pylori* are part of our ancient indigenous biota, but that they are disappearing due to modern lifestyles. As such, that part of human physiology related to its presence is changing, which has consequences for both health and disease and may not be limited to the proximal gastrointestinal tract. *H. pylori* populations in each host are varied and continue to diversify over the course of the colonization of that host. Carriage of *H. pylori* clearly has biological costs and benefits to humans. Perhaps most importantly, the disappearance of *H. pylori* may be a marker for the extinction of other less easily detectable indigenous bacteria. The data suggest that human microecology is changing, and that *H. pylori* is an indicator organism. I propose that the activities of the human genome together with our indigenous microbial genomes (to the nth power) determine both the instantaneous and long-term status of the metabolome (Figure 3-5B). It is the interactions between the host and its microbes that participate in human physiology and homeostasis.

INDUCTION OF PATHOGENIC IMMUNE RESPONSES IN SUSCEPTIBLE HOSTS BY COMMENSAL ENTERIC BACTERIA

R. Balfour Sartor[4]

We coexist with an exceedingly complex mass of interacting bacteria and fungi in the distal ileum and colon. These predominantly anaerobic organisms are in intimate contact with the intestinal epithelium where reciprocal regulation of microbial and host gene expression is evident, as eloquently discussed by Jeff Gordon (Bäckhed et al., 2005). These resident intestinal bacteria profoundly influence both pathogenic and regulatory mucosal and systemic immune responses (MacDonald and Gordon, 2005; Strober et al., 2004). Strong experimental evidence supports the *hypothesis* that homeostasis versus chronic intestinal inflammation is determined by the host's genetically determined innate and adaptive immunologic responses to luminal commensal microbial antigens and adjuvants (Sartor, 2004). This review discusses the bacterial components and the genetically programmed host responses that determine coexistence or aggressive responses to commensal bacteria. These concepts help explain the pathogenesis of chronic immune-mediated intestinal inflammation such as the idiopathic IBD, Crohn's disease, and ulcerative colitis, as well as differential host responses to enteric microbial pathogens.

Normal Host Responses

The normal host with appropriate regulated immune responses develops tolerance when confronted with commensal bacteria (Figure 3-12A). This state of relative nonresponsiveness is mediated by regulatory T cells, dendritic cells, and epithelial cells that produce transforming growth factor β (TGF β), interleukin 10 (IL-10), protective prostaglandins and PGJ2, interferon (IFN) α, and intracellular inhibitory molecules such as PPARγ and A20 (Strober et al., 2004). Some regulatory cells, such as CD4+CD25+ T cells, may display membrane-bound TGF β. In contrast, genetically susceptible hosts with dysregulated immune responses develop chronic relapsing intestinal inflammation mediated by macrophages, TH1, and possibly natural killer (NK) T cells that secrete IL-1β, tumor necrosis factor (TNF), IL-12, IL-13, IL-17, IL-23 and IFNγ. Homeostasis is mediated not only by the net immunosuppressive tone of the mucosal immune response, but also by the controlled uptake of luminal microbial antigens and adjuvants. This is accomplished by an intact mucosal barrier that consists of epithelial tight junctions, secreted immunoglobulin A (IgA), α and β defensins secreted by Paneth cells and activated epithelial cells, respectively, as well as by a complex biofilm composed of mucosally adherent mucus, intestinal trefoil factor, and bacteria that are adapted

---

[4]Departments of Medicine, Microbiology and Immunology, University of North Carolina.

A Normal Host: Induction of Tolerance

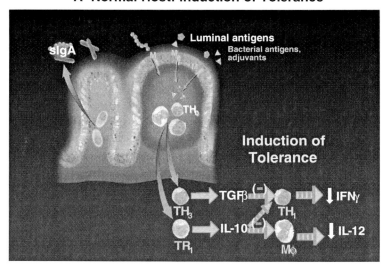

B IBD-Susceptible Host: Induction of Pathogenic Immune Responses

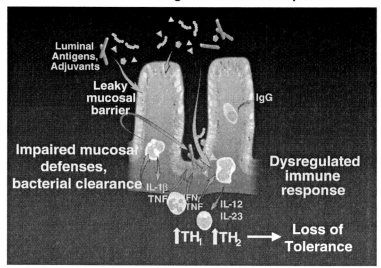

FIGURE 3-12 Induction of homeostatic or pathogenic immune responses by commensal bacteria. A: *Normal host*. Luminal bacteria are excluded by an impermeable epithelial barrier and biofilm. Controlled uptake of luminal antigens leads to regulatory immune responses in organized lymphoid aggregates. B: *Susceptible host*. A break in the mucosal barrier leads to activation of innate and acquired immune responses that progress to pathogenic TH1 or TH2 cell activation.
SOURCE: Sartor (2005).

to this ecologic niche. The net effect of this diverse mucosal shield is resistance to colonization and epithelial adherence by pathogens and a barrier to bacterial translocation. If this barrier is transiently broken by an acute infection or toxin, the epithelium of normal hosts almost instantly restores continuity through restitution, which is a rapid migration of epithelial cells along the intact basement membrane. This process is dependent on TGF β, other growth factors, and intestinal trefoil factor, and is independent of cellular proliferation. Furthermore, translocating microbial organisms are rapidly phagocytosed and killed by cytokine, NFκB-stimulated reactive oxygen metabolites, and nitric oxide. These multilayer defenses allow the distal small intestine and colon not only to maintain a relatively quiescent immunologic state while coexisting with commensal enteric bacteria, but also to appropriately respond to a variety of pathogens.

Pathogenic Mucosal Immune Responses to Bacteria in Genetically Susceptible Hosts

Hosts with a variety of genetic defects in mucosal barrier function, immune regulation, or bacterial killing can develop chronic relapsing intestinal inflammation when confronted with the same microbial environment present in normal hosts (Figure 3-12B). Either an intrinsic, genetically determined defect in the mucosal barrier, a transient breach of mucosal defenses by a self-limited pathogen, or exposure to an epithelial toxin such as a nonsteroidal anti-inflammatory drug (NSAID) can lead to increased bacterial translocation or uptake of antigens and adjuvants from commensal bacteria. Resident mucosal macrophages are relatively unresponsive to microbial adjuvants due to down regulated TLRs and CD14 (Smythies et al., 2005), but they can respond to pathogenic amounts of microbial stimulants. Liberation of chemokines induces immigration into the lamina propria of more highly responsive monocytes and neutrophils with full expression of TLRs and CD14. Activation of these cells by bacterial adjuvants through pattern recognition receptors such as TLR2, TLR4, and TLR5, which bind to bacterial peptidoglycan and lipoteichoic acid, then lipopolysaccharide (LPS) and flagellin, respectively, activate NFκB and a host of proinflammatory molecules including TNF, IL-1β, IL-6, chemokines, IL-12 and IL-23 (Sartor and Hoentjen, 2005). IL-12 activates TH1 cells to secrete IFNγ, while IL-23 induces IL-17. In concert with TNF, IFNγ lyses epithelial cells to cause mucosal ulceration. Similarly, IL-13, which increases in ulcerative colitis, can then increase mucosal permeability by interfering with epithelial tight junctions, inducing epithelial apoptosis and interfering with epithelial restitution (Heller et al., 2005). Tissue damage is further intensified by liberation of metalloproteases such as collagenase, elastase, and stromolysin that degrade the extracellular matrix. Normally, such pathogenic responses are rapidly down-regulated by appropriate induction of immunosuppressive molecules such as IL-10 and TGF β. However, hosts with genetic defects in immune regulation, bacterial killing, or mucosal barrier repair develop inflammatory responses that are perpetuated by continued uptake of microbial antigens and ligands of pattern recognition receptors. This leads to loss of tolerance to commensal bacteria and chronic immune-mediated inflammation.

The best evidence that commensal enteric bacteria have a role in the pathogenesis of chronic intestinal inflammation is provided by studies in gnotobiotic rodents (Sartor, 2004). In at least 10 different diverse models ranging from genetically engineered mice and rats to nonhuman primates, there is no immune activation and no colitis in the absence of bacterial stimulation (Figure 3-13). However, exposure of these susceptible hosts to nonpathogenic resident bacteria activates macrophage and effector T lymphocytes that cause colitis. For example, IL-10 knockout mice on a 129 SvEv background raised in a germ-free (sterile) environment exhibit no colitis, but develop histologic evidence of mild colitis within one week of colonization with specific pathogen-free (SPF) bacteria (Sellon et al., 1998). This progresses to moderate colitis after two weeks of bacterial colonization and to severe transmural TH1-mediated colitis by 3–4 weeks. The onset of histologically detectable colitis is preceded by colonic secretion of IL-12 p40 and enteric-specific IFNγ secretion by CD4+ T cells (Kim et al.,

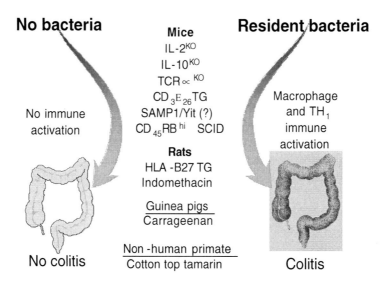

FIGURE 3-13 Immune activation and chronic intestinal inflammation depends on the presence of commensal luminal bacteria in multiple animal models.
SOURCE: Sartor (2005).

2005b). Although the timing is different in the other listed models, the net result is quite similar. In these models, broad spectrum antibiotics prevent the onset and treat established disease while more selective antibiotics that suppress a narrow bacterial spectrum of commensal bacteria can attenuate disease in prophylactic protocols but not reverse established colitis (Hoentjen et al., 2003; Rath et al., 2001).

A single model, colitis induced by dextran sodium sulfate (DSS),provides an exception to this rule. DSS is an epithelial toxin that induces rapid colonocyte apoptosis with shortening of crypts and eventually mucosal ulceration of the colon within one week of exposure to 3–5 percent DSS in drinking water. Initial studies by Axelsson showed enhanced rather than attenuated colitis in germ-free mice fed DSS (Axelsson et al., 1996). More recently, Rakoff-Nahoum et al. (2004) reported that MyD88-deficient mice showed enhanced mortality and mucosal inflammation after exposure to DSS relative to wild-type congenic mice. MyD88 is a key adapter protein that is necessary for all TLR signaling to NFκB. Depletion of commensal microbiota by broad-spectrum antibiotics did not alter the results in knockout mice and potentiated DSS-induced colonic injury in wild-type mice (Araki et al., 2005).

Resolution of these seemingly disparate data requires an understanding of the complexity of pro- and anti-inflammatory signals induced by intestinal bacteria. DSS induces colitis that is mediated by innate immune mechanisms that selectively target the epithelium. Dieleman et al. (1994) demonstrated in severe combined immune deficient (SCID) mice that the absence of T lymphocytes did not affect acute DSS-induced colitis. In an elegant series of studies, Greten et al. (2004) demonstrated that NFκB activation in epithelial cells versus myeloid cells led to differential effects on colitis. Targeted deletion of IKKβ in enterocyte villin-CRE/IKKβ$^{F/F}$ mice treated with the procarcinogen azoxymethane plus three cycles of DSS lost significantly more weight than wild-type controls and had increased mucosal injury. However, when IKKβ was deleted in myeloid cells (lysM-CRE/IKKβ$^{F/F}$), this led to markedly decreased colitis with the same dose of DSS. These results suggest that NFκB activation on epithelial cells, presumably by commensal enteric bacteria, induces homeostatic responses while myeloid cell NFκB activation induces colitis. This conclusion is supported by observations using the same epithelial and myeloid-targeted NFκB in activation through a radiation model (Egan et al., 2004) and ischemia/reperfusion (Chen et al., 2003).

We conclude from these gnotobiotic studies that normal luminal bacteria can induce and perpetuate chronic T cell-mediated colitis and gastroduodenitis and associated extraintestinal inflammation such as peripheral arthritis in genetically susceptible hosts. However, although luminal bacterial and genetic factors are essential, neither is sufficient to cause chronic inflammation. Colitis does not develop in the absence of either microbial stimulation or genetic susceptibility. Induction of chronic immune-mediated inflammation requires the interaction of

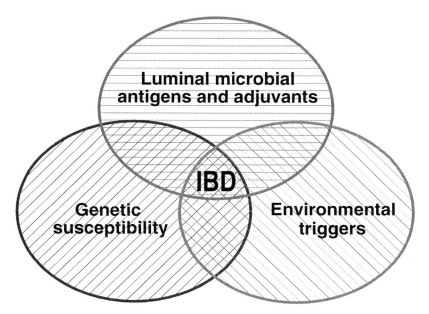

FIGURE 3-14 Interaction of genetic, environmental, and microbial factors in the pathogenesis of IBD.
SOURCE: Sartor (2005).

genetic and environmental factors (Figure 3-14). Finally, luminal bacteria can induce both detrimental and protective responses, with epithelial activation of NFκB by commensal bacteria being predominantly beneficial.

Microbial and Host-Specific Pathogenic Responses

We have demonstrated in gnotobiotic rodents that all bacterial species are not equal in their ability to induce colitis. Both bacterial and host specificity is evident in these studies. HLA B27 transgenic rats raised in a germ-free environment exhibit no colitis but develop active TH1-mediated inflammation in the colon, distal stomach, and duodenum within one month of being colonized with SPF (free of *Helicobacter species* and all demonstratable pathogens) enteric bacteria derived from feces of wild-type normal rats (Rath et al., 1996). Selective colonization (monoassociation) of transgenic rats with *Bacteroides vulgatus* leads to the onset of moderate T cell-mediated colitis within one month of colonization. However, equal luminal levels of *E. coli* do not cause colitis (Rath et al., 1999). Cocolonization with *Lactobacillus GG* and SPF bacteria attenuated colonic inflammation (Dieleman et al., 2003). These results indicate that some common enteric commensal bacteria are aggressive, some are neutral, and yet others are protective. *Bacteroides vulgatus* is not a traditional pathogen since colonization of nontransgenic (wild-type) littermates have no detectible inflammation despite equal luminal concentrations of *B. vulgatus* (Rath et al., 1999). We have demonstrated species specific responses within the *Bacteroides* genus. *Bacteroides vulgatus*, *Bacteroides thetaiotaomicron*, and *Bacteroides fragilis* cause colitis in HLA B27 transgenic—but not nontransgenic—controls. However, *Bacteroides distasonis* did not cause inflammation (Mann et al., 2003).

We then demonstrated host-specific responses to selective enteric commensal bacterial species. As mentioned, HLA B27 transgenic rats monoassociated with *B. vulgatus* develop a cecal-predominant colitis, but no disease with *E. coli* nor with *Enterococcus faecalis* (Kim et al., 2005a; Kim et al., 2005b). Exactly the opposite results were found in IL-10 deficient mice, in which *B. vulgatus* caused no inflammation and *E. coli* and *E. faecalis* induced chronic colitis. Yet another model, the bone marrow-transplanted CD3ε transgenic mouse, showed no inflammation when colonized with any of these three organisms. Of particular clinical interest, we demonstrated different phenotypes of disease in a single host colonized with two different bacterial species. *E. faecalis* induced slow onset (10–12 weeks) distal colitis in IL-10 deficient mice and duodenal inflammation leading to obstruction and gastric outlet obstruction with protracted monoassociation (26 or more weeks) (Kim et al., 2005b). In contrast, *E. coli* monoassociation induced a predominantly right-sided colitis three weeks after colonization. Dual association of germ-free IL-10 knockout mice with *E. coli* plus *E. faecalis* caused an aggressive pancolitis with onset one week after colonization (Kim et al., 2004).

These results indicate that certain commensal bacterial species can selectively induce disease in hosts with different genetic backgrounds and cause different phenotypes of disease in a single genetically susceptible host. Some bacterial species are aggressive, some protective, and some neutral, but no single species yet identified can induce as aggressive a colitis as the complex microflora of the distal intestine. These results have obvious therapeutic implications in that antibiotics, probiotics, and prebiotics with selective spectra of activity can be used to treat IBD patients, but each subset of patients may respond selectively to various agents. Thus, we will need to individualize treatments for each patient.

Mechanisms of Genetic Susceptibility to Intestinal Inflammation

These results clearly indicate that host susceptibility is a dominant determinant of experimental colitis. Likewise, IBD patients show increased concordance in monozygotic versus dizygotic twins. The concordance rate in Crohn's disease is 44–58 percent compared to 3–5 percent in dizygotic twins (Halfvarson et al., 2003). Ulcerative colitis exhibits less of a genetic influence with concordance in monozygotic twins at 6–18 percent. The search for IBD-related genes has consisted of two approaches. A genomewide search using single nucleotide polymorphism probes have found association in many chromosomes, with chromosome

1, 5, 6, 12, and 16 being replicated (Newman and Siminovitch, 2005; Schreiber et al., 2005). In 2001, two independent groups simultaneously identified NOD2/CARD 15 as the gene responsible for susceptibility to Crohn's disease (Hugot et al., 2001; Ogura et al., 2001). A single polymorphism in this gene enhances susceptibility 1.5 to 3 fold over incident ranges, but a homozygous polymorphism, or two independent (compound heterozygous), abnormalities enhances susceptibility approximately 30 fold. Similarly, polymorphisms in the organic cation transporter (OCTN) genes 1 and 2 on chromosome 5 have been associated with Crohn's disease (Peltekova et al., 2004). Genes responsible for susceptibility on the other identified chromosomes have not yet been recognized.

A second approach is to search for candidate genes in multiplex families. These types of studies have implicated the HLA region, polymorphisms in TLR4 and TLR5, as well as in IL-10, PPARγ, and IL-1 receptor antagonists (Newman and Siminovitch, 2005). The genes most commonly associated with IBD are listed in Table 3-1.

It is quite interesting, and potentially important, to note that the genes studied to date fall into several categories relating to either epithelial barrier function or response to bacteria. The first gene implicated in Crohn's disease, NOD2/CARD 15, is an intracellular bacterial sensor whose leucine-rich repeat (LRR) region binds to the bacterial peptidoglycan component muramyl dipeptide (Girardin et al., 2003). The three most common single nucleotide polymorphisms associated with Crohn's disease lie within, or very near, the LLR region. Several groups have demonstrated diminished NFκB activation in mutant NOD2/CARD 15, in-

TABLE 3-1 Genes Associated with IBD and Experimental Colitis

Gene	Chromosome (Human)	Function
A. *Crohn's disease*		
NOD 2 (CARD 15)	16	NFκB activation/regulation, killing intracellular pathogens, Paneth cell function (α defensin production)
OCTN 1/2	5	Organic cation, carnitine transporter, transports xenobiotic substances
DLG 5	10	Epithelial scaffolding protein
PPARγ		Intracellular inhibitor of NFκB and cellular activation
B. *Ulcerative colitis*		
Mdr-1	7	Efflux transporter drugs and possibly xenobiotic compounds

dicating that these common mutations lead to loss of function (Ogura et al., 2001). Recent data indicate that Crohn's related polymorphisms and NOD2/CARD 15 lead to decreased intracellular killing after epithelial invasion by *Salmonella* (Hisamatsu et al., 2003), decreased α defensin production (Wehkamp et al., 2004), and defective suppression of NFκB activation after peptidoglycan ligation of TLR2 (Watanabe et al., 2004). Decreased α defensin production is particularly intriguing in light of the knowledge that NOD2/CARD 15 is constitutively expressed in Paneth cells that are selectively found in the small intestine (Lala et al., 2003). NOD2 polymorphisms are highly associated with ileal Crohn's disease. In addition, Swidsinski et al. (2002) have demonstrated genetically enhanced mucosally associated bacterial populations in active Crohn's disease patients versus normal controls. Recent observations in NOD2-deficient mice indicate defective clearance of oral *Listeria monocytogenes* with defective cryptdin-like defensin 4 and 10 production (Kobayashi et al., 2005). These investigations support the concept that NOD2/CARD 15 protects the ileal mucosa by several mechanisms and is an important contributor to mucosal homeostasis of the ileum in response to commensal bacteria and possibly pathogens.

Conclusions

Mammals have involved multiple redundant mechanisms to protect themselves from the aggressive microbial milieu in the distal ileum and colon. Normally, the host lives in peaceful coexistence with these commensal organisms because of net tolerogenic mucosal immune responses mediated by production of immunosuppressive TGFβ and IL-10. However, intermittent exposure to pathogens and other environmental triggers, such as NSAIDs, can initiate acute injury in the intestines of all patients. Normal hosts rapidly restore homeostasis by clearing the bacterial invader, healing the mucosal barrier, and down-regulating the inflammatory response once the offending stimulus has been eliminated. In contrast, a genetically susceptible host fails to appropriately inhibit the inflammatory process, which can become self-perpetuating due to continued uptake of luminal bacterial products. Genetic susceptibility factors include defective mucosal barrier function, defective/incomplete bacterial clearance, and ineffective ability to down-regulate inflammation. Commensal bacteria provide the constant antigenic and adjuvant stimuli that perpetuate chronic intestinal inflammation in susceptible hosts, but induce homeostatic signals in normal hosts. Thus, we hypothesize that the inflammatory bowel diseases are the result of an overly aggressive cell-mediated immune response to a relatively small subset of commensal bacteria in a genetically susceptible host. Dominant microbial antigens may be unique for each individual. Genetic susceptibility is determined by defective genes that encode barrier function, bacterial clearance, and immunoregulation. The onset or activation of disease is triggered by environmental factors that injure the epithelial barrier and initiate inflammatory responses. These triggering factors include

NSAIDs or self-limited bacterial, viral, or parasitic infections. A more thorough understanding of the mechanisms of induction and perpetuation of intestinal inflammation should provide the means to selectively inhibit these responses and restore mucosal homeostasis. Based on our results, we predict that appropriate therapy will need to be individualized to each patient based on their genetic susceptibility, their enteric bacterial profiles, and their T-cell and serologic responses to these commensal bacteria.

Acknowledgments

These studies were supported by NIH grants, DK 40249 and DK 53347, as well as the Crohn's and Colitis Foundation of America and the Broad Research Foundation. The author thanks Susie May for her excellent secretarial assistance.

HOW DO CHANGES IN MICROECOLOGY AFFECT THE HUMAN HOST?

María G. Domínguez-Bello[5]

In a living world that has been microbial since its origins, all other forms of life have evolved in interaction with microorganisms. Therefore not only pathogens but also microbial mutualists must have shaped animals' immunity. Self-recognition and recognition of indigenous microbes is key to the function of the immune system, which should act specifically against pathogenic invaders. This implies that there has to be some degree of resistance of indigenous microbes to host innate and adaptive immunity.

Germs have had a great impact on human perception of microbes, and it is recently that indigenous microbes are being recognized to have an important physiological function. The perception of microbes as entities capable of causing disease has triggered a cultural and technological antimicrobial response. The effect of hygiene practices and use of broad-spectrum antimicrobials is nonspecific. Modern practices have become arms of microbial mass destruction, to which, of course, many infectious disease agents have succumbed. Yet, as infectious diseases disappear in modern societies, autoimmune disorders and obesity are increasing.

This paper discusses some aspects of the interaction between animals and their microbiomes and points out the importance of recognizing that prokaryotes and eukaryotes naturally colonizing human surfaces and cavities have shaped our evolution. They are likely to play a role in promoting health and protecting from disease.

---

[5]Department of Biology, University of Puerto Rico. Rio Piedras, San Juan, PR.

Beneficial Microbes: The Rumen as an Example of True Mutualism

Microbes interact with all other forms of life. Animals have coevolved with bacteria, responding to their selective pressures and also driving bacterial evolution. In certain animals, some microbes became so closely associated with their hosts, that together they establish a functional unit, an organ, vital for both microbes and hosts. The rumen is one of these examples of "true mutualism." Indigestible plant cell walls and dietary toxins have exerted the evolutionary pressure for the appearance of symbiotic foregut fermentative digestion. Microbes contribute with digestive enzymes the host animal lacks, expanding the animal's nutritional niche by fermenting plant structural carbohydrates and other dietary components into short-chain fatty acids (Figure 3-15), the most important energy source for the animal (Van Soest, 1994).

Because dietary protein is also fermented, the main amino acids source for a ruminant on a natural diet comes from the microbial biomass itself. Because bacterial cell walls—enclosing proteins—are also indigestible, foregut fermenters have multiplied the lysozyme gene and recruited the enzyme to act as a digestive enzyme (Dobson et al., 1984). Rather than feeding on plants, ruminants and other foregut fermenters really feed on the microbes they farm in the foregut.

Foregut fermentative digestion evolved convergently in mammals—ruminants, howler monkeys, sloth—and in at least one bird, the hoatzin, that ferments in the crop and also harbors a complex microbiota (Domínguez-Bello et al., 1993; Grajal et al., 1989).

The rumen ecosystem is populated by a high diversity of microorganisms, including bacteria, archaea, fungi, protozoa, (Hungate, 1972; Nelson et al., 2003; Ogimoto and Imai, 1981; Tajima et al., 2001a,b; Van Soest, 1994) and viruses (Klieve and Bauchop, 1988; Klieve and Swain, 1993; Klieve et al., 1989; Nemcova et al., 1993). Ribosomal DNA sequence data has recently revealed that gastrointestinal bacterial communities in cattle appear to be dominated by Firmicutes, particularly those related to the genus *Clostridium* (Nelson et al., 2003; Tajima et al., 2001a; Whitford et al., 1998). Novel rumen Archaea, not associated with known rumen methanogens, have also been recently discovered (Tajima et al., 2001b).

Culturable anaerobic bacteria from the rumen have been intensively studied over the past 40 years (Hungate, 1966; Ogimoto and Imai, 1981). Much work on this subject was published between 1960 and 1980. In those days, there were crowded scientific meetings about the rumen—such as the Chicago Conference on Rumen Function (now Conference on Gastrointestinal Function) started in 1951. Rumen studies have been seminal to the understanding of digestive processes in other animals and in humans. Unfortunately, since research on animal nutrition has become a low funding priority, scientists who previously worked on rumen microbiology have now moved to other fields. The rumen represents a case of true microbial mutualism and should be viewed as a model to further the understanding of the function of human colonic fermentation.

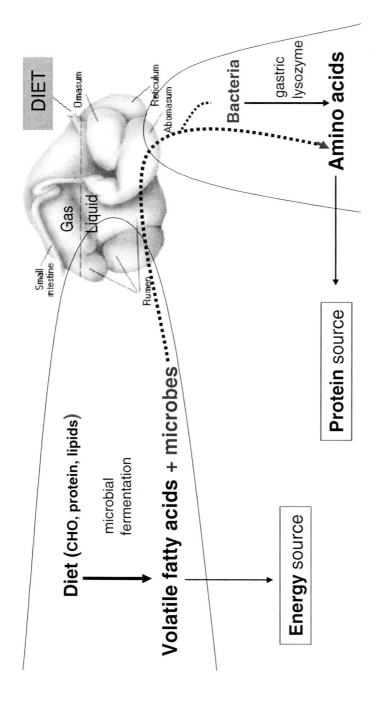

FIGURE 3-15 Fate of dietary products in the rumen, providing microbial products and biomass for the nutrition of the host. Similar fermentation of plant fiber takes place in the colon of mammals, including humans.
SOURCE: Domínguez-Bello (2005).

Changes in the Human Gastrointestinal Microbiome: Indigenous Microbes in Indigenous Peoples

Bacteria are important in the bowel function and for the correct function of the gut immune system (Cash and Hooper, 2005; Hooper et al., 2001, 2003; Stappenbeck et al., 2002). As a consequence, disrupting intestinal host-bacterial relationships may lead to immune disorders. Diversity and population structure of intestinal bacteria is dynamic and complex. They are influenced by niche resources, diet, antimicrobials, competing sympatric species, and mucosal immunity. Innate and adaptive immunity are important to reach a healthy equilibrium of the microbial ecosystem. Paneth cells in the small intestine secrete microbicidal peptides (lysozyme, Ang4), and Peyer's patch dendritic cells present microbial antigens to lymphocytes (Figure 3-16).

Host immunity and indigenous microbes may protect against the assault of primary pathogens through what is known as colonization resistance, while host immunity acts specifically against invaders. Resistance of indigenous microbes to innate immunity is still a poorly understood phenomenon, but some rumen bacteria can develop resistance to cow gastric lysozyme (Domínguez-Bello et al., 2004). Also, *Bacteroides thetaiotaomicron* is resistant to the antimicrobial peptide Ang4 whose secretion is induced by the intestinal presence of the bacterium (Hooper et al., 2003).

When we think of intestinal microbes, we still think of bacteria. Recent molecular methods have unveiled an unexpected diversity of 500 bacterial species, with 30 to 40 of them accounting for 99 percent of the total intestinal population (Harmsen et al., 2002) and a great number of novel sequences (Eckburg et al., 2005). We know little about the ecological role of Archaea in the human intestine (Bäckhed et al., 2005), and nothing about the role of viruses, except that phages are the most abundant entity, with a total of 1,200 viral genotypes in the intestinal community (Breitbart and Rohwer, 2005; Edwards and Rohwer, 2005). Parasites and phages surely modulate bacterial populations in the intestine, but what are their effects on our immunity and health? (Figure 3-16).

Quantitative and qualitative changes in our indigenous bacteria brought by our modern life are unknown, but the disappearance of *H. pylori* from the stomach of people in modern societies (Pérez-Pérez et al., 2002) might be a marker for other bacteria as well. The degree of alterations of modern human microbiomes can only be studied by comparison with more natural human microbial ecosystems in primitive human societies.

Lack of intestinal parasites is perhaps the most noticeable example of microbiome alteration in modern humans. Science currently regards intestinal parasites as harmful (Dreyfuss et al., 2001). Of course we know the diseases they can produce, but we do not understand why most colonized persons remain asymptomatic. The fact that we call "parasites" these intestinal protozoa and helminths that have evolved in the human intestine, reflects our own prejudices.

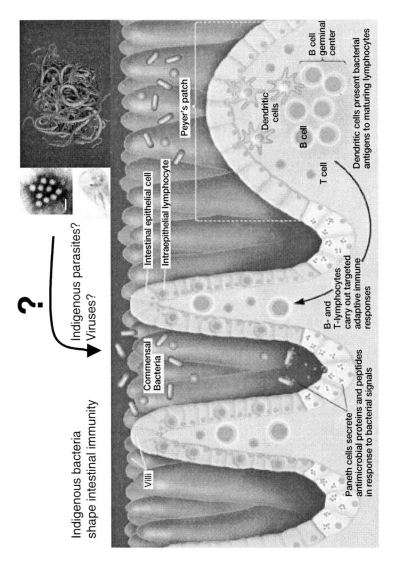

FIGURE 3-16 Model of modulation of adaptive and innate immunity by indigenous bacteria, showing the unknown effect of other microbes on mucosal immunity.
SOURCE: Cash and Hooper (2005).

Preliminary results from our studies in Venezuelan Amerindian villages (Dominguez-Bello et al., 2005) show some unexpected associations between gastrointestinal microbes and health. Living in areas of malaria risk, people in these villages do not suffer from food shortage—they fish from the river and eat seasonal fruits—but morbidity and mortality due to infant diarrhea is high. All but one of 72 asymptomatic children and adults of these communities carried parasites. Most people had *Ascaris lumbricoides*, *Trichiura trichuris*, and *Entamoeba* sp in their intestines, and multiparasitism had no effect on body mass index ($P = .593$). Other studies have also found high prevalence of asymptomatic intestinal parasitism. In Ecuador, 93 percent of pregnant women participating in a study carried at least one species of intestinal parasite, and 88 percent had *Entamoeba histolytica* (Dreyfuss et al., 2001). The possibility that some degree of parasitism might be beneficial for humans cannot be ruled out. Perhaps the optimal degree of parasitism varies according to local conditions. For example, anemia-inducing parasites might be beneficial in regions where malaria is endemic (Domínguez-Bello and Blaser, 2005; Kucik et al., 2004; Murray et al., 1978; Nacher et al., 2003; Oppenheimer, 2001).

In addition to parasites, most adults in our study had *H. pylori* (82 percent of adults and half the children). Interestingly, *H. pylori*-colonized children had higher cell mass and better nutritional status than *H. pylori*-negative children (Dominguez-Bello et al., 2005); ($P < .05$; subjects were 43 *H. pylori* positive and 29 *H. pylori* negative). The lack of detrimental effect of microbes on nutritional status supports the hypothesis of a mutualistic nature of the relation between some intestinal "parasites" and us. Which ones are our beneficial microbes? Which ones should children carry to optimize health? Which ones threaten to become opportunistic pathogens and when?

Microbial-Related Diseases and Modernity

Evolution of microbiomes and their protective function in concert with host immunity has taken nature a long evolutionary time. The "intelligent" use of antimicrobials by man, outside the pace of evolution, lacks selectivity. Although the fight against infectious diseases has increased human well-being and life expectancy, nature's trade-off imposes a cost to this success: new diseases as a consequence of microbiome alterations. When microbes face a lethal force, they either die or compensate with changes conferring survival that are selected for. The wide use of antibiotics has resulted in increased resistance among indigenous and pathogenic bacteria. In the last 50 years, tetracycline has been used broadly as an antibiotic for the treatment of bacterial and protozoal infections in humans, as a growth promoter in animals, and as an immunosuppressant. A variety of tetracycline resistance genes are present in the oral (Pantoja et al., 2005; Villedieu et al., 2003) and intestinal (Salyers et al., 2004) microflora of healthy adults. Compounds other than antibiotics could also exert positive selection on antibiotic resistance genes. Salicylate modulates multiple antibiotic resistance via *mar* genes, influencing bacterial multidrug resistance. In addition, copper selects for bacterial antibiotic resistance in agricultural soils (Berg et al., 2005).

According to the hygiene hypothesis, our antimicrobial behavior is linked to the appearance of new diseases. As societies develop and adopt Western lifestyles, the risk of some emergent and reemergent diseases, autoimmune diseases, and obesity increases (Figure 3-17). Developing countries still fall in the descendent region of the bimodal curve in Figure 3-17, suffering from primary pathogens, but perhaps keeping their normal microbiota less altered than modern societies. What are the actual changes in human microbiota as we get modern? What are their effects on immunity and health? Do we have mutualistic relations with parasites, fungi, or viruses? The gastrointestinal microbiomes of people living in primitive societies can probably help in unveiling what we have lost and what we can still gain in terms of our microbiomes.

An integration of concepts of host-microbe interactions is presented in the model of Figure 3-18. The newborn baby leaves a germ-free uterus and the external environment provides an initial colonization that leads to others in a successional way. In the mammalian colon, breast milk containing special oligosaccharides—inulin-type fructans—bypass the small intestine and enrich for bifidobacteria and lactobacilli (Forchielli and Walker, 2005). The nature of this fermentation dictates proliferation of the host tissue cells and of the microbial

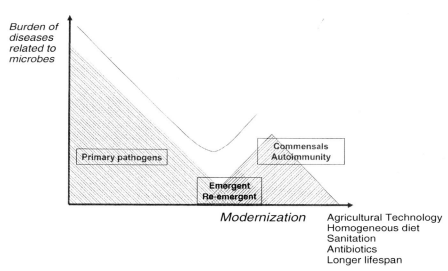

FIGURE 3-17 Evolution of human societies and their diseases.
SOURCE: Domínguez-Bello (2005).

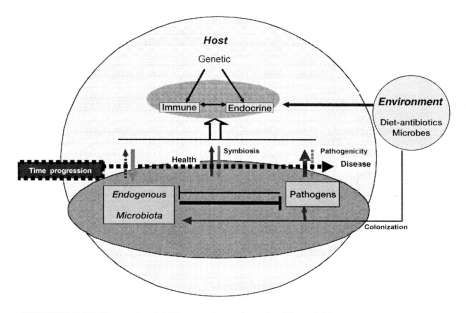

FIGURE 3-18 Host-microbial interactions shape health and disease
SOURCE: Dominguez-Bello (2005).

community in the colon. Signals emitted in the "crosstalk" between microbes and host shape the course of colonization.

The immune signals from the newborn are strong because of maternal immunity, but the actual protective function of the gut develops by microbial stimulation. As time progresses, there is a "balanced" signaling between host and indigenous microbes. Time of acquisition of microbes and a particular succession of colonization may be very important to reach a healthy equilibrium.

Host responses to microbes, either immune (adaptive, innate) or endocrine (leptin, ghrelin), are influenced by genetic factors, but as the human microbiota is reduced in its diversity, it may contribute to changes in endocrine responses that might be involved in higher obesity risk. Although without an apparent effect on blood levels, eradication of *H. pylori* increases ghrelin and reduces leptin expression in the stomach (Azuma et al., 2001; Nwokolo et al., 2003). The fact that *H. pylori*-positive children had better nutritional status than noncolonized children in the Brazilian state of Amazonas (Dominguez-Bello et al., 2005) also supports this hypothesis. It has also been hypothesized that exposure to microbes—both exogenous pathogens and endogenous biota—might be critical environmental determinants of the expression of human height (Beard and Blaser, 2002).

Finally, in our model of Figure 3-18, endogenous microbiota exert colonization resistance, but when pathogens break the barrier, they can disturb the ecological equilibrium. Ecologic disturbances can lead to monopolization of the niche by a primary pathogen or by indigenous microbes that become opportunistic pathogens. As the host grows old, the impairment of the immune response leads to disturbance of this dynamic equilibrium and to disease.

Adequate and complete identification of the indigenous human microbiome is the first step in elucidating its role in the physiology of our colonized organs and in the maintenance of health.

REFERENCES

Akopyants NS, Clifton SW, Kersulyte D, Crabtree JE, Youree BE, Reece CA, Bukanov NO, Drazek ES, Roe BA, Berg DE. 1998. Analyses of the cag pathogenicity island of *Helicobacter pylori*. *Molecular Microbiology* 28(1):37–53.

Amieva MR, Vogelmann R, Covacci A, Tompkins LS, Nelson WJ, Falkow S. 2003. Disruption of the epithelial apical-junctional complex by *Helicobacter pylori* CagA. *Science* 300(5624):1430–1434.

Araki A, Kanai T, Ishikura T, Makita S, Uraushihara K, Iiyama R, Totsuka T, Takeda K, Akira S, Watanabe M. 2005. MyD88-deficient mice develop severe intestinal inflammation in dextran sodium sulfate colitis. *Journal of Gastroenterology* 40(1):16–23.

Aras RA, TakataT, Ando T, Van der Ende A, Blaser NJ. 2001. Regulation of the HpyII restriction-modification system of *Helicobacter pylori* by gene deletion and horizontal reconstitution. *Molecular Microbiology* 42(2):369–382.

Aras RA, Small AJ, Ando T, Blaser MJ. 2002. *Helicobacter pylori* interstrain restriction-modification diversity prevents genome subversion by chromosomal DNA from competing strains. *Nucleic Acids Research* 30(24):5391–5397.

Aras RA, Kang J, Tschumi A, Harasaki Y, Blaser MJ. 2003a. Extensive repetitive DNA facilitates prokaryotic genome plasticity. *Proceedings of the National Academy of Science USA* 100(23):13579–13584.

Aras RA, Lee Y, Kim S-K, Israel D, Peek RM, Blaser MJ. 2003b. Natural variation in populations of persistently colonizing bacteria affect human host cell phenotype. *Journal of Infectious Diseases* 188(4):486–96.

Axelsson LG, Midtvedt T, Bylund-Fellenius AC. 1996. The role of intestinal bacteria, bacterial translocation and endotoxin in dextran sodium sulphate-induced colitis in the mouse. *Microbial Ecology in Health and Disease* 9:225–37

Azuma T, Suto H, Ito Y, Ohtani M, Dojo M, Kuriyama M, Kato T. 2001. Gastric leptin and *helicobacter pylori* infection. *Gut* 49(3):324–329.

Azuma T, Yamakawa A, Yamazaki S, Fukuta K, Ohtani M, Ito Y, Dojo M, Yamazaki Y, Kuriyama, M. 2002. Correlation between variation of the 3' region of the *cagA* gene in *Helicobacter pylori* and disease outcome in Japan. *Journal of Infectious Diseases* 186(11):1621–1630.

Bäckhed F, Ley RE, Sonnenburg JL, Peterson DA, Gordon JI. 2005. Host-bacterial mutualism in the human intestine. *Science* 307(5717):1915–1920.

Beard, AS, Blaser MJ. 2002. The ecology of height: The effect of microbial transmission on human height. *Perspectives in Biology and Medicine* 45(4):475–498.

Berg, JA, Tom-Petersen A, Nybroe O. 2005. Copper amendment of agricultural soil selects for bacterial antibiotic resistance in the field. *Letters in Applied Microbiology* 40(2):146–151.

Blaser MJ. 1990. *Helicobacter pylori* and the pathogenesis of gastroduodenal inflammation. *Journal of Infectious Diseases* 161(4):626–633.

Blaser MJ. 1992. Hypotheses on the pathogenesis and natural history of Helicobacter pylori-induced inflammation. *Gastroenterology* 102(2):720–727.
Blaser MJ. 1997. Ecology of *Helicobacter pylori* in the human stomach. *Journal of Clinical Investigation* 100(4):759–762.
Blaser MJ. 1998. Helicobacters are indigenous to the human stomach: Duodenal ulceration is due to changes in gastric microecology in the modern era. *Gut* 43(5):721–727.
Blaser MJ. 1999. The changing relationships of *Helicobacter pylori* and humans: Implications for health and disease. *Journal of Infectious Diseases* 179(6):1523–1530.
Blaser MJ. 2005 (March 16). *Session I: Host-Pathogen Interactions: Defining the Concepts of Pathogenicity, Virulence, Colonization, Commensalism, and Symbiosis.* Presentation at the Forum on Microbial Threats Workshop Ending the War Metaphor: The Changing Agenda for Unraveling the Host-Microbe Relationship, Washington, D.C., Institute of Medicine. Forum on Microbial Threats.
Blaser MJ, Atherton JC. 2004. *Helicobacter pylori* persistence: Biology and disease. *Journal of Clinical Investigation* 113(3):321–333.
Blaser MJ, Kirschner D. 1999. Dynamics of *Helicobacter pylori* colonization in relation to the host response. *Proceedings of the National Academy of Sciences USA* 96(15):8359–8364.
Blaser MJ, Chyou PH, Nomura A. 1995a. Age at establishment of *Helicobacter pylori* infection and gastric carcinoma, gastric ulcer, and duodenal ulcer risk. *Cancer Research* 55(3):562–565.
Blaser MJ, Pérez-Pérez GI, Kleanthous H, Cover TL, Peek RM, Chyou PH, Stemmermann GN, Nomura A. 1995b. Infection with *Helicobacter pylori* strains possessing cagA associated with an increased risk of developing adenocarcinoma of the stomach. *Cancer Research* 55(10):2111–2115.
Breitbart M, Rohwer F. 2005. Here a virus, there a virus, everywhere the same virus? *Trends in Microbiology* 13(6):278–284.
Calam J. 1995. *Helicobacter pylori*, acid and gastrin. *European Journal of Gastroenterology and Hepatology* 7:310–317.
Cash HL, Hooper LV. 2005. Commensal bacteria shape intestinal immune system development. *American Society of Microbiology News* 71(2):77–83.
Censini S, Lange C, Xiang ZY, Crabtree JE, Ghiara P, Borodovsky M, Rappuoli R, Covacci A. 1996. Cag, a pathogenicity island of *Helicobacter pylori*, encodes type I-specific and disease-associated virulence factors. *Proceedings of the National Academy of Sciences USA* 93(25):14648–14653.
Chen LW, Egan L, Li ZW, Greten FR, Kagnoff MF, Karin M. 2003. The two faces of IKK and NF-kappaB inhibition: Prevention of systemic inflammation but increased local injury following intestinal ischemia-reperfusion. *Nature Medicine* 9(5):575–581.
Chow WH, Blaser MJ, Blot WJ, Gammon MD, Vaughan TL, Risch HA, Pérez-Pérez GI, Schoenberg JB, Stanford JL, Rotterdam H, West AB, Fraumeni JF. 1998. An inverse relation between cagA+ strains of *Helicobacter pylori* infection and risk of esophageal and gastric cardia adenocarcinoma. *Cancer Research* 58(4):588–590.
Cockburn TA. 1971. Infectious diseases in ancient populations. *Current Anthropology* 12:45–62.
Correa P, Haenszel W, Cuello C, Tannenbaum S, Archer M. 1975. A model for gastric cancer epidemiology. *Lancet* 2(7924):58–60.
Covacci A, Censini S, Bugnoli M, Petracca R, Burroni D, Macchia G, Massone A, Papini E, Xiang Z, Figura N, Rappuoli. 1993. Molecular characterization of the 128-kDa immunodominant antigen of *Helicobacter pylori* associated with cytotoxicity and duodenal ulcer. *Proceedings of the National Academy of Sciences USA* 90(12):5791–5795.
Cover TL, Dooley CP, Blaser MJ. 1990. Characterization and human serologic response to proteins in *Helicobacter pylori* broth culture supernatants with vacuolizing cytotoxin activity. *Infection and Immunity* 58(3):603–610.

Crabtree JE, Taylor JD, Wyatt JI, Heatley RV, Shallcross TM, Tompkins DS, Rathbone BJ. 1991. Mucosal IgA recognition of *Helicobacter pylori* 120 kDa protein, peptic ulceration, and gastric pathology. *Lancet* 338(8763):332–335.

de Martel C, Llosa AE, Farr SM, Friedman GD, Vogelman JH, Orentreich N, Corley DA, Parsonnet J. 2005. Helicobacter pylori infection and the risk of development of esophageal adenocarcinoma. *Journal of Infectious Diseases* 191(5):761–767.

Devesa SS, Blot WJ, Fraumeni JK Jr. 1998. Changing patterns in the incidence of esophageal and gastric carcinoma in the United States. *Cancer* 83(10):2049–2053.

Dieleman LA, Ridwan BU, Tennyson GS, Beagley KW, Bucy RP, Elson CO. 1994. Dextran sulfate sodium-induced colitis occurs in severe combined immunodeficient mice. *Gastroenterology* 107(6):1643–1652.

Dieleman LA, Goerres M, Arends A, Sprengers D, Torrice C, Hoentjen F, Grenther WB, Sartor RB. 2003. *Lactobacillus GG* prevents recurrence of colitis in HLA-B27 transgenic rats after antibiotic treatment. *Gut* 52(3):370–376.

Dobrindt U, Hochhut B, Hentschel U, Hacker J. 2004. Genomic islands in pathogenic and environmental microorganisms. *National Review of Microbiology* 2(5):414–424.

Dobson, DE, Prager EM, Wilson AC. 1984. Stomach lysozymes of ruminants. I. Distribution and catalytic properties. *Journal of Biological Chemistry* 259(18):11607–11616.

Dominguez-Bello MG, Blaser MJ. 2005. Are iron-scavenging parasites protective against malaria? *Journal of Infectious Diseases* 191(4):646.

Dominguez-Bello MG, Ruiz MC, Michelangeli F. 1993. Evolutionary significance of foregut fermentation in the hoatzin (*Opisthocomus hoazin*; Aves, Opisthocomidae). *Journal of Comparative Physiology B* 163:594–601.

Dominguez-Bello MG, Pacheco MA, Ruiz MC, Michelangeli F, Leippe M, de Pedro MA. 2004. Resistance of rumen bacteria murein to bovine gastric lysozyme. *BioMed Central Ecology* 4:7.

Dominguez-Bello MG, Marini GE, Maldonado AL, Hidalgo G, Cabras S, Buffa R, Marini E, Floris G, Racugno W, Pericchi LR, Castellanos ME, Blaser MJ, Gröschl M. 2005. *No Evidence of Detrimental Effect of* Helicobacter pylori *and Intestinal Parasites on the Nutritional Status of Amerindians in Venezuela*. ASM Conference on Beneficial Microbes, Lake Tahoe, Nevada.

Dreyfuss ML, Msamanga GI, Spiegelman D, Hunter DJ, Urassa EJ, Hertzmark E, Fawzi WW. 2001. Determinants of low birth weight among HIV-infected pregnant women in Tanzania. *American Journal of Clinical Nutrition* 74(6):814–826.

Eckburg PB, Bik EM, Bernstein CN, Purdom E, Dethlefsen L, Sargent M, Gill SR, Nelson KE, Relman DA. 2005. Diversity of the human intestinal microbial flora. *Science* 308(5728):1635–1638.

Edwards RA, Rohwer F. 2005. Viral metagenomics. *Nature Reviews Microbiology* 3(6):504–510.

Egan LJ, Eckmann L, Greten FR, Chae S, Li ZW, Myhre GM, Robine S, Karin M, Kagnoff MF. 2004. IkappaB-kinasebeta-dependent NF-kappaB activation provides radioprotection to the intestinal epithelium. *Proceedings of the National Academy of Sciences USA* 101(8):2452–2457.

El-Omar EM, Carrington M, Chow WH, McColl KE, Bream JH, Young HA, Herrera J, Lissowska J, Yuan CC, Rothman N, Lanyon G, Martin M, Fraumeni JF Jr, Rabkin CS. 2000. Interleukin-1 polymorphisms associated with increased risk of gastric cancer. *Nature* 412(6842):99.

Falkow S. 1998. Who speaks for the microbes? *Emerging Infectious Diseases* 4(3):495–497.

Falkow S. 2005 (March 17). *Session III:Understanding the Dynamic Relationships of Host-Microbe Interactions*. Presentation at the Forum on Microbial Threats Workshop Ending the War Metaphor: The Changing for Unraveling the Host-Microbe Relationship, Washington, D.C., Institute of Medicine, Forum on Microbial Threats.

Falush D, Kraft C, Taylor NS, Correa P, Fox JG, Achtman M, Suerbaum S. 2001. Recombination and mutation during long-term gastric colonization by *Helicobacter pylori*: Estimates of clock rates, recombination size, and minimal age. *Proceedings of the National Academy of Sciences USA* 98(26):15056–15061.

Falush D, Wirth T, Linz B, Pritchard JK, Stephens M, Kidd M, Blaser MJ, Graham DY, Vacher S, Perez-Perez GI, Yamaoka Y, Negraud F, Otto K, Reichard U, Katzowitsch E, Wang X, Achtman M, Suerbaum S. 2003. Traces of human migration in *Helicobacter pylori* populations. *Science* 299(5629):1582–1585.

Forchielli ML, Walker WA. 2005. The role of gut-associated lymphoid tissues and mucosal defence. *British Journal of Nutrition* 93(Suppl 1):S41–S48.

Ghose C, Perez-Perez GI, Dominguez-Bello MG, Pride DT, Bravi CM, Blaser MJ. 2002. East Asian genotypes of *Helicobacter pylori*: Strains in Amerindians provide evidence for its ancient human carriage. *Proceedings of the National Academy of Sciences USA* 99(23):15107–15111.

Ghose C, Perez-Perez GI, van Doorn LJ, Dominguez-Bello MG, Blaser MJ. 2005. High frequency of gastric colonization with multiple *Helicobacter pylori* strains in Venezuelan subjects. *Journal of Clinical Microbiology* 43(6):2635–2641.

Girardin SE, Boneca IG, Viala J, Chamaillard M, Labigne A, Thomas G, Philpott DJ, Sansonetti PJ. 2003. Nod2 is a general sensor of peptidoglycan through muramyl dipeptide (MDP) detection. *Journal of Biological Chemistry* 278(11):8869–8872.

Goodman KJ, Correa P. 2000. Transmission of *Helicobacter pylori* among siblings. *Lancet* 355(9201): 358–362.

Goodman KJ, Correa P, Tengana Aux HJ, Ramirez H, DeLany JP, Guerrero Pepinosa O, Lopez Quinones M, Collazos Parra T. 1996. *Helicobacter pylori* infection in the Colombian Andes: A population-based study of transmission pathways. *American Journal of Epidemiology* 144(3): 290–299.

Govoni G, Gros P. 1998. Macrophage NRAMP1 and its role in resistance to microbial infections. *Inflammation Research* 47(7):277–284.

Grajal A, Strahl S, Parra R, Dominguez MG, Neher A. 1989. Foregut fermentation in the hoatzin, a Neotropical leaf-eating bird. *Science* 245(4923):1236–1238.

Greten FR, Eckmann L, Greten TF, Park JM, Li ZW, Egan LJ, Kagnoff MF, Karin M. 2004. IKKbeta links inflammation and tumorigenesis in a mouse model of colitis-associated cancer. *Cell* 118(3):285–296.

Halfvarson J, Bodin L, Tysk C, Lindberg E, Jarnerot G. 2003. Inflammatory bowel disease in a Swedish twin cohort: A long-term follow-up of concordance and clinical characteristics. *Gastroenterology* 124(7):1767–1773.

Harford WV, Barnett C, Lee E, Perez-Perez G, Blaser MJ, Peterson WL. 2000 Acute gastritis with hypochlorhydria: Report of 35 cases with long-term follow-up. *Gut* 47(4) 467–472.

Harmsen, HJ, Raangs GC, He T, Degener JE, Welling GW. 2002. Extensive set of 16S rRNA-based probes for detection of bacteria in human feces. *Applied Environmental Microbiology* 68(6): 2982–2990.

Hatakeyama M. 2004. Oncogenic mechanisms of the *Helicobacter pylori* CagA protein. *Nature Reviews Cancer* 4(9):688–694.

Hayes W. 1968. *Genetics of Bacteria and Their Viruses: Studies in Basic Genetics and Molecular Biology.* 2nd ed. New York: John Wiley & Sons, Inc.

Hazell SL, Lee A, Brady L, Hennessy W. 1986. Campylobacter pyloridis and gastritis: Association with intercellular spaces and adaptation to an environment of mucus as important factors in colonization of the gastric epithelium. *Journal of Infectious Diseases* 153(4):658–663.

Heller F, Florian P, Bojarski C, Richter J, Christ M, Hillenbrand B, Mankertz J, Gitter AH, Burgel N, Fromm M, Zeitz M, Fuss I, Strober W, Schulzke JD. 2005. Interleukin-13 is the key effector Th2 cytokine in ulcerative colitis that affects epithelial tight junctions, apoptosis, and cell restitution. *Gastroenterology* 129(2):550–64.

Hentschel E, Brandstatter G, Dragosics B, Hirschl AM, Nemec H, Schutze K, Taufer M, Wurzer H. 1993. Effect of ranitidine and amoxicillin plus metronidazole on the eradication of *Helicobacter pylori* and the recurrence of duodenal ulcer. *New England Journal of Medicine* 328(5):308–312.

Higashi H, Tsutsumi R, Muto S, Sugiyama T, Azuma T, Asaka M, Hatakeyama M. 2001. SHP-2 tyrosine phosphatase as an intracellular target of *Helicobacter pylori* CagA protein. *Science* 295(5555):683–686.

Hisamatsu T, Suzuki M, Reinecker HC, Nadeau WJ, McCormick BA, Podolsky DK. 2003. CARD15/NOD2 functions as an anti-bacterial factor in human intestinal epithelial cells. *Gastroenterology* 124(4):993–1000.

Hoentjen F, Harmsen HJ, Braat H, Torrice CD, Mann BA, Sartor RB, Dieleman LA. 2003. Antibiotics with a selective aerobic or anaerobic spectrum have different therapeutic activities in various regions of the colon in interleukin-10 gene deficient mice. *Gut* 52(12):1721–1727.

Hooper, LV, Wong MH, Thelin A, Hansson L, Falk PG, Gordon JI. 2001. Molecular analysis of commensal host-microbial relationships in the intestine. *Science* 291(5505): 881–884.

Hooper LV, Stappenbeck TS, Hong CV, Gordon JI. 2003. Angiogenins: A new class of microbicidal proteins involved in innate immunity. *Nature Immunology* 4(3):269–273.

Horvath TL, Diano S, Sotonyi P, Heiman P, Tschöp M. 2001. Minireview: Ghrelin and the regulation of energy balance—a hypothalamic perspective. *Endocrinology* 142(10):4163–4169.

Howson CP, Hiyama T, Wynder EL. 1986. The decline in gastric cancer: Epidemiology of an unplanned triumph. *Epidemiology Review* 8:1–27.

Hugot JP, Chamaillard M, Zouali H, Lesage S, Cezard JP, Belaiche J, Almer S, Tysk C, O'Morain CA, Gassull M, Binder V, Finkel Y, Cortot A, Modigliani R, Laurent-Puig P, Gower-Rousseau C, Macry J, Colombel JF, Sahbatou M, Thomas G. 2001. Association of NOD2 leucine-rich repeat variants with susceptibility to Crohn's disease. *Nature* 411(6837):599–603.

Hungate RE. 1966. *The rumen and its microbes*. New York: Academic Press.

Hungate RE. 1972. Relationships between protozoa and bacteria of the alimentary tract. *American Journal of Clinical Nutrition* 25(12):1480–1484.

IARC (International Agency for Research on Cancer). 1994. Infection with *Helicobacter pylori*. *IARC Monograph Evaluation of Carcinogenic Risks in Humans* 61: 77–240.

Isomoto H, Nakazato M, Ueno H, Date Y, Nishi Y, Mukae H, Mizuta Y, Ohtsuru A, Yamashita S, Kohno S. 2004. Low plasma ghrelin levels in patients with *Helicobacter pylori*-associated gastritis. *American Journal of Medicine* 117(6):429–432.

Israel D, Lou A, Blaser MJ. 2000. Characteristics of *Helicobacter pylori* natural transformation. *FEMS Microbiology Letters* 186(2):275-280.

Israel D, Salama N, Krishna U, Rieger UM, Atherton JC, Falkow S, Peek RM. 2001. *Helicobacter pylori* genetic diversity within the gastric niche of a single human host. *Proceedings of the National Academy of Sciences USA* 98(25):14625–14630.

Karnes WE Jr, Samloff IM, Siurala M, Kekki M, Sipponen P, Kim SW, Walsh JH. 1991. Positive serum antibody and negative tissue staining for *Helicobacter pylori* in subjects with atrophic body gastritis. *Gastroenterology* 101(1):167–174.

Kersulyte D, Chalkauskas H, Berg DE. 1999. Emergence of recombinant strains of *Helicobacter pylori* during human infection. *Molecular Microbiology* 31(1):31–43.

Kim SC, Tonkonogy SL, Bower M, Sartor RB. 2004. Dual-association of gnotobiotic IL-10-/- mice with two nonpathogenic commensal bacterial species accelerates colitis [abstract]. *Gastroenterology* 126:A291.

Kim SC, Tonkonogy SL, Albright CA, Sartor RB. 2005a. Different host genetic backgrounds determine disease phenotypes induced by selective bacterial colonization [abstract]. *Gastroenterology* 128:A512.

Kim SC, Tonkonogy SL, Albright CA, Tsang J, Balish EJ, Braun J, Huycke MM, Sartor RB. 2005b. Variable phenotypes of enterocolitis in interleukin 10-deficient mice monoassociated with two different commensal bacteria. *Gastroenterology* 128(4):891–906.

Kirschner DE, Blaser MJ. 1995. The dynamics of *Helicobacter pylori* infection of the human stomach. *Journal of Theoretical Biology* 176(2):281–290.

Klein PD, Graham DY, Gaillour A, Opekun AR, Smith EO. 1991. Water source as risk factor for *Helicobacter pylori* infection in Peruvian children. Gastrointestinal Physiology Working Group. *Lancet* 337(8756):1503–1506.

Klieve AV, Bauchop T. 1988. Morphological diversity of ruminal bacteriophages from sheep and cattle. *Applied Environmental Microbiology* 54(6):1637–1641.

Klieve AV, Swain RA. 1993. Estimation of ruminal bacteriophage numbers by pulsed-field gel electrophoresis and laser densitometry. *Applied Environmental Microbiology* 59:2299–2303.

Klieve AV, Hudman JF, Bauchop T. 1989. Inducible bacteriophages from rum nal bacteria. *Applied Environmental Microbiology* 55:1630–1634.

Kobayashi KS, Chamaillard M, Ogura Y, Henegariu O, Inohara N, Nunez G, Flavell RA. 2005. Nod2-dependent regulation of innate and adaptive immunity in the intestinal tract. *Science* 307(5710): 731–734.

Kucik CJ, Martin GL, Sortor BV. 2004. Common intestinal parasites. *American Family Physician* 69(5):1161–1168.

Kuipers EJ, Uyterlinde AM, Peña AS, Roosendaal R, Pals G, Nelis GF, Festen HP, Meuwissen SG. 1995a. Long-term sequelae of *Helicobacter pylori* gastritis. *Lancet* 345(8964):1525–1528.

Kuipers EJ, Pérez-Pérez GI, Meuwissen SGM, Blaser MJ. 1995b. *Helicobacter pylori* and atrophic gastritis: Importance of the cagA status. *Journal of the National Cancer Institute* 87(23):1777–1780.

Kuipers EJ, Israel DA, Kusters JG, Gerrits MM, Weel J, van der Ende A, van der Hulst RWM, Wirth H-P, Hôôk-Nikanne J, Thompson SA, Blaser MJ. 2000. Quasispecies development of *Helicobacter pylori* observed in paired isolates obtained years apart in the same host. *Journal of Infectious Diseases* 181(1):273–282.

Lagergren J, Bergström R, Lindgren A, Nyrén O. 1999. Symptomatic gastroesophageal reflux as a risk factor for esophageal adenocarcinoma. *New England Journal of Medicine* 340(11): 825–831.

Lala S, Ogura Y, Osborne C, Hor SY, Bromfield A, Davies S, Ogunbiyi O, Nunez G, Keshav S. 2003. Crohn's disease and the NOD2 gene: A role for Paneth cells. *Gastroenterology* 125(1):47–57.

Lederberg J. 2000. Infectious history. *Science* 288(5464):287–293.

Lee HM, Wang G, Englander EW, Kojima M, Greeley Jr. GH. 2002. Ghrelin, a new gastrointestinal endocrine peptide that stimulates insulin secretion: Enteric distribution, ontogeny, influence of endocrine, and dietary manipulations. *Endocrinology* 143(1):185–190.

Loffeld RJLF, Werdmuller BFM, Kusters JG, Blaser MJ, Pérez-Pérez GI, Kuipers EJ. 2000. Colonization with cagA-positive *H. pylori* strains inversely associated with reflux oesophagitis and Barrett's oesophagitis. *Digestion* 62(2-3):95–99.

Lu X, Francois F, Yang L, Zhou M, Bini E, Blaser MJ, Pei Z. 2005 (June). Alteration of the bacterial biota in reflux esophagitis. Paper presented at: 105th General Meeting of the American Society of Microbiology; Atlanta, GA.

MacDonald TT, Gordon JN. 2005. Bacterial regulation of intestinal immune responses. *Gastroenterology Clinic of North America* 34(3):401-412.

Machado JC, Figueiredo C, Canedo P, Pharoah P, Carvalho R, Nabais S, Castro Alves C, Campos ML, Van Doorn LJ, Caldas C, Seruca R, Carneiro F, Sobrinho-Simoes M. 2003. A pro-inflammatory genetic profile increases the risk for chronic atrophic gastritis and gastric carcinoma. *Gastroenterology* 125(2):364–371.

Mackowiak PA. 1982. The normal microbial flora. *New England Journal of Medicine* 307(2):83–93.

Mann BA, Kim SC, Sartor RB. 2003. Selective induction of experimental colitis by monoassociation of HLA-B27 transgenic rats with various enteric *Bacteroides species* [abstract]. *Gastroenterology* 124:A322.

Matson CA, Reid DF, Cannon TA, Ritter RC. 2000. Cholecystokinin and leptin act synergistically to reduce body weight. *American Journal of Physiology, Regulatory, Integrative and Comparative Physiology* 278(4):R882–R890.

McNeill WH. 1976. *Plagues and Peoples*. Garden City, NY: Anchor Books.
Moss SF, Calam J. 1993. Acid secretion and sensitivity to gastrin in patients with duodenal ulcer: Effect of eradication of *Helicobacter pylori*. *Gut* 34(7):888–892.
Moss SF, Legon S, Bishop AE, Polak JM, Calam J. 1992. Effect of *Helicobacter pylori* on gastric somatostatin in duodenal ulcer disease. *Lancet* 340(8825):930–932.
Murray J, Murray A, Murray M, Murray C. 1978. The biologicalsuppression of malaria: An ecological and nutritional interrelationship of a host and two parasites. *American Journal of Clinical Nutrition* 31(8):1363–1366.
Nacher M, McGready R, Stepniewska K, Cho T. Looareesuwan S, White NJ, Nosten F. 2003. Haematinic treatment of anaemia increases the risk of *Plasmodium vivax* malaria in pregnancy. *Transactions of the Royal Society of Tropical Medicine and Hygiene* 97(3):273–276.
Naumann M, Wessler S, Bartsch C, Wieland B, Covacci A, Haas R, Meyer TF. 1999. Activation of activator protein 1 and stress response kinases in epithelial cells colonized by *Helicobacter pylori* encoding the cag pathogenicity island. *Journal of Biological Chemistry* 274(4):31655–31662.
Nelson KE, Zinder SH, Hance I, Burr P, Odongo D, Wasawo D, Odenyo A, Bishop R. 2003. Phylogenetic analysis of the microbial populations in the wild herbivore gastrointestinal tract: Insights into an unexplored niche. *Environmental Microbiology* 5(11):1212–1220.
Nemcova R, Styriak I, Stachova M, Kmet V. 1993. Isolation and partial characterization of three rumen *Lactobacillus plantarum* bacteriophages. *New Microbiology* 16(2):177–180.
Newman B, Siminovitch KA. 2005. Recent advances in the genetics of inflammatory bowel disease. *Current Opinions in Gastroenterology* 21(4):401–407.
Nomura AM, Stemmermann GN, Chyou P-H, Pérez-Pérez GI, Blaser MJ. 1994. *Helicobacter pylori* infection and the risk for duodenal and gastric ulceration. *Annals of Internal Medicine* 120(12):977–981.
Nomura AM, Perez-Perez GI, Lee J, Stemmermann G, Blaser MJ. 2002a. Relationship between *H. pylori cagA* status and risk of peptic ulcer disease. *American Journal of Epidemiology* 155(11):1054–1059.
Nomura AM, Lee J, Stemmermann G, Nomura RY, Perez-Perez GI, Blaser MJ. 2002b. *Helicobacter pylori cagA* seropositivity and gastric carcinoma risk in a Japanese American population. *Journal of Infectious Diseases* 186(8):1138–1144.
Nwokolo CU, Freshwater DA, O'Hare P, Randeva HS. 2003. Plasma ghrelin following cure of *Helicobacter pylori*. *Gut* 52(5):637–640.
Occhialini A, Marais A, Urdaci M, Sierra R, Munoz N, Covacci A, Megraud F. 2001. Composition and gene expression of the *cag* pathogenicity island in *Helicobacter pylori* strains isolated from gastric carcinoma and gastritis patients in Coast Rica. *Infection and Immunity* 69(3):1902–1908.
Odenbreit S, Püls J, Sedlmaier B, Gerland E, Fischer W, Haas R. 2000. Translocation of *Helicobacter pylori* CagA into gastric epithelial cells by type IV secretion. *Science* 287(5457):1497–1500.
Ogimoto K, Imai S. 1981. *Atlas of Rumen Microbiology*. Tokyo, Japan: Scientific Society Press.
Ogura Y, Bonen DK, Inohara N, Nicolae DL, Chen FF, Ramos R, Britton H, Moran T, Karaliuskas R, Duerr RH, Achkar JP, Brant SR, Bayless TM, Kirschner BS, Hanauer SB, Nunez G, Cho JH. 2001. A frameshift mutation in NOD2 associated with susceptibility to Crohn's disease. *Nature* 411(6837):603–606.
Oliveira AM, Queiroz DM, Rocha GA, Mendes EN. 1994. Seroprevalence of Helicobacter pylori infection of children of low socioeconomic level in Belo Horizonte, Brazil. *American Journal of Gastroenterology* 89(12):2201–2204.
Oppenheimer SJ. 2001. Iron and its relation to immunity and infectious disease. *Journal of Nutrition* 131(2S-2):616S-633S.
Pantoja, I, Mojica M, Vargas-Pinto G, Scott K, Patterson A, Flint H, Blaser M, Dominguez-Bello MG. 2005. *Tetracycline Resistance Genes in Bolivian Amerindians with Low Antibiotic Exposure*. San Francisco, CA: Infectious Diseases Society of America.

Parsonnet J. 1995. The incidence of *Helicobacter pylori* infection. *Alimentary Pharmacology and Therapeutics* 9(Suppl 2):45–51.
Parsonnet J, Friedman GD, Orentreich N, Vogelman H. 1997. Risk for gastric cancer in people with CagA positive or CagA negative *Helicobacter pylori* infection. *Gut* 40(3):297–301.
Peek RM, Blaser MJ. 2002. *Helicobacter pylori* and gastrointestinal tract aderocarcinomas. *Nature Reviews Cancer* 2(1):28–37.
Peek RM Jr, Peek RM, Vaezi MF, Falkow S, Goldblum JR, Pérez-Pérez GI, Richter JE, Blaser MJ. 1999. The role of *Helicobacter pylori cagA$^+$* strains and specific host immune responses on the development of premalignant and malignant lesions of the gastric cardia. *International Journal of Cancer* 82:520–524.
Pei Z, Bini EJ, Yang L, Zhou M, Francois F, Blaser MJ. 2004. Bacterial biota in the human distal esophagus. *Proceedings of the National Academy of Sciences USA* 101(12):4250–4255.
Pei Z, Yang L, Peek RM, Levine SM, Pride DT, Blaser MJ. 2005. Bacterial biota in reflux esophagitis and Barrett's esophagus. *World Journal of Gastroenterology* In press.
Peltekova VD, Wintle RF, Rubin LA, Amos CI, Huang Q, Gu X, Newman B, Van Oene M, Cescon D, Greenberg G, Griffiths AM, St George-Hyslop PH, Siminovitch KA. 2004. Functional variants of OCTN cation transporter genes are associated with Crohn disease. *Nature Genetics* 36(5):471–475.
Perez-Perez GI, Salomaa A, Kosunen TU, Daverman B, Rautelin H, Aromaa A, Knekt P, Blaser MJ. 2002. Evidence that *cagA+Helicobacter pylori* strains are disappearing more rapidly than *cagA-* strains. *Gut* 50(3):295–298.
Perez-Perez GI, Sack RB, Reid R, Santosham M, Croll J, Blaser MJ. 2003. Transient and persistent *Helicobacter pylori* colonization in Native American children. *Journal of Clinical Microbiology* 41(6):2401–2407.
Pohl H, Gilbert H. 2005. The role of overdiagnosis and reclassification in the marked increase of esophageal adenocarcinoma incidence. *Journal of the National Cancer Institute* 97(2):142–146.
Queiroz DM, Guerra JB, Rocha GA, Rocha AM, Santos A, De Oliveira AG, Cabral MM, Nogueira AM, De Oliveira CA. 2004. IL1B and IL1RN polymorphic genes and *Helicobacter pylori cagA* strains decrease the risk of reflux esophagitis. *Gastroenterology* 127(1):73–79.
Rakoff-Nahoum S, Paglino J, Eslami-Varzaneh F, Edberg S, Medzhitov R. 2004. Recognition of commensal microflora by toll-like receptors is required for intestinal homeostasis. *Cell* 118(2):229–241.
Rath HC, Herfarth HH, Ikeda JS, Grenther WB, Hamm TE Jr, Balish E, Taurog JD, Hammer RE, Wilson KH, Sartor RB. 1996. Normal luminal bacteria, especially *Bacteroides* species, mediate chronic colitis, gastritis, and arthritis in HLA-B27/human beta2 microglobulin transgenic rats. *Journal of Clinical Investigation* 98(4):945-953.
Rath HC, Wilson KH, Sartor RB. 1999. Differential induction of colitis and gastritis in HLA-B27 transgenic rats selectively colonized with *Bacteroides vulgatus* and *Escherichia coli*. *Infection and Immunity* 67(6):2969-2974.
Rath HC, Schultz M, Freitag R, Dieleman LA, Li F, Linde HJ, Scholmerich J, Sartor RB. 2001. Different subsets of enteric bacteria induce and perpetuate experimental colitis in rats and mice. *Infection and Immunity* 69(4):2277–2285.
Rauws EA, Langenberg W, Houthoff HJ, Zanen HC, Tytgat GN. 1998. Campylobacter pyloridis-associated chronic active antral gastritis: A prospective study of its prevalence and the effects of antibacterial and antiulcer treatment. *Gastroenterology* 94(1):33–40.
Rehnberg-Laiho L, Rautelin H, Koskela P, Sarna S, Pukkala E, Aromaa A, Knekt P, Kosunen TU. 2001. Decreasing prevalence of helicobacter antibodies in Finland, with reference to the decreasing incidence of gastric cancer. *Epidemiology and Infection* 126(1):37–42.
Rosebury T. 1962. *Microorganisms Indigenous to Man*. New York: McGraw Hill.
Rothenbacher D, Blaser MJ, Bode G, Brenner H. 2000. An inverse relationship between gastric colonization by *Helicobacter pylori* and diarrheal illnesses in children: Results of a population-based cross-sectional study. *Journal of Infectious Diseases* 182(5):1446–1449.

Salyers A, Gupta A, Wang Y. 2004. Human intestinal bacteria as reservoirs for antibiotic resistance genes. *Trends in Microbiology* 12(9):412–416.

Sartor RB. 2004. Microbial influences in inflammatory bowel disease: Role in pathogenesis and clinical implications. In: Sartor RB, Sandborn WJ, eds. *Kirsner's Inflammatory Bowel Diseases.* Philadelphia, PA: Elsevier Publishers; Pp. 138–162.

Sartor RB. 2005 (March 16). *Session I: Host-Pathogen Interactions: Defining the Concepts of Pathogenicity, Virulence, Colonization, Commensalism, and Symbiosis.* Presentation at the Forum on Microbial Threats Workshop Ending the War Metaphor: The Changing Agenda for Unraveling the Host-Microbe Relationship, Washington, D.C., Institute of Medicine, Forum on Microbial Threats.

Sartor RB, Hoentjen F. 2005. Proinflammatory cytokines and signaling pathways in intestinal innate immune cells. In: Mestecky J, Lamm ME, Strober W, Bienenstock J, McGhee JR, Mayer L, eds. *Mucosal Immunology.* London: Elsevier Academic Press; Pp. 681–701.

Savage DC. Microbial ecology of the gastrointestinal tract. 1977. *Annual Review of Microbiology* 31:107–133.

Schreiber S, Rosenstiel P, Albrecht M, Hampe J, Krawczak M. 2005. Genetics of Crohn disease, an archetypal inflammatory barrier disease. *Nature Reviews Genetics* 6(5):376–388.

Segal ED, Cha J, Lo J, Falkow S, Tompkins LS. 1999. Altered states: Involvement of phosphorylated CagA in the induction of host cellular growth changes by *Helicobacter pylori. Proceedings of the National Academy of Sciences USA* 96(25):14559–14564.

Segal S, Hill AV. 2003. Genetic susceptibility to infectious disease. *Trends in Microbiology* 11(9): 445–448.

Sellon RK, Tonkonogy S, Schultz M, Dieleman LA, Grenther W, Balish E, Rennick DM, Sartor RB. 1998. Resident enteric bacteria are necessary for development of spontaneous colitis and immune system activation in interleukin-10-deficient mice. *Infection and Immunity* 66(11): 5224–5231.

Smythies LE, Sellers M, Clements RH, Mosteller-Barnum M, Meng G, Benjamin WH, Orenstein JM, Smith PD. 2005 Human intestinal macrophages display profound inflammatory anergy despite avid phagocytic and bacteriocidal activity. *Journal of Clinical Investigation* 115(1):66–75.

Sobhani I, Buyse M, Goiot H, Weber N, Laigneau JP, Henin D, Soul JC, Bado A. 2002. Vagal stimulation rapidly increases leptin secretion in human stomach. *Gastroenterology* 122(2): 259–263.

Stappenbeck TS, Hooper LV, Gordon JI. 2002. Developmental regulation of intestinal angiogenesis by indigenous microbes via Paneth cells. *Proceedings of the National Academy of Sciences USA* 99(24):15451–15455.

Strober W, Fuss I, Boirivant M, Kitani A. 2004. Insights into the mechanism of oral tolerance derived from the study of models of mucosal inflammation. *Annual of the New York Academy of Sciences* 1029:115–131.

Suerbaum S, Smith JM, Bapumia K, Morelli G, Smith NH, Kunstmann E, Dyrek I, Achtman M. 1998. Free recombination with *Helicobacter pylori. Proceedings of the National Academy of Sciences USA* 95(21):12619–12624.

Swidsinski A, Ladhoff A, Pernthaler A, Swidsinski S, Loening-Baucke V, Ortner M, Weber J, Hoffmann U, Schreiber S, Dietel M, Lochs H. 2002. Mucosal flora in inflammatory bowel disease. *Gastroenterology* 122(1):44–54.

Tajima K, Aminov RI, Nagamine T, Ogata K, Nakamura M, Matsui H. 2001a. Rumen bacterial diversity as determined by sequence analysis of 16S rDNA libraries. *FEMS Microbiology Ecology* 29:159–169.

Tajima K, Nagamine T, Matsui H, Nakamura M, Aminov RI. 2001b. Phylogenetic analysis of archaeal 16S rRNA libraries from the rumen suggests the existence of a novel group of archaea not associated with known methanogens. *FEMS Microbiology Letters* 200(1):67–72.

Tham KT, Peek RM, Atherton JC, Cover TL, Perez-Perez GI, Shyr Y, Blaser MJ. 2001. *Helicobacter pylori* genotypes, host factors, and gastric mucosal histopathology in peptic ulcer disease. *Human Pathology* 32(3):264–273.

Tomb JF, White O, Kerlavage AR, Clayton RA, Sutton GG, Fleischmann RD, Ketchum KA, Klenk HP, Gill S, Dougherty BA, Nelson K, Quackenbush J, Zhou L, Kirkness EF, Peterson S, Loftus B, Richardson D, Dodson R, Khalak HG, Glodek A, McKenney K, Fitzegerald LM, Lee N, Adams MD, Hickey EK, Berg DE, Gocayne JD, Utterback TR, Peterson JD, Kelley JM, Cotton MD, Weidman JM, Fujii C, Bowman C, Watthey L, Wallin E, Hayes WS, Borodovsky M, Karp PD, Smith HO, Fraser CM, Venter JC. 1997. The complete genome sequence of the gastric pathogen *Helicobacter pylori*. *Nature* 388(6642):539–547.

Tummuru MKR, Cover TL, Blaser MJ. 1993. Cloning and expression of a high molecular weight major antigen of *Helicobacter pylori*: Evidence of linkage to cytotoxin production. *Infection and Immunity* 61(5):1799–1809.

Tummuru MKR, Sharma SA, Blaser MJ. 1995. *Helicobacter pylori picB*, a homologue of the *Bordetella pertussis* toxin secretion protein, is required for induction of IL-8 in gastric epithelial cells. *Molecular Microbiology* 18(5):867–876.

Vaezi MF, Falk GW, Peek RM, Vicari JJ, Goldblum JR, Perez-Perez GI, Rice TW, Blaser MJ, Richter JE. 2000. cagA-positive strains of *Helicobacter pylori* may protect against Barrett's esophagus. *American Journal of Gastroenterology* 95(9):2206–2211.

Van Soest PJ. 1994. *Nutritional Ecology of the Ruminant*. Ithaca, NY: Comstock.

Viala J, Chaput C, Boneca IG, Cardona A, Girardin SE, Moran AP, Athman R, Memet S, Huerre MR, Coyle AJ, DiStefano PS, Sansonetti PJ, Labigne A, Bertin J, Philpott DJ, Ferrero RL. 2004. Nod1 responds to peptidoglycan delivered by the *Helicobacter pylori cag* pathogenicity island. *Nature Immunology* 5(11):1166–1174.

Vicari JJ, Peek RM, Falk GW, Goldblum JR, Easley KA, Schnell J, Pérez-Pérez GI, Halter SA, Rice TW, Blaser MJ, Richter JE. 1998. The seroprevalence of cagA-positive *Helicobacter pylori* strains in the spectrum of gastroesophageal reflux disease. *Gastroenterology* 115(1):50–57.

Villedieu A, Diaz-Torres ML, Hunt N, McNab R, Spratt DA, Wilson M, Mullany P. 2003. Prevalence of tetracycline resistance genes in oral bacteria. *Antimicrobial Agents in Chemotherapy* 47(3): 878–882.

Warburton-Timmsa VJ, Charlettd A, Valorib RM, Uffc JS, Shepherdc NA, Barrb H, McNultya CAM. 2001. The significance of $cagA^+$ *Helicobacter pylori* in reflux oesophagitis *Gut* 49(3):341–346.

Warren JR, Marshall BJ. 1983. Unidentified curved bacilli on gastric epithelium in active chronic gastritis. *Lancet* 1(8336):1273–1275.

Watanabe T, Kitani A, Murray PJ, Strober W. 2004. NOD2 is a negative regulator of Toll-like receptor 2-mediated T helper type 1 responses. *Nature Immunology* 5(8):800–808.

Wehkamp J, Harder J, Weichenthal M, Schwab M, Schaffeler E, Schlee M, Herrlinger KR, Stallmach A, Noack F, Fritz P, Schroder JM, Bevins CL, Fellermann K, Stange EF. 2004. NOD2 (CARD15) mutations in Crohn's disease are associated with diminished mucosal alpha-defensin expression. *Gut* 53(11):1658–1664.

Whitford MF, Forster RJ, Beard CE, Gong J, Teather RM. 1998. Phylogenetic analysis of rumen bacteria by comparative sequence analysis of cloned 16S rRNA genes. *Anaerobe* 4:153–163.

Wirth HP, Yang M, Peek RM, Hook-Nikanne J, Fried M, Blaser MJ. 1999. Phenotypic diversity in Lewis expression of *Helicobacter pylori* isolates from the same host. *Journal of Laboratory and Clinical Medicine* 133(5):488–500.

Wu AH, Crabtree JE, Bernstein L, Hawtin P, Cockburn M, Tseng C, Forman D. 2003. Role of *Helicobacter pylori* $cagA^+$ strains and risk of adenocarcinoma of the stomach and esophagus. *International Journal of Cancer* 103(6):815–821.

Yamaji Y, Mitsushima T, Ikuma H, Okamoto M, Yoshida H, Kawabe T, Shiratori Y, Saito K, Yokouchi K, Omata M. 2001. Inverse background of *Helicobacter pylori* anti-cancer: Analysis of 5732 Japanese subjects. *Gut* 49(3):335–340.

Yamaoka Y, Kodama T, Kashima K, Graham DY, Sepulveda AR. 1998. Variants of the 3' region of the cagA gene in *Helicobacter pylori* isolates from patients with different *H. pylori*-associated diseases. *Journal of Clinical Microbiology* 36(8):2258–2263.

Ye W, Held M, Lagergren J, Engstrand L, Blot WJ, McLaughlin JK, Nyrén O. 2004. *Helicobacter pylori* infection and gastric atrophy: Risk of adenocarcinoma and squamous-cell carcinoma of the esophagus and adenocarcinoma of the gastric cardia. *Journal of the National Cancer Institute* 96(5):388–396.

4

The Host Response to Pathogens

OVERVIEW

A complete understanding of pathogenesis must consider not only how microorganisms inflict damage—the primary focus of research under the war metaphor—but also the mechanisms by which hosts discriminate among microbes and convert that information into an immune response. This expanded field of inquiry is yielding intriguing results, as illustrated in the two contributions that comprised by this chapter: the first characterizes the complex host-microbe interactions that establish mucosal immunity in the gut; the second describes insights gained from analyzing patterns of global host gene expression in response to infection.

Much of the intestinal epithelium features a combination of innate defenses, but these defenses are reduced in cells that lie between lymphoid follicles and the intestinal lumen. This follicle-associated epithelium, which serves as a key interchange in signaling between microbes on one side of the epithelial barrier and host immune and inflammatory cells on the other, is the focus of research in Marian Neutra's laboratory. She describes the structure and function of these rare and specialized regions of the intestinal epithelium and their vital role in the development of mucosal immunity; particular attention is paid to the role of M cells, which transport pathogens and antigens from the lumen to the lymphoid tissue. Understanding the molecular means by which M cells fulfill their gatekeeping role could inform the design of mucosal vaccines to prevent infection by pathogens such as human immunodeficiency virus (HIV) and provide insights on the prevention and treatment of inflammatory bowel disease (IBD) and associated immune disorders.

Researchers have greatly expanded our understanding of the complexities of host-microbe interactions through the use of molecular techniques that monitor microbial and host cell gene expression. In his contribution to this chapter, David Relman describes studies conducted in his laboratory that employ DNA microarrays to monitor host transcript abundance in blood cells following exposure to known bacterial and viral pathogens. Their findings illustrate variation in the indigenous microbial flora of healthy humans and the range of host transcriptional response to infection; Relman and colleagues also identify recurring patterns and possible sources of variability in that response. Relman also describes the use of rDNA polymerase chain reaction (PCR) to explore the possible pathogenic activity of archaea, focusing on their potential role in peridontitis.

One factor that has *not* been found to produce significant differences in host gene expression is the distinction between pathogen- versus commensal-associated stimuli. Detailed comparisons of host transcriptional responses to various pathogens over time are, however, revealing subtle transcriptional signatures upon the host response. Such variability—which is thought to result from pathogen-specific mechanisms that co-opt, subvert, or modify the stereotypical host response to microbial stimuli—offers the possibility of a new approach to disease prevention, diagnosis, and treatment.

THE INTESTINAL EPITHELIUM: AN INTERACTIVE BARRIER BETWEEN HOST AND MICROBE

Marian Neutra

Those of us who study mucosal immunity and mucosal protection are in the habit of using the war metaphor when we talk about the epithelial monolayer that lines the human gut. We have described it as a barrier and the mucus it secretes as our "front line" of defense. However, this impression is being revised as we discover that the intestinal epithelium also acts as a sensor of the contents of the lumen, and as an "intelligent" mediator of immune signaling between ourselves and the microbes we encounter.

By "intelligent," I mean that the intestinal epithelium appears capable of filtering a tremendous amount of information regarding the antigens borne by the huge and diverse population of microorganisms in the lumen. Specialized epithelial cells survey the contents of the gut and report it to a highly developed mucosal immune recognition system that resides in adjacent lymphoid cells—and, remarkably, this occurs without provoking all-out war in the form of chronic intestinal inflammation. The following essay recounts several recent discoveries that show how these specialized intestinal epithelial cells accomplish this critical balancing act.

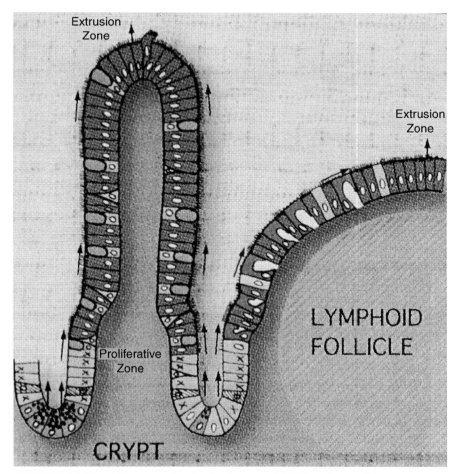

FIGURE 4-1 The follicle-associated epithelium and MALT: a close collaboration.
SOURCE: Neutra (2005).

Structure of the Follicle-Associated Epithelium

The sampling of luminal contents occurs in rare, specialized regions of the intestinal epithelium, as depicted in Figure 4-1. These include mucosa-associated lymphoid tissue (MALT) and associated epithelial cells. Because the epithelial cells in these immune induction sites are associated with underlying collections of lymphoid cells known as lymphoid follicles, they are known as the follicle-associated epithelium (FAE). In contrast to villus-associated epithelium, which covers the vast majority of the intestinal surface, FAE is sparsely distributed along the length of the gut. Peyer's patches, located in the ileum, contain the best-known example of lymphoid-associated epithelium in humans; these sites are most numerous in the colon and rectum, but they are also found in the oral cavities, the tonsils and adenoids, and perhaps also on minor salivary glands. The distribution of immune induction sites in the body generally reflects the local abundance of foreign material and microorganism (Neutra et al., 2001).

Villus-associated epithelium, which functions primarily to absorb nutrients, is heavily defended against microbial intrusion. Its cells secrete mucus, digestive enzymes, defensins,[1] and lysosyme, as well as IgA (which plays a role in both innate and adaptive immunity, as demonstrated below). Such defenses are significantly reduced in the FAE—in fact, rather than preventing microbial adherence or contact, specialized cells in the FAE, known as M cells, appear to invite microbes to enter. M cells appear to make their luminal surfaces readily accessible to microbes, which are then endocytosed and delivered to dendritic cells that lie just beneath the epithelial surface. The dendritic cells rapidly capture antigens and pathogens from the M cells and migrate to nearby deposits of T or B cells where the antigens are presented. Thus, the inductive system of the adaptive immune response, as well as that of innate immunity, occurs in these MALTs. The relative rarity of immune induction sites limits host exposure to potential pathogens.

Pathogen-M-Cell Interactions

Inevitably, some pathogens have evolved to exploit the FAE. Microbes—including *Salmonella, Shigella*, and poliovirus—gain entry to their hosts by selectively adhering to the M cell. A mouse reovirus that exclusively infects Peyer's patches causes a severe infection in newborn mice that spreads to the brain, but weaned mice with mature immune systems can clear such infections with a mucosal immune response. This reovirus provides a good model for examining how M cells select pathogens and how pathogens can select M cells.

To locate its target, the reovirus uses a carbohydrate "fingerprint" that is present on all the epithelial cells but is accessible to viral particles exclusively on the surface of M cells (Helander et al., 2003). We were able to show that one form of this reovirus (reovirus 1) targets a specific sialic acid-containing trisaccharide epitope, while another form of the reovirus (reovirus 3) uses a different

---

[1]Defensins are potent, small-peptide antibiotics made by neutrophils and macrophages that act by binding to the membranes of microbes and increasing membrane permeability. Defensin is also called human neutrophil peptide (HNP).

[2]Lectins are proteins, typically obtained from the seeds of leguminous plants, that have binding sites for specific mono- or oligosaccharides in cell walls or membranes. Lectin binding can alter cellular physiology to cause agglutination, mitosis, or other biochemical changes in the cell. Named originally for the ability of some to selectively agglutinate human red blood cells of particular blood groups, lectins are widely used as analytical and preparative agents in the study of glycoproteins.

epitope. The reovirus has extended attachment proteins on its surface that look like landing gear; these attachment proteins recognize the specific trisaccharide.

The carbohydrate epitope recognized by reovirus 1 is also bound by lectins[2] MAL I and MAL II, so we expected that the lectins would also specifically recognize M cells. However, when we applied MAL I and MAL II to mucosal tissue, they bound all epithelial cell surfaces readily and nonspecifically—until we displayed the lectins on particles. Clearly, the specificity for M-cell binding is a matter of accessibility, as well as carbohydrate recognition. As shown in Figure 4-2, M cells are differentiated by their lack of a thick glycoprotein coat, which

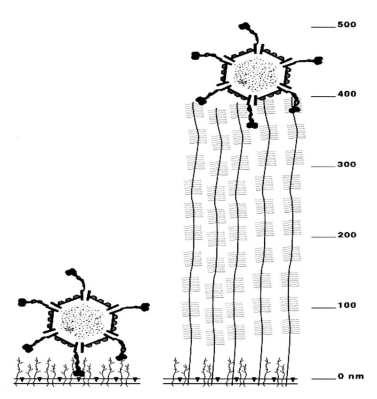

FIGURE 4-2 Reovirus has access to carbohydrate receptors on M cells. Drawn to (nanometer) scale, the virus is about 80 nm in diameter, and has 40-nm extensions ("landing gear") made of trimers of a protein called sigma-1. With its sigma 1 protein extended, the virus can reach through the M cell's glycoprotein coat (shown on the left), which is only about 30 nm thick. The absorptive epithelial cells that cover the intestinal mucosa bear a thick glycoprotein coat (as shown on the right) that cannot be penetrated by the extended sigma 1 "landing gear."
SOURCE: Helander et al. (2003).

renders certain carbohydrates on their surfaces accessible to binding by the reovirus surface protein, sigma-1. Moreover, the reovirus can only bind the M-cell if the viral sigma-1 protein is in an extended conformation. It achieves this structure through the action of gut proteases, which process the folded reoviral surface protein on the native virion into this infectious form.

Because we are interested in mucosal immunity, we wanted to determine an immune response that could protect M cells from attachment of the virus and prevent reinfection of the mucosa. We found that only antibodies against the head of the sigma-1 protein were successful, and that protection depended upon blocking the interaction between sigma-1 and the carbohydrate epitope it recognizes on M cells.

The Dual Role of IgA

Another series of studies on the FAE led us to discover how IgA is both an adaptive and an innate protective mechanism. Using a technique we call the *backpack tumor method*, we inject hybridoma tumor cells under the skin on the backs of syngeneic (genetically identical) mice. When the resulting tumor reaches about 1 centimeter in diameter, it starts producing large amounts of antibody. These mice produce only one type of monoclonal antibody, which is determined by the hybridoma used; otherwise, they have no means of immune protection against challenge with a specific pathogen. In mice with a tumor expressing anti-sigma-1 IgG, a great deal of IgG is produced by the hybridoma and enters the blood, but only a negligible amount of IgG is secreted into the intestine; thus there is no IgG in the gut lumens of such mice (Hutchings et al., 2004). We also made mice with tumors that expressed dimeric IgA. These animals secrete the monoclonal antibody, and it is also present in their blood. In addition, we examined control animals that expressed anticholera toxin IgG and anticholera toxin dimeric IgA, as well as some without tumors.

When we orally challenged all five of these types of mice (which are not transgenic) with reovirus, we found, as expected, that only the mice secreting the anti-sigma-1 IgA were completely protected against oral reovirus challenge (see Figure 4-3) (Hutchings et al., 2004). However, we also found that IgA knockout mice that have never been exposed to reovirus before had especially high viral levels in their mucosa compared with the normal mouse controls, indicating that IgA might act as a nonspecific defense mechanism. This view is supported by our finding that the irrelevant IgA (against cholera toxin) offered significant (but not complete) protection against reoviral entry. We have seen this with other pathogens as well, so we conclude that it is good to have IgA, whether it is specific or not. This nonspecific protective effect of IgA might be especially important early in life; for example, by permitting an innate immune response to a variety of pathogens or even as an adjuvant following exposure to a single pathogen.

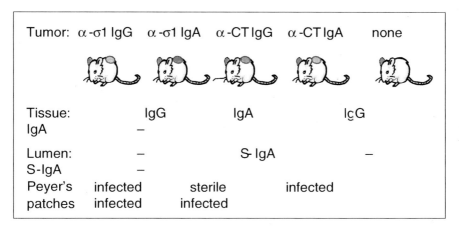

FIGURE 4-3 The "backpack" hybridoma tumor protocol.
SOURCE: Neutra (2005).

One might question what these mice, which secrete such excessive amounts of monoclonal IgA, could really tell us about what is going on in a normal human mucosa. However, when we actually captured IgA secreted by human tissues (with little wicks and sponges) and measured it, we found large amounts—for example, as much as three milligrams per milliliter of IgA, and some IgG as well—on the epithelial surface of the human rectum. After a local immunization in the rectum with a strong antigen, 10 to 15 percent of the secreted antibody may be antigen-specific IgA.

We also were surprised to discover that, when we labeled antigen-specific mouse monoclonal IgAs and introduced them into the lumen of a mouse or rabbit, they would adhere selectively to M cells. This was consistent with a previous report that newborn rabbits have collections of IgA on the surfaces of their M cells and nowhere else. Nick Mantis, a member of my laboratory, then showed that human IgA2 (but not IgA1) binds a unique receptor on M cells that has not yet been identified. This receptor is specific to antibody containing a constant domain 1 and domain 2 of the heavy chain in close proximity; if the domains are separated by a long linker region, as they are in human IgA1, the antibody can no longer be recognized by the M-cell receptor. M cells also did not bind hybrid antibody containing homologous constant domains 1 and 2 of IgG.

What advantages might the display of IgA on the FAE confer upon the host? Our current hypothesis is that IgA interacts specifically or nonspecifically with gut microbes, then brings them back to be sampled or promotes further sampling by the organized mucosal lymphoid tissues.

Toll-Like Receptors in the FAE

Another unique feature of the FAE concerns the display and function of toll-like receptors (TLRs). Villus-associated epithelial cells bear TLRs that can send signals either directly or via subepithelial macrophages, as shown by Jeffrey Gordon and others to dampen inflammation and, at the same time, promote epithelial health and renewal (Bäckhed et al., 2004; Rakoff-Nahoum et al., 2004). Signaling through these TLRs, which occurs in response to the commensal flora, prompts the constant migration and turnover of epithelial cells in the intestine. Given the role of the FAE in mucosal immunity, it would seem paradoxical that it would bear receptors that repress the immune response, yet we found that several types of TLRs are indeed displayed in these sites.

To explore this conundrum, Sophie Chabot, in my laboratory, examined how TLRs in the FAE respond to various ligands. Her studies focused on TLR2, which recognizes peptidoglycans and several other bacterial molecules. When she labeled the FAE with a fluorescent lectin to identify M cells and also with a fluorescent antibody against TLR2 this is what she saw: the FAE cells bearing TLR2 appear largely distinct from the M cells, although a few M cells displayed TLR2. Interestingly, we also found that TLR2 is displayed on both the apical and basolateral surfaces of the FAE, whereas it is only present on the apical surfaces of villus and crypt cells. The purpose of the basolateral receptors has not yet been determined.

Little is known about the non-M cells of the FAE, which are called FAE enterocytes, but it is known that these cells produce chemokines that attract dendritic cells. When we injected peptidoglycan, a TLR2 ligand, to the intestinal lumen, the apical TLR2s disappeared from the FAE enterocytes within 90 minutes, but not from the M cells. We therefore suspect that the binding of the ligand caused the enterocyte TLR2s to be endocytosed and degraded, and we hypothesize that these events resulted in release of signaling molecules by the FAE. By staining the dendritic cells just below the FAE with a specific fluorescent marker, we could also visualize what happened to them: after the FAE was exposed to the TLR2 ligand, some dendritic cells rushed into the epithelial layer. Because we know that dendritic cells can enter M-cell pockets, and we know that dendritic cells are involved in antigen capture, these observations suggest to us that TLR2 binding sets off a signaling cascade that alerts the underlying dendritic cells to prepare for subsequent antigen delivery by M cells.

Antigen Transfer in the FAE

Another effect we observed following exposure of the FAE to peptidoglycan was a dramatic increase in the rate of transcytosis of particles across the epithelium. We noted similar reactions (both the increased rate of transcytosis and the migration of dendritic cells into the epithelium) after exposing the FAE to cholera toxin; this suggests that a number of different compounds may signal the FAE to increase transport of antigens to the dendritic cells. We have also seen that over longer periods of time adjuvants, or bacterial products similar to toxins, can influence the further movement of the dendritic cells.

We monitored these phenomena using virus-sized polystyrene fluorescent particles, which, if fed to mice, are taken up exclusively by their M cells. A postdoctoral student in my laboratory, Vijay Shreedhar, found that when he did this, the particles accumulated, as expected, in the dendritic cells. However, contrary to our expectations, those dendritic cells did not proceed to deliver their cargo to the nearby T-cell areas. Instead, the particles remained in the FAE indefinitely (we stopped checking after two weeks). Suspecting that another signal was needed to complete antigen transfer to the T cells, he fed the mice cholera toxin; the dendritic cells then moved to the T-cell areas. The same thing happened when the mice were fed *Salmonella* instead of cholera toxin.

Summary and Conclusion

As demonstrated by this gallery of recent snapshots of the MALT and the associated FAE in action, these sites are the focus of intense communication between the outside world and the mucosal immune system, between microbe and host. M cells, which act as gatekeepers at this boundary, have reduced antimicrobial defenses and instead promote contact with antigens and potential pathogens in the lumen. Many details of the mechanisms of signaling in the FAE remain to be determined, but it appears that the FAE is especially sensitive to TLR ligands (e.g., peptidoglycan). This localization may allow the host to respond to pathogens without creating havoc throughout the intestinal epithelium.

Understanding the differences between the FAE and the rest of the intestinal epithelium, between antigen sampling sites and nutrient absorption sites, is likely to be critical to the design of mucosal vaccines. The gut will generally not mount an immune response to a nutrient peptide or a noninfectious particle alone. Mucosal immune responses clearly require extra signals, such as ligands recognized by TLRs, enterotoxins, and probably others yet unknown; such information is being used to boost the effectiveness of mucosal vaccines. However, much more needs to be learned about how these signals work and how they might be manipulated to promote human health.

HOW THE HOST "SEES" AND RESPONDS TO PATHOGENS

David A. Relman[3]

Traditional perspectives of human responses to infection suggest that these responses are dominated by a limited number of effector molecules, such as

---

[3]Stanford University.

cytokines and a limited number of signaling pathways such as those associated with TLRs. Genomic tools now allow a more comprehensive assessment of human responses to infectious agents. DNA microarrays, in particular, permit one to examine human genomewide RNA transcript abundance patterns during the course of an infectious disease. Although this effort is in its early days, the resulting data reveal previously unappreciated sterotyped patterns, suggesting choreography and great complexity. The following set of observations on these kinds of data comes with several disclaimers. First, complexity and subtlety will be described at a superficial level. Second, these observations are based on transcript abundance patterns, which provide only one prism for viewing host-microbe interactions. Third, the data discussed in this essay were derived from blood, and are, therefore, limited to one anatomic compartment, albeit highly distributed, within the highly compartmentalized human host. Nevertheless, some early and important lessons have been learned concerning the variability of the host response to different kinds of microbial stimuli and the possible sources of that variability.

Conserved Response Structures and Pathways

Given that hosts have prominent mechanisms for recognizing conserved patterns among microbes (see previous contribution from Marian Neutra), one might expect to find evidence of shared responses to pathogens and commensals. To obtain a genomic perspective on the question of whether hosts can distinguish pathogen from commensal, we and other groups have conducted a broad variety of experiments in which human cells are exposed to various kinds of microbial stimuli *in vitro*, and their RNA transcripts are then monitored with DNA microarrays. Many of these experiments have employed human blood cells and subsets thereof, such as peripheral blood mononuclear cells (PBMCs). Although there have been many such studies with a variety of methodological and biological nuances, they seem to convey a common message: much of the response by human cells to microbial components, and to microorganisms themselves, is in fact shared. The most dominant responses are similar across time and fairly similar across different kinds of agents.

Some of the mechanisms that govern these common patterns result from well-known response systems in host cells, such as the NF-kappa-B regulon, and are probably mediated by conserved microbial pattern recognition systems. As demonstrated by Rakoff-Nahoum et al. (2004), the TLR system, an important pattern-recognition system, also recognizes commensal organisms. In fact, it is the constant stimulation by commensals that imparts or stimulates a protective, health-associated response at the mucosal barrier. The same system that recognizes pathogen-associated patterns also recognizes these same patterns in non-pathogenic microbes. The NOD-LRR family of conserved pattern-recognition receptors also recognizes both commensals and pathogens (Eckmann and Karin, 2005; Kobayashi et al., 2005). However, we (and others) have also noted that there are differences in the response of human cells *in vitro* to different intact or live pathogens that cannot be explained by simple corrections for equivalent dose or time (Boldrick et al., 2002). These differences have supported the concept that the human host is capable of discrimination among pathogens. But, are the responses observed *in vitro* necessarily similar to those that occur *in vivo*?

How Conserved and Shared Are the Responses Seen in a Primate Host?

These observations lead to the question of disease mechanism from the perspective of host response systems. There are lessons to be learned from examining changes in transcript abundance patterns triggered by conserved signaling systems such as the NF-kappa-B regulon. Stress, infection, cytokines, and other factors trigger transcriptional responses in a large set of common genes with some variation based on the nature of the stimulus and set of cognate receptors. Yet, we know that a diverse set of pathogens have evolved the means of perturbing or subverting the NF-kappa-B response system. We have worked with several groups of collaborators in order to explore established *in vivo* models of disease in nonhuman primates caused by five diverse, overwhelming systemic infectious agents, all of which cause similar, fulminant disease in humans: Marburg and Ebola viruses, anthrax, smallpox, and monkeypox. Macaques were deliberately infected with these microbes, so that we could establish time points for infection and standardize sampling procedures, and their PBMCs were sampled over many time points, until death, which was the most common outcome in all of these infections. The overall transcriptional patterns, over time, suggested some degree of conservation among the responses to diverse stimulating agents. Yet there was also evidence of variability. At least one source of variability appears to be the infectious agent (see below). Changes in the relative abundance of blood cell subsets can also affect the apparent abundance of cell type-specific gene transcripts. However, the source of variability is often difficult to resolve due to confounding, biologically important parameters such as time and dose.

Based on the "30,000-foot view" of host transcriptional response that we obtained from these primate model hosts, we now suspect that, although the set of host responses to all microbes is largely conserved, disease—a specific host response to pathogens—acquires its agent-specific features when conserved responses are triggered at a time point, or at a location within the host, or to a magnitude, that is not usually seen when the same responses are triggered by commensals. Thus, pathogens may set off host response programs when the host recognizes that microbes are present at an inappropriate location or at concentrations higher than normally found with commensals.

Can Archaea Act as Pathogens?

Archaea are the most abundant of the three domains of life on earth, and yet it is curious that they have not been frequently implicated in human disease. These organisms do not possess the microbial patterns—such as lipopolysaccharides and peptidoglycans—that are recognized by pattern-recognition receptors such as the TLRs and NOD-LRRs. Perhaps humans (and other higher organisms) do not interface with or confront archaea with the necessary cell types or at the proper sites, or perhaps the archaea do not present the necessary patterned molecules or virulence factors to allow them to cause disease. On the other hand, it is also possible that the archaea do cause disease. However, because they are difficult to detect, we are not aware of them as the causal factors in these cases. To pursue some of these possibilities, we have focused on a common disease, chronic (adult) periodontitis (Lepp et al., 2004). In this disease, deep pockets form between the gums and teeth. The bacterial communities in these pockets may include 500 or more species and strains, a number that has been associated with the severity of disease. We wanted to determine whether archaea are present in these pockets, as some have previously suggested, and if so, identify them and examine whether they are associated in any meaningful way with the disease state. Using broad range archaeal rDNA PCR, we detected archaeal sequences only at sites with moderate or severe disease. The relative abundance of the archaeal sequences was significantly higher in severe disease than in lesser degrees of disease, and decreased in association with favorable responses to treatment (scaling and root planing) at diseased sites.

The archaeal sequences we obtained were restricted to a discrete number of clades of methanogenic archaea, suggesting that there is limited archaeal diversity in such communities. We, therefore, suspected that these particular methanogens play a role in some (but not all) cases of periodontitis. As noted by Jeffrey Gordon (see paper by Bäckhed et al. in Chapter 1), methanogenic archaea represent the "final microbial link" in the polysaccharide processing chain. In the human mouth, archaea may participate in syntropic relationships with secondary bacterial fermentors, resulting in benefits for all participants. At sites of severe peridontitis without methanogens, other syntropic partners, such as the treponemes, may substitute for the methanogens; for example, we found an inverse relationship between treponeme ribosomal DNA abundance and methanogen ribosomal DNA abundance at sites of moderate and severe disease. This suggests that treponemes—and possibly other organisms—can take the place of methanogens in the community enterprise that is periodontitis. Thus, this pathologic host response appears to be generated by a disturbed community structure, one component of which may be archaeal. This example illustrates the complexity and variability of the microbial stimuli that are capable of eliciting the same gross pathology, and emphasizes how much we still need to learn about the microbial ecology and synergy of molecular mechanisms responsible for some common forms of pathology.

Sources of Variation in Host Response to Pathogens

From a simple, conceptual framework, there are three factors that might help to determine the nature of the host response to a pathogen: host genetics, environmental factors that condition the host response, and pathogens. A recent study, which compared patterns of transcript abundance in the PBMCs of 77 healthy people, found relatively little variation among them (Whitney et al., 2003). Sources of variability among these subjects included gender, age of host, and time of the day (see Figure 4-4). Some of the most "host-intrinsic" genes may turn out to be previously unrecognized determinants of human individuality. In comparison, among individuals with hematologic malignancies, there was a high degree of variability in these patterns.

Individuals with fever and systemic infection caused by different known microbial agents displayed an intermediate degree of variability in their blood-associated transcript abundance patterns (between that associated with health and cancer). Although our analysis of patients from one study of fever and infection is so far only preliminary, the data suggest that microbiological diagnosis is an important source of this intermediate variability (Personal Communication, Popper SJ, Brown PO, Relman DA, Department of Microbiology and Immunology,

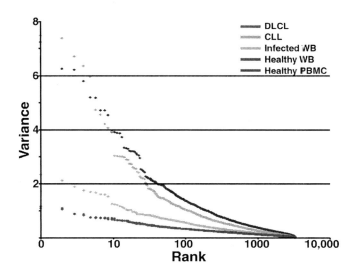

FIGURE 4-4 Variation in gene expression in health and disease. Global gene expression was measured in 45 samples from each of five studies. See text for details on each sample set. Of the well-measured microarray elements, 3,826 were randomly selected from each group and variance was calculated for each. Variance was plotted in rank order (highest to lowest) for the genes in each of the specimen groups. DLCL, diffuse large B-cell lymphomas; CLL, chronic lymphocytic leukemia; WB, whole blood.
SOURCE: Whitney et al. (2003).

Stanford University School of Medicine, March 17, 2005). Similarly, detailed analysis of the *in vivo* responses of nonhuman primates to the five systemic infectious agents described earlier reveals significant numbers of genes with transcript abundance patterns that distinguish otherwise similar responses of macaques infected with smallpox from those infected with monkeypox, and a similar general finding when any two of the infections are compared to each other. One of these distinguishing features in smallpox appears to be down-regulation of the NF-kappa-B regulon (Rubins et al., 2004). In contrast, Ebola produces a very strong NF-kappa-B response in the same host, as do many kinds of fulminant infectious disease agents. Thus, it appears that one of the sources of variability in host transcriptional response to pathogens results from pathogen-specific mechanisms that co-opt, subvert, or modify the stereotypical host response to microbial stimuli. These subtle signatures could potentially be exploited for diagnostic purposes, even during the early, asymptomatic stages of overwhelming diseases such as Ebola.

Among the other environmental factors that may determine the nature of variability in host responses to noxious stimuli (and influence the set-point of any given individual, prior to infection, for example) is the composition and structure of the host indigenous microbial communities.

Variation in the Indigenous Microbial Flora Among Healthy Humans

In my laboratory, we recently undertook a large-scale survey of the surface-adherent colonic and fecal microbial communities in a small number of healthy individuals (Eckburg et al., 2005). Microbes at six different colonic mucosal sites, ranging from the cecum to the rectum, were sampled in each of three healthy people, as were feces. Using broad-range rDNA PCR, we analyzed more than 11,000 bacterial and 1,500 archaeal sequences from these samples. Every archaeal sequence was identical, and corresponded to the known rDNA sequence from *Methanobrevibacter smithii*. Among the bacteria, we found great diversity, but concentrated within seven phyla, with a preponderance of members from the phyla *Bacteroidetes* and *Firmicutes*. Among the latter, the enormously diverse *Clostridia* class and the *Molicutes* and *Bacilli* classes were highly abundant. About 60 percent of the sequences we discovered were novel, and about 80 percent corresponded to bacteria that have not apparently yet been cultivated in the laboratory, or at least have not been recognized as having been cultivated. Among the surprises were some *Cyanobacteria*-like sequences, as well as sequences from *Verrucomicrobia*.

We looked at a number of analytical approaches for comparing microbial diversity within and between these different specimens and subjects. When we analyzed the species-level abundance of the various bacterial taxa for each individual by sample location, we found that the greatest degree of variability existed between individuals, rather than between the various sampling sites. We employed double principle coordinate analysis to assess the relative magnitude and sources of differences in community diversity between and among subjects. Once again, we found distinct clustering by individual. Although the community composition of the mucosal samples within any given individual resembled each other more than they did the fecal community from that same individual, the latter specimens were collected one month after the mucosal specimens. Thus, the distinct microbial communities that are in constant contact with the human host at sites such as the intestines and the mouth may prove to be another important source of human individuality, and may precondition the host for the subsequent responses that occur when confronted with a pathogen.

Future Inquiries

A prerequisite to answering some of the questions that I have raised in the above discussion is the generation of more complete time- and anatomic site-dependent profiles of genomewide transcript abundance in humans with natural infectious disease of various kinds, as well as during various states of health. To be most useful, such data sets should include analyses from patients infected by closely related microbial pathogens (by taxonomy or by virulence mechanism), and patients with the same clinical syndrome—but caused by different microbial agents, or patients with defined genetic differences who have been infected with the same agent. It will also be important to develop relevant animal models of disease in order to control such variables.

Concurrent analyses of host mucosal transcript abundance patterns and the composition of the adjacent microbial community might reveal the degree to which host and community determine the responses and physiological state of the other, as well as the mechanisms behind these responses. An understanding of these issues might lead to novel approaches for preserving human health, predicting disease, and treating the latter with much more meaningful end points.

REFERENCES

Bäckhed F, Ding H, Wang T, Hooper LV, Koh GY, Nagy A, Semenkovich CF, Gordon JI. 2004. *Proceedings of the National Academy of Sciences USA* 101(44):15718–15723.

Boldrick JC, Alizadeh AA, Diehn M, Dudoit S, Liu CL, Belcher CE, Botstein D, Staudt LM, Brown PO, Relman DA. 2002. Stereotyped and specific gene expression programs in human innate immune responses to bacteria. *Proceedings of the National Academy of Sciences USA* 99(2): 972–977.

Eckburg PB, Bik EM, Bernstein CN, Purdom E, Dethlefsen L, Sargent M, Gill SR, Nelson KE, Relman DA. 2005. Diversity of the human intestinal microbial flora *Science* 308(5728): 1635–1638.

Eckmann L, Karin M. 2005. NOD2 and Crohn's disease: Loss or gain of function? *Cell* 118(2): 229–241.

Helander A, Silvey KJ, Mantis NJ, Hutchings AB, Chandran K, Lucas WT, Nibert ML, Neutra MR. 2003. The viral sigma1 protein and glycoconjugates containing alpha2-3-linked sialic acid are involved in type 1 reovirus adherence to M cell apical surfaces. *Journal of Virology* 77(14): 7964–7977.

Hutchings AB, Helander A, Silvey KJ, Chandran K, Lucas WT, Nibert ML, Neutra MR. 2004. Secretory immunoglobulin A antibodies against the sigma1 outer capsid protein of reovirus type 1 Lang prevent infection of mouse Peyer's patches. *Journal of Virology* 78(2):947–957.

Kobayashi KS, Chamaillard M, Ogura Y, Henegariu O, Inohara N, Nunez G, Flavell RA. 2005. Nod-2 dependent regulation of innate and adaptive immunity in the intestinal tract. *Science* 307(5710): 731–734.

Lepp PW, Brinig MM, Ouverney CC, Palm K, Armitage GC, Relman DA. 2004. Methanogenic Archaea and human periodontal disease. *Proceedings of the National Academy of Sciences USA* 101(16):6176–6181.

Neutra MR. 2005 (March 17). *Session II: Ecology of Host-Microbe Interactions.* Presentation at the Forum on Microbial Threats Workshop Ending the War Metaphor: The Changing Agenda for Unraveling the Host-Microbe Relationship, Washington, D.C., Institute of Medicine, Forum on Microbial Threats.

Neutra MR, Mantis NJ, Kraehenbuhl JP. 2001. Collaboration of epithelial cells with organized mucosal immune lymphoid tissues. *Nature Immunity* 2(11):1004–1009.

Rakoff-Nahoum S, Paglino J, Eslami-Varzaneh F, Edberg S, Medzhitov R. 2004. Recognition of commensal microflora by toll-like receptors is required for intestinal homeostasis. *Cell* 118(2): 22–41.

Rubins KH Hensley LE, Jahrling PB, Whitney AR, Geisbert TW, Huggins JW, Owen A, Leduc JW, Brown PO, Relman DA. 2004. The host response to smallpox: Analysis of the gene expression program in peripheral blood cells in a nonhuman primate model. *Proceedings of the National Academy of Sciences USA* 101(42):15190–15195.

Whitney A, Diehn M, Popper SJ, Alizadeh AA, Boldrick JC, Relman DA, Brown PO. 2003. Individuality and variation in gene expression patterns in human blood. *Proceedings of the National Academy of Sciences USA* 100(4):1896–1901.

5

Addressing Complexity in Microbial and Host Communities

OVERVIEW

In keeping with the goal of placing host-microbe relationships within an ecological context, the two contributions that make up this chapter discuss important sources of complexity in host-microbiota ecosystems: the biodiversity of endogenous microbial communities and the networks of host-microbe relationships among pathogens that typically infect multiple hosts (which are in turn infected by multiple pathogens).

In his workshop presentation, microbial ecologist David Stahl predicted that a better understanding of the natural history of microbes—their diversity, as well as their phylogenetic and ecological relationships to each other and to other living things—will improve researchers' ability to develop questions and hypotheses that probe host-microbe relationships at the molecular level (see Summary and Assessment). His paper, which describes the use of DNA microarrays to characterize endogenous oral microbes in humans, speaks to the promise of pursing this research strategy.

Stahl and coworkers demonstrate how links between human health status and oral microbiota composition can be explored with microarray-based tools that detect oral microorganisms and monitor their responses to environmental changes. In the near future, microarray-based diagnostics may allow dentists and clinicians to detect microbial sentinels of disease in the oral cavity, permitting earlier and more definitive diagnosis, as well as improved treatment. Such diagnostics could play a key role in elucidating the apparent relationships between oral microbes and such chronic conditions as cardiovascular disease, diabetes, and arthritis, and potentially in the detection and treatment of such ailments.

The second paper, contributed by veterinary biologist Mark Woolhouse, expands the ecological perspective to address the relationships among all hosts colonized by the same microbial species, and in particular, the web of relationships surrounding the transmission and survival of zoonotic pathogens in novel hosts. Woolhouse and coworker Sonya Gowtage-Sequeira present quantitative data on the diversity of human pathogens, investigate the association between emerging infectious diseases and host range, and examine the implications of having multiple hosts for pathogen evolution. Their findings reveal the importance of taking a broad, multidisciplinary, and ecological approach to the study of infectious disease rather than focusing on the interactions between individual host and microbe species.

DNA MICROARRAYS AS SALIVARY DIAGNOSTIC TOOLS FOR CHARACTERIZING THE ORAL CAVITY'S MICROBIAL COMMUNITY[1]

Laura M. Smoot, James C. Smoot, Hauke Smidt, Peter A. Noble, Martin Könneke, Z. A. McMurry, David A. Stahl[2]

The interest in using saliva as a diagnostic medium has increased during the last decade, and recent technological developments are responsible for the advancement of its use as a diagnostic fluid (Streckfus and Bigler, 2002). There are several advantages to using saliva as a diagnostic fluid. Saliva is easy to collect, store, and ship, and, compared with the collection of blood, saliva collection is inexpensive and noninvasive, which is much safer for health-care workers (Slavkin, 1998). In the near future, salivary diagnostic devices based on highly parallel data collection methods (e.g., DNA microarrays) will be very useful tools for health-care professionals. DNA microarrays are now used as tools for developing a comprehensive characterization of oral diseases. For example, Li et al. (2004) used high-density oligonucleotide microarrays to profile transcripts found in saliva from head and neck cancer patients, and found that thousands of human mRNAs are present in cell-free saliva. In conjunction with collaborators, our laboratory is using DNA microarrays to detect microorganisms from the human oral cavity and, ultimately, to develop a microarray-based device for clinical applications.

---

[1]Reprinted with permission from *Advances in Dental Research.* 2005;18:6–11.

[2]LM Smoot, JC Smoot, PA Noble, M Könneke, ZA McMurry, and DA Stahl are from the Civil and Environmental Engineering, 302 More Hall, Box 352700, University of Washington, Seattle, WA 98195. H Smidt is from Wageningen University, Wageningen, Netherlands. DA Stahl is also the corresponding author, dastahl@u.washington.edu.

The Oral Cavity's Microbiota and Human Health

The oral microbiota play critical roles in human health and are directly linked to diseases such as dental caries and periodontitis. Although it is clear that microorganisms are intimately involved in disease, studies are revealing that the composition of the complex microbial assemblages resident in the human oral cavity is strongly associated with pathology, resistance, and predisposition to dental caries and periodontal diseases, which remain the most common chronic illnesses in humans. For example, *Actinobacillus actinomycetemcomitans* is strongly associated with juvenile periodontitis, and *Streptococcus mutans* is the primary etiologic agent of dental caries. In addition, the structure and activity of oral microbial populations may serve as sentinels of human systemic diseases. Evidence is accumulating that periodontal microbiota are involved in the development of various systemic diseases (Greenstein and Lamster, 2000; Kinane and Marshall, 2001; Scannapieco, 1998; Teng et al., 2002), including cardiovascular disease (Beck et al., 1998; Glurich et al., 2002; Kinane and Lowe, 2000), pneumonia (Scannapieco et al., 1998; Terpenning et al., 2001), arthritis (Mercado et al., 2001), diabetes (Grossi and Genco, 1998; Miller et al., 1992), and preterm low-weight birth (Madianos et al., 2001; Offenbacher et al., 1998, 2001).

More than 600 microbial species are known to inhabit the human oral cavity (Kolenbrander, 2000; Moore and Moore, 1994; Paster et al., 2001). The oral microbiota are broadly distributed among many taxonomically distinct groups, and all domains of life have representatives in the oral cavity (Figure 5-1). Only about half of the oral microorganisms have been successfully cultured (Paster et al., 2001), and the identification of uncultured and novel microbial phylotypes from oral biofilms with small subunit ribosomal DNA (rDNA) clone libraries highlights the need for culture-independent methods for the accurate description of oral microbial communities (Kroes et al., 1999; Paster et al., 2001; Relman, 1999; Sakamoto et al., 2000).

Most of the oral microbiota are organized in complex multispecies biofilms attached to hard and soft surfaces of teeth and oral tissues. Characterization of microbial population structure within oral biofilms has been studied on a spatial, temporal, and disturbance basis with a variety of strategies, including chemostat studies of oral mixed cultures (Bradshaw and Marsh, 1998), fluorescent in situ visualization of microorganisms in native and artificial biofilms with confocal laser scanning microscopy (Guggenheim et al., 2001; Kolenbrander et al., 1999; Wecke et al., 2000), and checkerboard DNA-DNA hybridization (Haffajee and Socransky, 2001; Haffajee et al., 2001; Socransky et al., 1998). Oral biofilm structure and microbial virulence are influenced by various host-associated factors, such as genetic predisposition, activity of the immune system, diabetes, and estrogen deficiency (Greenstein and Lamster, 2000). Although human health status and oral microbiota appear to be linked, the ecology of the oral microbiota (i.e., interactions of microbes with biotic and abiotic factors in the mouth) is not yet

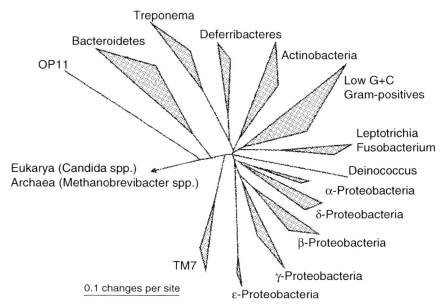

FIGURE 5-1 Phylogenetic tree generated from small subunit rRNA sequences of oral microorganisms. Sequences not yet present in the latest available ARB database [http://www.arbhome.de/] were added from public databases. Alignment and phylogenetic analysis were performed with the ARB software (Strunk and Ludwig, 1995), and the tree was constructed with the use of the "neighbor joining" method (*E. coli* position 40-1406, Olsen correction) (Saitou and Nei, 1987). The reference bar indicates 10 nucleotide exchanges *per* 100 nucleotides. Eukaryotic Archaeal (*Methanobrevibacter* sp.) branches were removed.
SOURCE: Smoot et al. (2005).

fully understood. Thus, it is essential that tools be developed for the detection of microorganisms and the monitoring of their responses to factors important in the relationship with their host, such as physical and chemical changes (e.g., pH and anaerobiosis) or perturbations (e.g., brushing and smoking) in the local environment. Ultimately, associating these responses with disease development and progression is paramount to human oral cavity research.

Whole saliva provides a convenient and reliable means to sample the oral cavity microbiota. However, salivary flow rates vary based on an individual's circadian rhythms and factors such as stress and exercise (Lawrence, 2002). Many bacteria survive and grow in saliva (de Jong et al., 1984; Palmer et al., 2001; Rudney, 2000), despite the important antimicrobial functions of saliva (Rudney, 2000; Tenovuo, 1998). Microorganisms attached to the surfaces of the mouth are continuously shed into the salivary fluid, and bacteria residing in the periodontal pockets are constantly washed into saliva by the gingival crevicular fluids (Umeda et al., 1998). The presence of these micro-organisms can be indicative of health status (e.g., salivary levels of periodontal pathogens reflect the periodontal status of the patient) (Sakamoto et al., 2000; Umeda et al., 1998; von Troil-Linden et al., 1995). Thus, the development of salivary diagnostic tools to monitor and detect microbes in the human oral cavity will provide significant benefits to the field of clinical dentistry.

Highly sensitive instruments and highly parallel methods of analysis are needed to identify the microbial sentinels of disease and to listen to their messages. Conventional microbiological approaches that rely on cultivation for the detection of microorganisms in the oral cavity are not sufficient for such comprehensive and intensive monitoring. These techniques are time consuming, require many specialized and complex growth media, capture only a minor fraction of the oral microbiota, and do not provide in vivo data of gene expression during infection and subsequent disease. Molecular techniques such as clone libraries, quantitative polymerase chain reaction (PCR), and fluorescent in situ hybridization analyses, although informative, are labor intensive and impractical for routine patient monitoring. Thus, the field needs to develop tools that provide high-fidelity data in a high-throughput format to characterize the complex microbial communities of the human oral cavity.

Application of DNA Microarray Technology to Dentistry and Oral Diagnostics

The genetic information of all living organisms is present in the nucleic acid polymers DNA and RNA. This information identifies an organism, its genotype, and its potential phenotype. DNA microarrays, ordered displays of genetic material deposited on a surface or matrix, provide a highly parallel means for the analysis of genetic information. For instance, from hundreds to hundreds of thousands of ordered DNA oligonucleotide probes may be present on a single microarray. Several types of DNA microarrays have been developed, and many reviews of the technology and its application exist (e.g., there are 34 citations for reviews of microarray technology in the PubMed database for the first half of 2004). DNA oligonucleotide microarrays are assemblages of short (from 8 to 70 bases long) nucleic acid sequences (probes) linked to a matrix. Sources of target nucleic acids (RNA or DNA molecules with sequences complementary to the probe) include reference or model organisms in pure culture, clinical specimens, and environmental samples. Target nucleic acids are isolated from a sample, labeled, and hybridized to the microarray. The nucleic acid target may be an amplified product of a gene of interest that is either labeled directly or indirectly during the PCR, or it may be directly isolated from a sample and labeled. Hybridization occurs when target nucleic acids bind to their complementary oligonucleotide probes.

DNA microarray analysis is an emerging technology that is being used in a diverse set of molecular applications (Cummings and Relman, 2000; Stears et al., 2003; Zhou, 2003). DNA microarrays were first used for the simultaneous measurement of differential gene expression of 45 *Arabidopsis* genes (Schena et al., 1995). Since the seminal work of Schena et al., multitudes of studies incorporating microarray analysis have been done (e.g., when the PubMed database was queried on *microarray and expression*, there were 1055 citations for the first half of 2004). These types of experiments provide information about what genes are up-regulated and down-regulated under certain environmental conditions, under regulator control, or in specific tissue samples. Additional applications of microarrays include the examination of pathogen genetic diversity (Cummings et al., 2004; Fitzgerald et al., 2001; Smoot et al., 2002) and the detection of single nucleotide polymorphisms (SNPs). Microarray SNP analysis provides a simultaneous analysis of thousands of genetic loci and provides insight on chromosomal regions associated with particular diseases (Kuo et al., 2003). For example, high-density DNA microarrays can be used as molecular screens for certain cancers and tumor subtypes. Specific examples include the evaluation of genes involved in head and neck squamous cell carcinoma of the oral cavity (Kuo et al., 2002). In addition to the study of oral cancers, microarrays can be used to study infectious diseases of the oral cavity. In fact, the National Institute of Dental and Craniofacial Research recently funded the Institute of Genomic Research to produce oligonucleotide microarrays (70mers) for *S. mutans* and *Porphyromonas gingivalis*. Studies with these arrays will undoubtedly lead to the discovery of novel disease-causing attributes, identification of targets for novel therapeutics, and characterization of the genetic network that allows for biofilm formation on the hard and soft surfaces in the oral cavity.

Another example of DNA microarrays is those composed of DNA oligonucleotide probes complementary to different regions of the rRNA molecules. Typically, these types of microarrays contain oligonucleotide probes designed to regions that vary in conservation, providing a phylogenetic hierarchy to probe specificity (e.g., species, genus, division, domain). Two strategies have been used to detect specific rRNA gene sequences with DNA oligonucleotide microarrays. In both cases, target rRNA hybridizes to multiple hierarchically nested probes, thereby providing a high level of information redundancy, which is an essential design feature required for confident data interpretation (Amann et al., 1995; Stahl, 1995). Using a rational probe design approach, Guschin et al. (1997) used a microarray composed of oligonucleotide probes complementary to a region of the rRNA molecule spanning bases 156–1390. In contrast, Wilson et al. (2002) used a high-density hierarchical microarray composed of over 60,000 oligonucleotide probes complementary to bases 1409–1491 of the rRNA molecule. A significant feature of these types of microarrays is that they provide the phylogenetic signature of an organism. Hence, they can be used in applications that simultaneously detect specific pathogens and characterize entire microbial populations, such as flora resident in the human oral cavity.

Our laboratory is currently using rRNA phylogenetic microarrays in the MAGIChip (MicroArray of Gel-immobilized Compounds) format (Figure 5-2B). In this format, oligonucleotide probes are covalently immobilized in three-dimensional polyacrylamide gel pads (Yershov et al., 1996). This format provides specific advantages over conventional glass microarrays with respect to microbial detection: (1) higher probe density, and thus larger dynamic range of target sequence capture; (2) a local environment suitable for performing real-time measurements of probe-target duplex stability; and (3) a reusable format that may reduce experimental variation and cost (Guschin et al., 1997). In the current format, target RNA is fragmented with a hydroxyl radical-based reaction and is simultaneously end-labeled with a fluorescent dye (Figure 5-2A; Bavykin et al., 2001). Following hybridization and washing at room temperature, the fluorescent signal from each gel element is quantified with the use of a custom-designed epifluorescence microscope equipped with a charge-coupled device camera. Nonequilibrium dissociation curves are determined with the use of image analysis software to capture intensity readings for each array element during controlled heating on a temperature-controlled stage (Figure 5-2C; Fotin et al., 1998; Yershov et al., 1996).

Although microarray technology is currently used primarily by the biomedical research community to identify disease-related genes and to characterize gene targets for clinical intervention and novel therapeutic discovery, its use in an applied setting such as clinical dentistry is imminent. Microarrays hold great promise for the analysis of oral cavity diseases, and with the continued evolution and improvement of the technology, dentists will be able to use these tools to better manage patients' health care. There are several advantages to the use of DNA microarrays in the dental setting. The ability to screen simultaneously for infectious disease agents, cancer markers, and other common oral disorders, as well as monitor general oral health over time, is clearly an advantage. The technique is sensitive, and the assay is relatively quick. Both of these issues are very important in the detection and/or monitoring of oral cavity microorganisms, especially those that are uncultivable or difficult to grow in the laboratory. Furthermore, microarray technology will allow the dentist to fingerprint a patient's oral cavity and monitor changes. This focus on preventive and personalized medicine should result in healthier patients and, in the long run, reduced health care costs.

Despite the many advantages and capabilities of microarrays, the dental community has several challenges to face before microarray-based assays are used routinely in the dental office. Once the device is developed, individuals will need training on the new technique and instruction on data interpretation and analysis. Other challenges include the high costs associated with start-up of the technology and the management and analysis of data generated by the assays. Technical promise does exist for overcoming these obstacles. For example, costs for per-

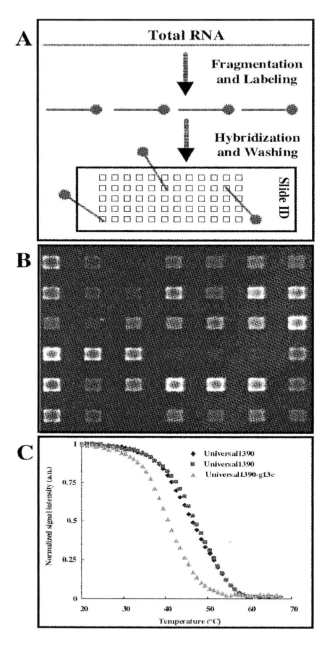

FIGURE 5-2 Description of the MAGIChip DNA oligonucleotide microarray technology used in the Stahl laboratory. (A) Simplified schematic overview of the protocol used
caption continues at right

forming microarray analyses have dropped significantly since their inception, and the competition among, and continuous establishment of, new manufacturers of microarray equipment and reagents keep costs on the decline. Scientists are also now developing and using integrated databases to store the massive amounts of raw microarray data from multiple laboratories. These databases, which are typically Internet-accessible, are invaluable resources, as they allow for the storage, retrieval, and cross-comparison of data from experiments that were conducted in different laboratories.

Technology Integration Required for Point-of-Care Instruments

Recent reviews of microfluidic technology used in point-of-care and molecular diagnostic devices highlight the advances made in microelectromechanical systems (MEMS) (Cunningham, 2001; Gardeniers and van den Berg, 2004; Huang et al., 2002). To produce microarray-based in vitro diagnostic devices for clinical use, scientists must couple DNA microarray technology with microfluidics. Microfluidics enables small sample sizes to be used, avoids reagent and waste costs, and allows for new types of assays that are impossible at macroscopic scales. Practical use of the technology in the clinical setting will require cost-effective integration of several microfluidic processes. This integrated circuitry of fluidic processes will overcome several limitations in microarray technology and move microarrays from basic science tools to devices suitable for application in the clinic. In fact, several different strategies have been used to improved hybridization kinetics and microarray fabrication with microfluidics (e.g., Cheek et al., 2001; Dill et al., 2004; Santacroce et al., 2000). However, few have attempted to manufacture fully integrated systems (Anderson et al., 2000; Baum et al., 2003; Liu et al., 2004). The merger of these technologies produces new challenges. Use of microarrays and their corresponding microfluidic support systems as diagnostic devices requires robust design and validation strategies, traditional quality assurance process control, and quality control testing. Devel-

---

to fragment and end-label total RNA directly from saliva. The RNA pool is complex, and targets can range in size from 100 bases to several kilobases. Fragmentation is a chemical nuclease reaction, where the average desired size of molecules ranges from 80–50 bases. (B) Image from a MAGIChip. DNA oligonucleotide microarray following hybridization with total RNA isolated from a human saliva sample. Total RNA was isolated from 300 μL of a human saliva sample. RNA was fragmented, labeled, and hybridized to the microarray. A portion of the microarray image is shown. Individual gel pads are $100 \times 100 \times 20$ μm. Gel pads are arrayed in a 26×26 matrix and have 300 μm center-to-center spacing. (C) Example of nonequilibrium thermal dissociation curves measured from 3 gel pads (replicate perfectly matched probes designed to detect all life, and a probe with a SNP that is used as a reference mismatch hybridization).
SOURCE: Smoot et al. (2005).

opment of point-of-care devices that interrogate oral microbiota nucleic acid targets will incorporate the economy of scale provided by microfluidics, a high-fidelity DNA microarray readout, and a highly integrated system consisting of components to miniaturize and automate cell lysis, target isolation, and target detection.

The initial steps in sample preparation are critical to the success of microfluidic microarray devices, and the variability in saliva viscosity, particle load, and microbial biomass makes these processes quite challenging. Preparation of saliva samples for DNA microarray analysis requires concentration of cells and disruption of microbe cell envelopes to make the RNA or DNA target molecules available for processing. An overview of different lysis and purification strategies is presented in a recent molecular diagnostics MEMS review (Huang et al., 2002). However, to date, no single universal cell lysis protocol exists for the quantitative extraction and purification of cellular nucleic acids from microorganisms. Integration of efficient lysis and extraction processes within a microfluidic component is essential for the development of a point-of-care microarray-based device for use in dental applications.

The method of detection and desired assay specifications dictate what processes are performed within the microfluidic component of the device. For example, if the goal is to detect a specific gene, which is present in low copy in the chromosome or is expressed at low levels, amplification strategies such as PCR will likely need to be incorporated. The current reported limit of detection with microarray technology is approximately 10^7 microorganisms, with direct detection of rRNA (El Fantroussi et al., 2003; Small et al., 2001) and with PCR-amplification of functional genes (Taroncher-Oldenburg et al., 2003). Based on recent quantitative PCR amplification studies with subgingival samples (Lepp et al., 2004), this level of detection may not detect subtle changes in the microbial community in response to changes in health status. Currently, in our laboratory, we can detect on the order of 10^6 microorganisms with direct detection of rRNA using improved labeling techniques. Further advancements in detection are enabled by microfluidic technology via increased target movement and hybridization buffer-mixing (Adey et al., 2002; Asbury et al., 2002; Liu et al., 2003).

Microarrays provide great promise for advancements in oral cavity biology for dentists in the 21st century. They should be especially useful for the diagnosis of microbes in the oral cavity because they have a high probe density that allows for the simultaneous detection of multiple microbes. As the technology matures, pivotal issues in the sample collection and processing component of point-of-care microfluidic devices include: (1) cell lysis efficiency, (2) target-labeling reactions in MEMS, (3) material compatibility with solvents and reagents, and (4) integration of multiple microfluidic processes. Key areas of future development for microarrays and detection instrumentation include: (1) improved methods of discrimination between perfectly matched hybridizations and cross-hybridization events, (2) heightened sensitivity and dynamic range of microarrays and detectors, and (3) miniaturization of detectors. The use of microarray-based devices in the dental field will allow dentists and clinicians to detect microbial sentinels in the oral cavity and provide improvements in diagnoses, prevention, and monitoring methods, which will lead to better management of patients' dental care.

Acknowledgments

The research of DA Stahl and PA Noble is supported by NIH grant U01 DE 14955-02. We thank our collaborators, J. Jackman, D. Relman, R. Lamont, and P. Milgrom. We are particularly indebted to M. Donlon, DARPA, and the Biosensor group at ANL, led by D. Chandler, for supporting our MAGIChip studies.

POPULATION BIOLOGY OF MULTIPLE HOSTS AND MULTIPLE PATHOGENS

Mark E. J. Woolhouse and Sonya Gowtage-Sequeira[3]

Introduction

Humans can be infected by many different pathogen species, and the majority can also infect other host species (Taylor et al., 2001). The same is true for those pathogens associated with emerging or reemerging human diseases (Morse, 1995). Moreover, the majority of human pathogens have probably been acquired by jumping into humans from a nonhuman reservoir (Diamond, 2002; Woolhouse et al., 2005). Hence if, as the title of this workshop demands, we are to successfully unravel the host-microbe relationship it seems obvious that we need to understand how multiple pathogens interact with multiple hosts, from pathological to evolutionary time scales and from the molecular level to the population level.

As a step towards this goal, we present some quantitative data on numbers of human pathogens, investigate the association between emerging infectious diseases and host range, and briefly review the implications of having multiple hosts for pathogen evolution. The message to take will be that it is often insufficient to consider the interaction between a single host and a single pathogen in isolation. Consequently, a broad, multidisciplinary approach that cuts across the traditional divides between human and veterinary medicine and between virology, bacteriology, and parasitology will be needed to tackle many infectious disease problems.

Numbers of Pathogens

We define a human pathogen as "a species infectious to and capable of causing disease in humans under natural transmission conditions." We confine atten-

---

[3]Centre for Infectious Diseases, University of Edinburgh, United Kingdom.

tion to the major pathogen groups: viruses and prions, bacteria and rickettsia, fungi, and protozoa. Helminths we do not consider ectoparasites. We include pathogens that have only been reported as causing human disease in a single case, and those which only cause disease in immunocompromised people. We also include instances of accidental laboratory infection, but exclude deliberate laboratory infections (of which a disturbingly large number have been reported in the scientific literature).

We obtain counts of pathogen species using an updated version of a previously published database (Taylor et al., 2001). Novel pathogens listed online by the Centers for Disease Control and Prevention (CDC), the World Health Organization (WHO) and ProMED were added to the database. Taxonomic changes were sourced from the online *Index virum* (International Committee on Taxonomy of Viruses) and its published updates (Mayo, 2002), the online National Centre for Biotechnology Information (NCBI) taxonomy browser, the online CABI bioscience database of fungal names, and standard texts (Collier et al., 1998; Schmidt and Roberts, 2000).

Total number of pathogen species in the major groups are given in Table 5-1. The grand total is 1406, which differs slightly from Taylor et al. (2001) due to new species recognition (e.g., metapneumovirus, SARS coronavirus) and of classification changes. The most diverse group is the bacteria with over 500 species known to be pathogenic to humans. We note that the definition of a *species* is problematic for many microorganisms, and so these numbers represent fairly crude measures of pathogen diversity: much of the diversity relevant to pathogenicity exists within species rather than between species.

Only a subset of these pathogens are associated with emerging or reemerging disease problems. There are several published definitions of emerging or reemerging infectious diseases. The CDC suggest: "diseases of infectious origin whose incidence in humans has increased within the past two decades or threatens to

TABLE 5-1 Counts of All, Emerging or Reemerging and Zoonotic Species of Human Pathogens and Comparison of the Relative Risks of Emergence for Zoonotic and Nonzoonotic Species for Each of the Major Pathogen Groups

	No. Species (%)	No. (Re-)Emerging Species (%)	No. Zoonotic Species (%)	No. (Re-)Emerging Zoonotic Species (%)	Relative Risk*
Viruses	208 (15)	77 (44)	143 (18)	56 (43)	1.2
Bacteria	538 (38)	53 (30)	253 (31)	42 (32)	4.3
Fungi	317 (23)	22 (13)	113 (14)	14 (11)	3.2
Protozoa	56 (4)	13 (7)	42 (5)	10 (8)	1.1
Helminths	287 (20)	10 (6)	266 (33)	8 (6)	0.3
Total	1406 (100)	175 (100)	817 (100)	130 (100)	2.1

*Risk of emergence for zoonotic species relative to risk of emergence for nonzoonotic species.

SOURCE: Woolhouse (2005).

increase in the near future." Woolhouse and Dye (2001) suggest: "an infectious disease whose incidence is increasing following its first introduction into a new host population or whose incidence is increasing in an existing population as a result of long-term changes in its underlying epidemiology." In practice, pathogens are usually regarded as emerging or reemerging based on the more subjective judgments of individual investigators, and this must be kept in mind when interpreting any apparent patterns in the data on these organisms.

We obtain counts of emerging and reemerging pathogen species using the updated version of the Taylor et al. (2001) database, as described above.

Total numbers of (re-)emerging pathogen species in the major groups are given in Table 5-1. The grand total is 175, which again differs slightly from the previously published value. The largest group is the viruses and prions, and these, together with the protozoa, are overrepresented in the list of emerging species. An obvious question is whether this reflects genuine differences in the biology and epidemiology of these groups or whether it merely reflects definition bias within the scientific community. But, at the very least, this is a potentially interesting observation that merits further investigation (Woolhouse, 2002).

Zoonotic Pathogens

Zoonoses are defined by the WHO as: "diseases or infections which are naturally transmitted between vertebrate animals and humans." It has often been noted (e.g., Morse, 1995) that most emerging and reemerging pathogens are zoonotic, but the hypothesis that being zoonotic is in some way associated with emergence cannot be tested formally without also knowing what fraction of *non*emerging species are zoonotic.

We can test this hypothesis using the updated version of the Taylor et al. (2001) database. Some care is required in the use of the WHO definition of zoonoses: for example, we do not consider pathogens with complex life cycles, with vertebrate intermediate hosts, and with humans as the only known definitive host as zoonotic. Nor do we consider pathogens—with recent zoonotic origins, but with animal-human transmission no longer being important—as zoonotic, such as the human immunodeficiency viruses (HIV). However, we do include as zoonotic the so-called anthroponoses where the main reservoir is in humans, but other vertebrates can play a minor role in their epidemiology.

Total numbers of zoonotic pathogen species and of zoonotic (re-)emerging pathogen species in the major groups are given in Table 5-1. There are several key observations. Firstly, the number of zoonotic pathogen species is large, comprising 58 percent of the total, over 800 in all. In other words, most human pathogens have a zoonotic component to their epidemiology. Secondly, the zoonotic fraction varies between the major pathogen groups; it is highest for the helminths, over 90 percent of which also infect other vertebrates. Thirdly, it is true that zoonotic species are overrepresented in the list of emerging and reemerging pathogens: 74 percent of these are zoonotic, corresponding to a relative risk of 2.1. However, the association is most marked in certain groups, notably the bacteria and the fungi; zoonotic helminths are, in fact, less likely to emerge (Table 5-1).

Cleaveland et al. (2001) looked at the nature of the nonhuman hosts of zoonotic pathogens and for (re-)emerging zoonotic pathogens (noting that many zoonotic pathogens have multiple nonhuman hosts). Perhaps the most striking observation is the breadth of possible nonhuman hosts. Across all zoonotic species the most common nonhuman hosts are carnivores and ungulates (both associated with over 300 species of human pathogen), followed by rodents, primates and nonmammals (all over 100), and then marine mammals and bats (both less than 50). The rank order is very similar for the (re-)emerging species, although these tend to have broader host ranges. Cleaveland et al. also noted that human pathogens were as likely to be associated with wildlife as they were with domestic animals, perhaps reflecting that emerging infectious diseases are often associated with human incursions into previously undeveloped regions.

Species Jumps

So far we have not distinguished between genuinely novel pathogens (emerging) and established pathogens undergoing a resurgence (reemerging). Novel pathogens can be acquired from a variety of sources (e.g., the environmental origins of *Legionella pneumophila*), but by far the most common source appears to be by jumping into humans from a nonhuman host. Recent examples of species jumps (reviewed in Woolhouse et al., 2005) include: monkeypox virus from prairie dogs (first reported in 2003); SARS coronavirus from (possibly) palm civets (2003); Nipah virus from bats (1999); H5N1 influenza A virus from chickens (1997); Australian bat lyssavirus from bats (1996); the variant Creutzfeldt-Jakob disease agent from cows (1996); Hendra virus from bats (1994); HIV-1 and HIV-2 from primates (1983 and 1986 respectively); *Borrelia burgdorferi* from (possibly) rodents or birds (1982); and *Escherichia coli* O157 from cattle (1982).

We can make several observations about this list. First, species jumps appear to be remarkably frequent. If the data are taken at face value then the human species has acquired at least 11 new pathogens from nonhuman reservoirs in the last 25 years. It may be that some of these pathogens are not truly novel and/or that they will quickly disappear from the human population. Even so, it seems highly unlikely that species jumps could have been occurring at this rate over evolutionary time scales. It is, however, more consistent with the idea that most human infectious diseases have been acquired relatively recently (Diamond, 2002). Second, humans can acquire novel pathogens from a wide range of vertebrate hosts—the taxonomic relatedness of host species does not appear to be a major factor constraining jumps. Third, the pathogens in this list are disproportionately single-stranded RNA viruses. We discuss a possible explanation for this below.

A species jump requires several steps to be successfully completed. These have been described as exposure, infection, spread, and adaptation (Antia et al., 2003; Woolhouse et al., 2005). Exposure refers to potentially infectious contacts between the new and existing host populations. This will reflect their geographic distributions, ecologies, and behaviors, as well as the modes of transmission of the pathogen (e.g., vector-borne pathogens do not require close contact between the two hosts).

Infection refers to the ability of the pathogen to invade, survive, and reproduce within the new host—sometimes termed *and expression compatibility*. Compatibility in turn reflects the pathogen's host range and the magnitude of any species barriers that inhibit transmission from one host species to another. The determinants of host range are, in general, quite poorly understood. However, for viruses one important determinant is the nature of the receptor that the virus uses to gain access to host cells. Receptors are known for approaching 100 virus species covering most families. Robertson (2002) defined *conserved* receptors as those with at least 85 percent amino acid sequence homology between humans and mice (as obtained from GenBank) and found a strong association between use of conserved receptors (e.g., vitronectin, coxsackie-adenovirus, and epidermal growth factor receptors) and breadth of host range. This is consistent with the hypothesis that use of conserved receptors predisposes a virus to jump between host species.

Spread refers to the transmission potential of the pathogen in the new host and is usually expressed in terms of the basic reproduction number, R_0, defined as the average number of secondary cases produced by a primary case of infection introduced into a large population of previously unexposed hosts. Knowledge of R_0 provides a basis for assessing the probability that a pathogen is capable of invading the new host population and causing a major epidemic (May et al., 2001). If R_0 is greater than one then each primary case is more than capable of replacing itself and can cause a major epidemic (and will do so provided it does not go extinct through chance events while the number of cases is still low). However, if R_0 is less than one then each primary case will, on average, fail to replace itself and the pathogen will die out, although short chains of transmission corresponding to minor outbreaks may still occur. In practice, only a minority of pathogens with zoonotic origins (such as HIV and SARS coronavirus) appear capable of causing major epidemics in humans; the majority (e.g., rabies and, so far, H5N1 influenza A) are not sufficiently transmissible, and most human cases are acquired from the animal reservoir rather than from other humans.

Finally, adaptation refers to genetic changes in the pathogen that occur soon after it enters the new host population and increase its transmission potential and/or its pathogenicity. Adaptive genetic change can occur via a variety of mechanisms: nucleotide substitutions (e.g., canine parvovirus); gene capture (e.g., *Salmonella enterica*); recombination or reassortment (e.g., influenza virus); or hybridization (e.g., the plant fungal pathogen *Phytophthora alni*). Adaptations which increase R_0 are of special interest when R_0 in the new host population is initially below one. A theoretical analysis by Antia et al. (2003) shows that the probability that the pathogen will successfully invade now becomes a race between how fast the pathogen goes extinct and how rapidly it can adapt to its new host. Pathogens with high rates of genetic change are expected to be far more likely to establish themselves in the new host. This may explain or partly explain why single-stranded RNA viruses appear to be overrepresented among pathogens jumping into the human population: their mutation rate is orders of magnitude greater than that of most DNA-based pathogens.

Pathogen Evolution

The expected course of pathogen evolution, once it has successfully invaded a new host population, is a much discussed topic. A particularly problematic issue is the evolution of virulence (which we take here to be broadly equivalent to pathogenicity, meaning the degree of harm that a pathogen does to its host). The naive expectation that a pathogen should evolve to be less virulent to its host is no longer accepted as a valid generalization; evolutionary biologists prefer to think in terms of an optimum level of virulence that maximizes the chances of successful transmission to other hosts (e.g., Ewald, 1994; Stearns,1999). Even so, in a one-pathogen-one-host system reduced virulence may indeed be favored in many circumstances. However, that is less likely to be the case when dealing with more complex systems (Woolhouse et al., 2001). For a pathogen which coexists in two or more host species, the optimum evolutionary strategy may well be to become more virulent in one of them. If one host is a dead end from which no further transmission occurs, then there are no evolutionary constraints on virulence in that host at all. Emerging pathogens that have jumped from a reservoir host will not have been subject to any evolutionary constraints in the novel host either, and therefore may well, at least initially, be unusually virulent.

In the longer term, pathogen evolution does not happen in isolation; the pathogen and host will coevolve. There are a number of conceptual models of coevolution. These include "arms races" in which genetic changes accumulate in both host and pathogen, and "Red Queen dynamics" in which genetic changes take the form of cycles (see Woolhouse et al., 2002). There are numerous examples of pathogen-host coevolution in the literature, but the majority of these involve invertebrate hosts. The most commonly cited example involving a vertebrate host is the myxoma virus-European rabbit interaction in Australia, in which evolution of the virus from extremely high to more moderate virulence was followed by increased host tolerance of infection and an associated partial recovery of pathogen virulence (Fenner and Fantini, 1999). There are no definitive examples of coevolution involving humans and their pathogens, but evidence consistent with coevolution has been reported for both *Plasmodium falciparum* and

HIV infections in humans. Even so, the ingredients for coevolution have frequently been reported: there are numerous examples of polymorphisms in genes involved on both sides of human-pathogen interactions and some examples of positive selection in those genes. It seems probable that many features of the human genome (including some genetic polymorphisms that predispose to noninfectious diseases) have been influenced by coevolution with pathogens.

Although pathogens do not evolve independently of their hosts, neither do they do so independently of other pathogens. Pathogens interact in various ways (Woolhouse et al., 2002). Within the host, viruses may share receptors (e.g., sialic acid is used by influenza viruses, reoviruses, and others). Some infections may predispose hosts to other infections; for example, the immunosuppressive effects of HIV or *P. falciparum* can result in other, opportunistic infections. Conversely, infections may inhibit one another; for example, GB virus C may inhibit the progression of HIV to AIDS. Pathogen interactions can also be indirect, mediated by cross-immunity, such as the smallpox and monkeypox viruses. The interactions can even be at the population level; for example, depletion of the population of susceptible children in the prevaccination era may have led to asynchronous epidemics of measles and whooping cough (Rohani et al., 2003).

Conclusions

We live in a multiple pathogen-multiple host world. A single host species—humans—has over 1,400 recognized pathogen species, over 12 percent of which are regarded as novel and/or causing increasing disease problems. Over half of all human pathogens, and three-quarters of emerging and reemerging pathogens, are shared with at least one other vertebrate host species. Moreover, pathogens not previously known to affect humans apparently make the jump from a nonhuman reservoir every few years.

All of this influences the way we need to think about host-pathogen interactions. Having multiple host species can have a major impact on pathogen epidemiology, as can sharing a single host species with other pathogens. What is more, pathogens evolve, sometimes very rapidly, but they do not evolve in isolation either from their hosts or other pathogens of those hosts. In such circumstances, we cannot view a single host-pathogen interaction in isolation, and any changes that occur, whether unplanned or as a result of human interventions, may have complex and perhaps unexpected effects.

Finally, taking a multihost-multipathogen perspective underlines the importance of a multidisciplinary approach to infectious disease problems. This in turn requires better communication, whether between medical, veterinary, and biological scientists, between virologists, bacteriologists, mycologists, and parasitologists, or between molecular geneticists, immunologists, pathologists, epidemiologists, and evolutionary biologists.

HOST RANGE AND EMERGING AND REEMERGING PATHOGENS[4]

Mark E.J. Woolhouse[5] *and Sonya Gowtage-Sequeria*[6]

An updated literature survey identified 1,407 recognized species of human pathogen, 58% of which are zoonotic. Of the total, 177 are regarded as emerging or reemerging. Zoonotic pathogens are twice as likely to be in this category as are nonzoonotic pathogens. Emerging and reemerging pathogens are not strongly associated with particular types of nonhuman hosts, but they are most likely to have the broadest host ranges. Emerging and reemerging zoonoses are associated with a wide range of drivers, but changes in land use and agriculture and demographic and societal changes are most commonly cited. However, although zoonotic pathogens do represent the most likely source of emerging and reemerging infectious disease, only a small minority have proved capable of causing major epidemics in the human population.

A recent, comprehensive literature survey of human pathogens listed >1,400 different species (Taylor et al., 2001), more than half known to be zoonotic, i.e., able to infect other host species (Taylor et al., 2001; Woolhouse et al., 2001). The survey data showed that those pathogens regarded as emerging and reemerging were more likely to be zoonotic than those that are not (Cleaveland et al., 2001; Taylor et al., 2001), confirming an association between these characteristics which had long been suspected (IOM, 2003; Morse, 1995), but which could not be formally demonstrated without denominator data as well as numerator data.

Here, we revisit these calculations, using updated information on the biology and epidemiology of recognized human pathogens. We pay close attention to possible differences between the major pathogen groups—viruses, bacteria, fungi, protozoa, and helminths. We also examine in detail the relationship between host range and pathogen emergence or reemergence, considering both the type and diversity of nonhuman hosts. We catalog the kinds of proximate factors or drivers that have been linked with pathogen emergence and reemergence and ask whether these differ between the major pathogen groups or between zoonotic and nonzoonotic pathogens.

We focus mainly on pathogen diversity (as numbers of species) rather than on the effects of disease that they impose, noting that many diseases, e.g., infant

---

[4]Reprinted from Woolhouse, MEJ and S. Gowtage-Sequeria. 2005. Host Range and Emerging and Reemerging Pathogens. *Emerging Infectious Diseases* 11(12):1842–1847. Available online at http://www.cdc.gov/ncidod/EID/vol11no12/pdfs/05-0997.pdf

[5]Centre for Infectious Diseases, University of Edinburgh, Edinburgh, United Kingdom. Address for correspondence: M.E.J. Woolhouse, Centre for Infectious Diseases, University of Edinburgh, Ashworth Laboratories, Kings Buildings, West Mains Rd. Edinburgh EH9 3JT, UK; fax: 44-131-650-6564; email: mark.woolhouse@ed.ac.uk

[6]Centre for Infectious Diseases, University of Edinburgh, Edinburgh, United Kingdom.

diarrhea, can be caused by more than one species of pathogen. However, we comment on the transmissibility of pathogens once they have been introduced into the human population because transmissibility is an important determinant of the potential public health problem.

Methods

We obtained counts of pathogen species from an updated version of the previously published database (Taylor et al., 2001). As before, we defined a human pathogen as "a species infectious to and capable of causing disease in humans under natural transmission conditions." We included pathogens that have only been reported as causing a single case of human disease and those that only cause disease in immunocompromised persons. We also included instances of accidental laboratory infection but excluded infections resulting from deliberate exposure in the laboratory. We added recently recognized pathogens listed online by the Centers for Disease Control and Prevention, ProMED, and elsewhere (CDC, 2003; Ecker et al., 2005; ProMed, 2001; WHO, 2006). We obtained taxonomic classifications online from the International Committee on Taxonomy of Viruses, the National Centre for Biotechnology Information, the CAB International Bioscience database of fungal names, and from standard texts (CAB International Bioscience, 2004; Center for Biotechnology Information, 2000; Collier et al., 1998; International Committee on the Taxonomy of Viruses, 2005; Schmidt and Roberts, 2000).

Pathogen species were categorized as emerging or reemerging based on previously published reviews of the literature (Cleaveland et al., 2001; Taylor et al., 2001), again updated from online sources (CDC, 2003; ProMed, 2001; WHO, 2006). A species was regarded as emerging or reemerging if any recognized variant fell into this category (e.g., *Escherichia coli* O157, H5N1 influenza A).

We considered the following pathogen groups: viruses (including prions), bacteria (including rickettsia), fungi (including microsporidia), protozoa, and helminths. We did not consider ectoparasites (ticks and lice). Each group was further divided into subgroups (families) to test whether biases existed in numbers of emerging and reemerging species at this level. The viruses were also divided according to genome type (e.g., negative single stranded RNA viruses).

We examined three aspects of host range, both for all pathogens combined and separately for each of the viruses, bacteria, fungi, protozoa, and helminths. First, we distinguished pathogen species according to whether they were known to be zoonotic, using the WHO definition "diseases or infections which are naturally transmitted between vertebrate animals and humans" (WHO, 1959). Note that this definition includes pathogens for which humans are the main host and other vertebrates are only occasional hosts, as well as the opposite, but excludes purely human pathogens that recently evolved from nonhuman pathogens, e.g., HIV. We then compared the fraction of emerging or reemerging species that were or were not zoonotic across the major pathogen groups and within each group by family.

Second, for all zoonotic species we identified the types of nonhuman vertebrate host they are known to infect, using the following broad categories: bats, carnivores, primates, rodents, ungulates, and other mammals and nonmammals (including birds, reptiles, amphibians, and fish). We excluded vertebrate intermediate hosts of parasites with complex life cycles. Host types were ranked by the number of zoonotic pathogen species associated with them, and rankings were compared by using Spearman rank correlation coefficient.

Third, we obtained a crude index of the breadth of host range by counting the number of the host types that each pathogen species is known to infect: 0 (i.e., not zoonotic), 1, 2, and 3 or more. We compared the fraction of emerging and re-emerging species across these four classes.

For the emerging and reemerging pathogen species, we identified the main factors believed to drive their increased incidence, geographic range, or both, by conducting a systematic review of the emerging diseases literature. We allocated these drivers to 1 or more broad categories (Table 5-2). Note that although we chose categories that we considered to be useful and informative for our immediate purposes, and which were similar to those listed elsewhere (IOM, 2003), this is inevitably a subjective procedure and alternative categorizations may be equally valid. We then ranked the drivers (by number of emerging and reemerging pathogen species associated with each) and compared the ranking of drivers for the major pathogen groups and for zoonotic versus nonzoonotic pathogens.

For the zoonotic species, we distinguished those known to be transmissible between humans, allowing that this might be through an indirect route (e.g., a vector or an intermediate host), from those for which humans can only acquire infection (directly or indirectly) from a nonhuman source. For the transmissible

TABLE 5-2 Main Categories of Drivers Associated with Emergence and Reemergence of Human Pathogens

Rank*	Driver
1	Changes in land use or agricultural practices
2	Changes in human demographics and society
3	Poor population health (e.g., HIV, malnutrition)
4	Hospitals and medical procedures
5	Pathogen evolution (e.g., antimicrobial drug resistance, increased virulence)
6	Contamination of food sources or water supplies
7	International travel
8	Failure of public health programs
9	International trade
10	Climate change

*Ranked by the number of pathogen species associated with them (most to least).

zoonotic species, we further distinguished those that are sufficiently transmissible to cause major epidemics in human populations from those that cause only relatively minor outbreaks. This classification was intended to distinguish between pathogens with $R_0>1$ in humans from those with $R_0<1$, where R_0 is the basic reproduction number, i.e., the average number of secondary infections produced by a single primary infection introduced into a large population of previously unexposed hosts. Direct estimates of R_0 are unavailable for most zoonotic pathogens.

Throughout the study, we quantified associations as the relative risk (RR) and tested for statistical significance using a standard χ^2 test (with correction for small expected values). Although these statistical analyses are susceptible to bias introduced by related species (e.g., several species of hantavirus exist, most of which are zoonotic and many of which are regarded as emerging or reemerging), the analysis at the family level is an indication of the extent of any such bias.

Results

The survey of human pathogens produced a count of 1,407 human pathogen species, with 177 (13%) species regarded as emerging or reemerging (online Appendix, available at www.cdc.gov/ncidod/EID/vol11no12/05-0997_app.htm). Of all pathogen species, 208 are viruses or prions, including 77 (37%) regarded as emerging or reemerging. For bacteria, the counts were 538 and 54 (10%), respectively; for fungi, 317 and 22 (7%), respectively; for protozoa, 57 and 14 (25%), respectively; and for helminths, 287 and 10 (3%), respectively. These numbers differ slightly from those previously published (Cleaveland et al., 2001; Taylor et al., 2001) as a result of adjustments to taxonomies and the discovery of previously unknown pathogen species. Clear differences were found between the pathogen groups ($\chi^2_4 = 154.3$, p<<0.001), with viruses greatly overrepresented among emerging and reemerging pathogens and helminths underrepresented.

Pathogen Taximony

More than 20 virus families contain human pathogens, with just 4, the *Bunyaviridae*, *Flaviviridae*, *Togaviridae*, and *Reoviridae*, accounting for more than half of the species affecting humans and, likewise, more than half of the emerging and reemerging species. Overall, no significant difference was found between the nine largest families (pooling the remainder) in the fraction of species regarded as emerging or reemerging ($\chi^2_9 = 14.9$, p = 0.09). Nor were any significant differences found according to genome type, e.g., between RNA and DNA viruses ($\chi^2_1 = 0.77$, p = 0.38) or between positive and negative single-stranded RNA viruses ($\chi^2_1 = 3.1$, p = 0.08).

More than 60 bacteria families contain human pathogens; the enterobacteria and the mycobacteria account for the most species and for the most emerging and reemerging species. Overall, no significant difference was found between the six largest families (pooling the remainder) in the fraction of species regarded as emerging or reemerging ($\chi^2_6 = 13.6$, p = 0.14). Numbers of species of emerging and reemerging fungi, protozoa, and helminthes were too small for meaningful comparisons between families, but no indication was found that emerging and reemerging species are concentrated in any particular taxa.

Host Range

Of the 1,407 human pathogen species, 816 (58%) are known to be zoonotic. In comparison, of the 177 emerging or reemerging pathogens, 130 (73%) are known to be zoonotic. This corresponds to an RR of 2.0 and confirms the expectation that zoonotic pathogens are disproportionately likely to be associated with emerging and reemerging infectious diseases. This pattern varies somewhat across the different pathogen groups: for bacteria and fungi the association is strongest with RRs of 4.0 and 3.2, respectively; for viruses and protozoa, no obvious association was found, with RRs of 1.2 and 0.9, respectively; and for helminths (which are almost all zoonotic but very rarely emerging or reemerging), RR is 0.3. However, the numbers involved are small (particularly for protozoa and helminths), and these differences were not statistically significant ($\chi^2_4 = 4.03$, p = 0.40).

All the defined host types are potential sources of zoonotic infections, but differences occurred in their importance (ranked by number of pathogen species supported) across viruses, bacteria, fungi, protozoa, and helminths and no 1 type consistently dominates (Figure 5-3A), although ungulates are the most important overall, supporting over 250 species of human pathogen. Emerging and reemerging pathogens show similar trends (Figure 5-3B), with ungulates again the most important overall, supporting over 50 species. In general, ranking of host types in terms of numbers of species correlates well both overall ($r_s = 0.79$, n = 7, p<0.05) and individually for each pathogen group. The general impression is that the emerging and reemerging zoonotic pathogens are not unusual in the types of nonhuman hosts they infect.

However, when the fraction of emerging and reemerging species is compared with the breadth of host range (as the number of host types other than humans), a pattern becomes apparent (Figure 5-4). Overall, the fraction tends to increase with host range: >40% of pathogens with the broadest host ranges (3 or more types of nonhuman host) are emerging or reemerging (exact p = 0.042). However, this trend does not hold for the protozoa and helminthes (although the numbers for these groups are small).

Drivers of Emergence

We identified 10 main categories of drivers of emergence and reemergence and ranked these by the total number of pathogen species associated with them

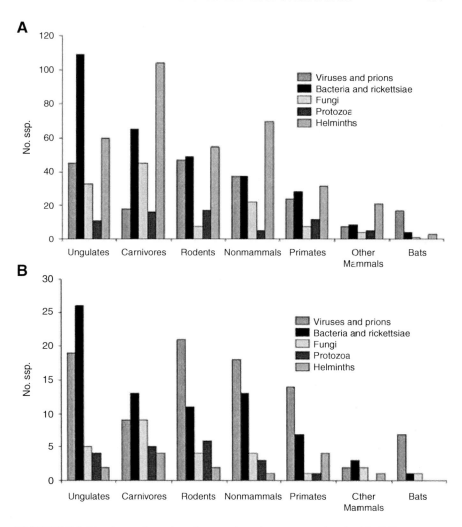

FIGURE 5-3 Numbers of species of zoonotic pathogens associated with different types of nonhuman host. Note that some pathogens are associated with >1 host. A) All zoonotic species. B) Emerging and reemerging zoonotic species only.

(Table 5-2). The ranking of drivers across different categories of pathogen showed poor concordance (e.g., Spearman rank correlation for bacteria vs. viruses, r_s = 0.41, n = 10, p = 0.24). The most striking discrepancies were as follows: (1) the marked association of emerging or reemerging fungi with hospitalization, poor population health, or both; (2) the greater importance of pathogen evolution and

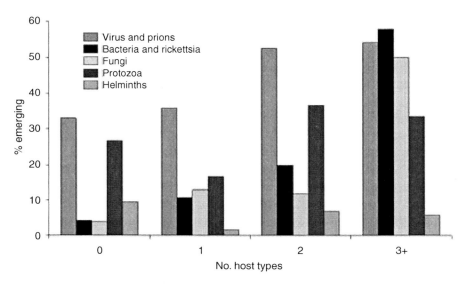

FIGURE 5-4 Relationship between breadth of host range (as number of nonhuman host types, as listed in Figure 5-3) and the fraction of pathogen species regarded as emerging or reemerging. A total of 122 zoonotic species (10 of them emerging or reemerging) for which the host range is unknown are omitted.

contaminated food and water and the lesser importance of international travel and changes in land use and agriculture for bacteria in comparison with viruses; and (3) the greater importance of changing land use and agriculture for zoonoses than for nonzoonoses.

Transmissibility

Overall, most zoonotic pathogens are either not transmissible (directly or indirectly) between humans at all (i.e., humans are a dead-end host) or are only minimally transmissible. Examples include rabies virus, Rift Valley fever virus, and *Borrelia burgdorferi* (the agent of Lyme disease). A small minority ($\approx 10\%$) of pathogen species that are technically zoonotic are, in fact, spread almost exclusively from person to person (e.g., *Mycobacterium tuberculosis* or measles virus) or can do so once successfully introduced from a nonhuman source (e.g., some strains of influenza A, *Yersinia pestis*, or severe acute respiratory syndrome (SARS) coronavirus). However, a substantial minority of zoonotic pathogens (about 25%, i.e., 200 species) are capable of some person-to-person transmission but do not persist without repeated reintroductions from a nonhuman reservoir (e.g., *E. coli* O157, *Trypanosoma brucei rhodesiense*, or Ebola virus). This pattern is fairly consistent across the major pathogen groups.

Discussion

Humans are affected by an impressive diversity of pathogens; 1,407 pathogenic species of viruses, bacteria, fungi, protozoa, and helminths are currently recognized. Of this total, 177 (13%) pathogen species are considered emerging or reemerging. This number must be viewed with some caution, given that these terms are still used somewhat subjectively. More rigorous definitions of emerging and reemerging have been proposed (IOM, 2003; OIE, 2006; Woolhouse and Dye, 2001), but these are difficult to apply universally because they require long-term data on distributions and incidences which are available for only a small subset of infectious diseases (e.g., malaria [Hay et al., 2004] and tuberculosis [Corbett et al., 2003]). Moreover, the counts of emerging and reemerging pathogen species reported here are subject to ascertainment bias. Despite these caveats, our results suggest that pathogens associated with emerging and reemerging diseases share some common features.

First, emerging and reemerging pathogens are disproportionately viruses, although they are not disproportionately different kinds of viruses. Numerically, RNA viruses dominate, comprising 37% of all emerging and reemerging pathogens. RNA viruses are also prominent among the subset of emerging pathogens that have apparently entered the human population only in the past few decades, such as HIV or the SARS coronavirus (Burke, 1998; Woolhouse et al., 2005). A possible explanation for this observation is that much higher nucleotide substitution rates for RNA viruses permit more rapid adaptation, greatly increasing the chances of successfully invading a new host population (Burke, 1998; Woolhouse et al., 2005).

Second, emerging and reemerging pathogens are not strongly associated with particular nonhuman host types, although emerging and reemerging pathogens more often are those with broad host ranges that often encompass several mammalian orders and even nonmammals. This pattern is consistent across the major pathogen groups. The determinants of host range in general remain poorly understood, but among viruses for which the cell receptor is known, an association exists between host range and whether the receptor is phylogenetically conserved (as measured by the homology of the human and mouse amino acid sequences) (Woolhouse, 2002).

Emerging and reemerging pathogens have been likened to weeds (Dobson and Foufopoulos, 2001), and that the associations reported above are likely reflecting underlying "weediness," that is, a degree of biologic flexibility that makes certain pathogens adept at taking advantage of new epidemiologic opportunities. This characteristic seems to be reflected in the broad range of drivers of the emergence or reemergence of pathogens, ranging from changes in land use and agriculture, through hospitalization to international travel. Although some drivers are numerically more important than others, the overall impression is that pathogens are exploiting almost any change in human ecology that provides new opportunities for transmission, either between humans or to humans from a nonhuman source.

Even if a pathogen is capable of infecting and causing disease in humans, most zoonotic pathogens are not highly transmissible within human populations and do not cause major epidemics. The possible magnitude of an infectious disease outbreak is related to the basic reproduction number, R_0 (Figure 5-5). For pathogens that are minimally transmissible within human populations (R_0 close to 0), outbreak size is determined largely by the number of introductions from the reservoir. For pathogens that are highly transmissible within human populations ($R_0 >> 1$), outbreak size is determined largely by the size of the susceptible population. For pathogens that are moderately transmissible within human populations (corresponding to $R_0 \approx 1$), notable outbreaks are possible (especially if multiple introductions occur), but the scale of these outbreaks is very sensitive to small changes in R_0. In other words, small changes in the nature of the host-pathogen interaction can lead to large increases (or decreases) in the scale of the public health problem (Figure 5-5). Such pathogens may be likely sources of emerging infectious disease problems in the future. However, we currently have no way of predicting whether a novel human pathogen will behave like rabies (frequently introduced into the human population, but not capable of causing major epidemics) or HIV (probably rarely introduced, but capable of causing a global pandemic).

In conclusion, this study suggests that biologic and epidemiologic correlates of pathogen emergence or reemergence may be identified. However, the most striking feature of emerging and reemerging pathogens is their diversity (online Appendix). For this reason, surveillance and monitoring of infectious disease trends may have to be broadly targeted to be most effective. Given that three-fourths of emerging and reemerging pathogens are zoonotic, in many cases this targeting might usefully be extended beyond at-risk human populations to include populations of potential animal reservoirs.

Acknowledgments

We thank Louise Taylor and Sophie Latham for their work on the original database and Ben Evans for his contribution to the updated database.

Dr. Woolhouse is professor of infectious disease epidemiology in the Centre for Infectious Diseases at the University of Edinburgh. His research interests include foot-and-mouth disease, *E. coli* O157, scrapie, and sleeping sickness. He is an advisor to the UK government on issues relating to infectious disease epidemiology.

Dr. Gowtage-Sequeira is a postdoctoral research assistant in the Division of Animal Health and Welfare at the University of Edinburgh. Her doctoral research, for the Institute of Zoology in London, was on the epidemiology of viral infections of canids in Namibia. She is currently studying the ecology of wild dogs in eastern Kenya.

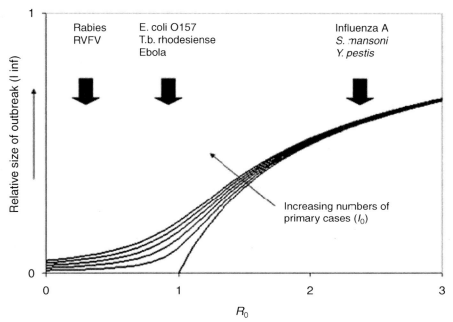

FIGURE 5-5 Expected relationship between outbreak size (as fraction of the population affected) and two key epidemiologic parameters: I_0 is the number of primary cases of infection introduced into the human population from an external source such as a zoonotic reservoir (increasing in the direction indicated); R_0 is the basic reproduction number, a measure of the transmissibility of the infection with the human population (see text). The curves are obtained from a modified version of the Kermack-McKendrick equation and show that expected outbreak size is particularly sensitive to small changes in I_0 or R_0 when R_0 is close to 1. Examples of zoonotic pathogens with $R_0 > 1$, $R_0 < 1$ and R_0 close to 1 are shown. RIVF, Rift Valley fever virus. (Reprinted with permission from [Woolhouse, 2002]).

REFERENCES

Adey NB, Lei M, Howard MT, Jensen JD, Mayo DA, Butel DL, Coffin SC, Moyer TC, Amann RI, Ludwig W, Schleifer KH. 1995. Phylogenetic identification and in situ detection of individual microbial cells without cultivation. *Microbiology Review* 59(1):143–169.

Anderson RC, Su X, Bogdan GJ, Fenton J. 2000. A miniature integrated device for automated multi-step genetic assays. *Nucleic Acids Research* 28(12):E60.

Antia R, Regoes RR, Koella JC, Bergstrom CT. 2003. The role of evolution in the emergence of infectious diseases. *Nature* 426(6967):658–661.

Asbury CL, Diercks AH, van den Engh G. 2002. Trapping of DNA by dielectrophoresis. *Electrophoresis* 23(16):2658–2666.

Baum M, Bielau S, Rittner N, Schmid K, Eggelbusch K, Dahms M, Schlauersbach A, Tahedl H, Beier M, Guimil R, Scheffler M, Hermann C, Funk JM, Wixmerten A, Rebscher H, Honig M, Andreae C, Buchner D, Moschel E, Glathe A, Jager E, Thom M, Greil A, Bestvater F, Obermeier F, Burgmaier J, Thome K, Weichert S, Hein S, Binnewies T, Foitzik V, Muller M, Stahler CF, Stahler PF. 2003. Validation of a novel, fully integrated and flexible microarray benchtop facility for gene expression profiling. *Nucleic Acids Research* 31(23):E151.

Bavykin SG, Akowski JP, Zakhariev VM, Barsky VE, Perov AN, Mirzabekov AD. 2001. Portable system for microbial sample preparation and oligonucleotide microarray analysis. *Applied Environmental Microbiology* 67(2):922–928.

Beck JD, Offenbacher S, Williams R, Gibbs P, Garcia R. 1998. Periodontitis: A risk factor for coronary heart disease? *Annals of Periodontology* 3(1):127–141.

Bradshaw DJ, Marsh PD. 1998. Analysis of pH-driven disruption of oral microbial communities in vitro. *Caries Research* 32(6):456–462.

Burke DS. 1998. Evolvability of emerging viruses. In: *Pathology of emerging infections 2*, Nelson AM and Horsburgh CR, ed. Washington, D.C: American Society for Microbiology. Pp. 1–12.

CAB International Bioscience. 2004. Index fungorum. [Online]. Available at: http://194.131.255.4/Names/Names.asp [accessed May 2, 2006].

CDC (Centers for Disease Control and Prevention). 2003. *Emerging Infectious Diseases.* [Online]. Available at: www.cdc.gov/ncidod/diseases/eid/index.htm [accessed May 2, 2006].

Cheek BJ, Steel AB, Torres MP, Yu YY, Yang H. 2001. Chemiluminescence detection for hybridization assays on the flow-thru chip, a three-dimensional microchannel biochip. *Analytical Chemistry* 73(24):5777–5783.

Cleaveland S, Laurenson MK, Taylor LH. 2001. Diseases of humans and their domestic mammals: Pathogen characteristics, host range and the risk of emergence. *Philosophical Transactions of the Royal Society of London Series B, Biological Sciences* 356(1411):991–999.

Collier L, Balows A, Sussman M. eds. 1998. *Topley and Wilson's Microbiology and Microbial Infection, Volume 4: Medical Mycology.* London, UK: Arnold.

Cummings CA, Relman DA. 2000. Using DNA microarrays to study host-microbe interactions. *Emerging Infectious Diseases* 6(5):513–525.

Cummings CA, Brinig MM, Lepp PW, van de Pas S, Relman DA. 2004. *Bordetella* species are distinguished by patterns of substantial gene loss and host adaptation. *Journal of Bacteriology* 186(5):1484–1492.

Cunningham DD. 2001. Fluidics and sample handling in clinical chemical analysis. *Analytica Chimica Acta* 429:1–18.

de Jong MH, van der Hoeven JS, van Os JH. 1984. Growth of oral *Streptococcus* species and *Actinomyces viscosus* in human saliva. *Applied Environmental Microbiology* 47(5):901–904.

Diamond J. 2002. Evolution, consequences and future of plant and animal domestication. *Nature* 418(6898):700–707.

Dill K, Montgomery DD, Ghindilis AL, Schwarzkopf KR. 2004. Immunoassays and sequence-specific DNA detection on a microchip using enzyme amplified electrochemical detection. *Journal of Biochemical and Biophysical Methods* 59(2):181–187.

Dobson A, Foufopoulos J. 2001. Emerging infectious pathogens of wildlife. *Philosophical Transactions of the Royal Society of London Series B, Biological Sciences* 356(1411):1001–1012.

Ecker DJ, Sampath R, Willett P, Wyatt JR, Samant V, Massire C, Hall TA, Hari K, McNeil JA, Büchen-Osmond C, Budowle B. 2005. The Microbial Rosetta Stone database: a compilation of global and emerging infectious microorganisms and bioterrorist threat agents. *BMC Microbiology* 5(1):19.

El Fantroussi S, Urakawa H, Bernhard AE, Kelly JJ, Noble PA, Smidt H, Yershov GM, Stahl DA. 2003. Direct profiling of environmental microbial populations by thermal dissociation analysis of native rRNAs hybridized to oligonucleotide microarrays. *Applied Environmental Microbiology* 69(4):2377–2382.

Ewald PW. 1994. *The Evolution of Infectious Diseases.* New York: Oxford University Press.
Fenner F, Fantini B. 1999. *Biological Control of Vertebrate Pests: The History of Myxomatosis—an Experiment in Evolution.* Wallingford, CT: CABI Publishing.
Fitzgerald JR, Sturdevant DE, Mackie SM, Gill SR, Musser JM. 2001. Evolutionary genomics of *Staphylococcus aureus:* Insights into the origin of methicillin-resistant strains and the toxic shock syndrome epidemic [online]. *Proceedings of the National Academy of Sciences USA* 98(15):8821–8826.
Fotin AV, Drobyshev AL, Proudnikov DY, Perov AN, Mirzabekov AD. 1998. Parallel thermodynamic analysis of duplexes on oligodeoxyribonucleotide microchips. *Nucleic Acids Research* 26(6):1515–1521.
Gardeniers JG, van den Berg A. 2004. Lab-on-a-chip systems for biomedical and environmental monitoring. *Analytical and Bioanalytical Chemistry* 378(7):1700–1703.
Glurich I, Grossi S, Albini B, Ho A, Shah R, Zeid M, Baumann H, Genco RJ, De Nardin E. 2002. Systemic inflammation in cardiovascular and periodontal disease: Comparative study. *Clinical and Diagnostic Laboratory Immunology* 9(2):425–432.
Greenstein G, Lamster I. 2000. Changing periodontal paradigms: Therapeutic implications. *International Journal of Periodontics and Restorative Dentistry* 20(4):336–357.
Grossi SG, Genco RJ. 1998. Periodontal disease and diabetes mellitus: A two-way relationship. *Annals of Periodontology* 3(1):51–61.
Guggenheim M, Shapiro S, Gmür R, Guggenheim B. 2001. Spatial arrangements and associative behavior of species in an in vitro oral biofilm model. *Applied Environmental Microbiology* 67(3):1343–1350.
Guschin DY, Mobarry BK, Proudnikov D, Stahl DA, Rittmann BE, Mirzabekov AD 1997. Oligonucleotide microchips as genosensors for determinative and environmental studies in microbiology. *Applied Environmental Microbiology* 63(6):2397–2402.
Haffajee AD, Socransky SS. 2001. Relationship of cigarette smoking to the subgingival microbiota. *Journal of Clinical Periodontology* 28(5):377–388.
Haffajee AD, Smith C, Torresyap G, Thompson M, Guerrero D, Socransky SS. 2001. Efficacy of manual and powered toothbrushes (II). Effect on microbiological parameters. *Journal of Clinical Periodontology* 28(10):947–954.
Huang Y, Mather EL, Bell JL, Madou M. 2002. MEMS-based sample preparation for molecular diagnostics. *Analytical and Bioanalytical Chemistry* 372(1):49–65.
International Committee on the Taxonomy of Viruses. 2005. Index virum. [Online]. Available at: http://life.anu.edu.au/viruses/Ictv/index.html [accessed May 10, 2005].
IOM (Institute of Medicine). 2003. *Microbial Threats to Health: Emergence, Detection, and Response.* Washington, D.C: The National Academies Press.
Kinane DF, Lowe GD. 2000. How periodontal disease may contribute to cardiovascular disease. *Periodontology* 23:121–126.
Kinane DF, Marshall GJ. 2001. Periodontal manifestations of systemic disease. *Australian Dental Journal* 46(1):2–12.
Kolenbrander PE. 2000. Oral microbial communities: Biofilms, interactions, and genetic systems. *Annual Reviews in Microbiology* 54:413–437.
Kolenbrander PE, Andersen RN, Kazmerzak K, Wu R, Palmer RJ Jr. 1999. Spatial organization of oral bacteria in biofilms. *Methods in Enzymology* 310:322–332.
Kroes I, Lepp PW, Relman DA. 1999. Bacterial diversity within the human subgingival crevice. *Proceedings of the National Academy of Sciences USA* 96(25):14547–14552.
Kuo WP, Whipple ME, Sonis ST, Ohno-Machado L, Jenssen TK. 2002. Gene expression profiling by DNA microarrays and its application to dental research. *Oral Oncology* 38(7):650–656.
Kuo WP, Whipple ME, Jenssen TK, Todd R, Epstein JB, Ohno-Machado L, Sonis ST, Park PJ. 2003. Microarrays and clinical dentistry. *Journal of the American Dental Association* 134(4):456–462; comment 134(4):1046.

Lawrence HP. 2002. Salivary markers of systemic disease: Noninvasive diagnosis of disease and monitoring of general health. *Journal of the Canadian Dental Association* 68(3):170–174.

Lepp PW, Brinig MM, Ouverney CC, Palm K, Armitage GC, Relman DA. 2004. Methanogenic *Archaea* and human periodontal disease. *Proceedings of the National Academy of Sciences USA* 101(16):6176–6181.

Li Y, Zhou X, St. John MA, Wong DT. 2004. RNA profiling of cell-free saliva using microarray technology. *Journal of Dental Research* 83(3):199–203.

Liu RH, Lenigk R, Druyor-Sanchez RL, Yang J, Grodzinski P. 2003. Hybridization enhancement using cavitation microstreaming. *Analytical Chemistry* 75(8):1911–1917.

Liu RH, Yang J, Lenigk R, Bonanno J, Grodzinski P. 2004. Self-contained, fully integrated biochip for sample preparation, polymerase chain reaction amplification, and DNA microarray detection. *Analytical Chemistry* 76(7):1824–1831.

Madianos PN, Lieff S, Murtha AP, Boggess KA, Auten RL Jr, Beck JD, Offenbacher S. 2001. Maternal periodontitis and prematurity. Part II: Maternal infection and fetal exposure. *Annals of Periodontology* 6(1):175–182.

May RM, Gupta S, McLean AR. 2001. Infectious disease dynamics: What characterizes a successful invader? *Philosophical Transactions of the Royal Society of London Series B, Biological Sciences* 356(1410):901–910.

Mayo MA. 2002. A summary of taxonomic changes recently approved by ICTV. *Archives of Virology* 147(8):1655–1663.

Mercado FB, Marshall RI, Klestov AC, Bartold PM. 2001. Relationship between rheumatoid arthritis and periodontitis. *Journal of Periodontology* 72(6):779–787.

Miller LS, Manwell MA, Newbold D, Reding ME, Rasheed A, Blodgett J, Kornman KS. 1992. The relationship between reduction in periodontal inflammation and diabetes control: A report of 9 cases. *Journal of Periodontology* 63(10):843–848.

Moore WE, Moore LV. 1994. The bacteria of periodontal diseases. *Periodontology 2000* 5:66–77.

Morse SS. 1995. Factors in the emergence of infectious diseases. *Emerging Infectious Diseases* 1(1):7–15.

National Center for Biotechnology Information. 2000. Taxonomy browser. [Online]. Available at: www.ncbi.nlm.nih.gov/Taxonomy/taxonomyhome.html/ [accessed May 2, 2006].

Offenbacher S, Jared HL, O'Reilly PG, Wells SR, Salvi GE, Lawrence HP, Socransky SS, Beck JD. 1998. Potential pathogenic mechanisms of periodontitis associated pregnancy complications. *Annals of Periodontology* 3(1):233–250.

Offenbacher S, Lieff S, Boggess KA, Murtha AP, Madianos PN, Champagne CM, McKaig RG, Jared HL, Mauriello SM, Auten RL Jr, Herbert WN, Beck JD. 2001. Maternal periodontitis and prematurity. Part I: Obstetric outcome of prematurity and growth restriction. *Annals of Periodontology* 6(1):164–174.

OIE (World Organization for Animal Health). 2006. Terrestrial animal health code. General definitions. [Online]. Available at: www.oie.int [accessed May 2, 2006].

Palmer RJ Jr, Kazmerzak K, Hansen MC, Kolenbrander PE. 2001. Mutualism versus independence: Strategies of mixed-species oral biofilms in vitro using saliva as the sole nutrient source. *Infection and Immunity* 69(9):5794–5804.

Paster BJ, Boches SK, Galvin JL, Ericson RE, Lau CN, Levanos VA, Sahasrabudhe A and Dewhirst FE. 2001. Bacterial diversity in human subgingival plaque. *Journal of Bacteriology* 183(12):3770–3783.

ProMED. 2001. The ProMED-mail archives. [Online]. Available at: www.promedmail.org [accessed May 2, 2006].

Relman DA. 1999. The search for unrecognized pathogens. *Science* 284(5418):1308–1310.

Robertson J. 2002. *Molecular biology of emerging diseases* [BSc thesis]. University of Edinburgh, Scotland.

Rohani P, Green CJ, Mantilla-Beniers NB, Grenfell BT. 2003. Ecological interference between fatal diseases. *Nature* 422(6934):885–888.
Rudney JD. 2000. Saliva and dental plaque. *Advances in Dental Research* 14:29–39.
Saitou N, Nei M. 1987. The neighbor-joining method: A new method for reconstructing phylogenetic trees. *Molecular Biology and Evolution* 4(4):406–425.
Sakamoto M, Umeda M, Ishikawa I, Benno Y. 2000. Comparison of the oral bacterial flora in saliva from a healthy subject and two periodontitis patients by sequence analysis of 16S rDNA libraries. *Microbiology and Immunology* 44(8):643–652.
Santacroce R, Ratti A, Caroli F, Foglieni B, Ferraris A, Cremonesi L, Margaglione M, Seri M, Ravazzolo R, Restagno G, Dallapiccola B, Rappaport E, Pollak ES, Surrey S, Ferrari M, Fortina P. 2000. Analysis of clinically relevant single-nucleotide polymorphisms by use of microelectronic array technology. *Clinical Chemistry* 48(12):2124–2130.
Scannapieco FA. 1998. Position paper of The American Academy of Periodontology: Periodontal disease as a potential risk factor for systemic diseases. *Journal of Periodontology* 69(7): 841–850.
Scannapieco FA, Papandonatos GD, Dunford RG. 1998. Associations between oral conditions and respiratory disease in a national sample survey population. *Annals of Periodontology* 3(1): 251–256.
Schena M, Shalon D, Davis RW, Brown PO. 1995. Quantitative monitoring of gene expression patterns with a complementary DNA microarray. *Science* 270(5235):467–470; comment 270(5235): 368–369, 371.
Schmidt GD, Roberts LS. 2000. *Foundations of Parasitology*. 6th ed. New York: McGraw Hill Higher Education.
Slavkin HC. 1998. Toward molecularly based diagnostics for the oral cavity. *Journal of the American Dental Association* 129(8):1138–1143.
Small J, Call DR, Brockman FJ, Straub TM, Chandler DP. 2001. Direct detection of 16S rRNA in soil extracts by using oligonucleotide microarrays. *Applied Environmental Microbiology* 67(10): 4708–4716.
Smoot JC, Barbian KD, Van Gompel JJ, Smoot LM, Chaussee MS, Sylva GL, Sturdevant DE, Ricklefs SM, Porcella SF, Parkins LD, Beres SB, Campbell DS, Smith TM, Zhang Q, Kapur V, Daly JA, Veasy LG, Musser JM. 2002. Genome sequence and comparative microarray analysis of serotype M18 group A *Streptococcus* strains associated with acute rheumatic fever outbreaks. *Proceedings of the National Academy of Sciences USA* 99(7):4668–4673.
Smoot LM, Smoot JC, Smidt H, Noble PA, Konneke M, McMurry ZA, Stahl DA. 2005. DNA microarrays as salivary diagnostic tools for characterizing the oral cavity's microbial community. *Advances in Dental Research* 18(1):6–11.
Socransky SS, Haffajee AD, Cugini MA, Smith C, Kent RL Jr. 1998. Microbial complexes in subgingival plaque. *Journal of Clinical Periodontology* 25(2):134–144.
Stahl DA. 1995. Application of phylogenetically based hybridization probes to microbial ecology. *Molecular Ecology* 4:535–542.
Stearns SC, ed. 1999. *Evolution in Health & Disease*. Oxford, UK: Oxford University Press.
Stears RL, Martinsky T, Schena M. 2003. Trends in microarray analysis. *Nature Medicine* 9(1): 140–145.
Streckfus CF, Bigler LR. 2002. Saliva as a diagnostic fluid. *Oral Diseases* 8(2):69–76.
Strunk O, Ludwig W. 1995. *A Software Environment for Sequence Data*. Munich, Germany: Department of Microbiology, Technical University of Munich.
Taroncher-Oldenburg G, Griner EM, Francis CA, Ward BB. 2003. Oligonucleotide microarray for the study of functional gene diversity in the nitrogen cycle in the environment. *Applied Environmental Microbiology* 69(2):1159–1171.

Taylor LH, Latham SM, Woolhouse MEJ. 2001. Risk factors for human disease emergence. *Philosophical Transactions of the Royal Society of London Series B, Biological Sciences* 356(1411):983–989.

Teng YT, Taylor GW, Scannapieco F, Kinane DF, Curtis M, Beck JD, Kogon S. 2002. Periodontal health and systemic disorders. *Journal of the Canadian Dental Association* 68(3):188–192.

Tenovuo J. 1998. Antimicrobial function of human saliva—how important is it for oral health? *Acta Odontologica Scandinavica* 56(5):250–256.

Terpenning MS, Taylor GW, Lopatin DE, Kerr CK, Dominguez BL, Loesche WJ. 2001. Aspiration pneumonia: Dental and oral risk factors in an older veteran population. *Journal of American Geriatrics Society* 49(5):557–563.

Umeda M, Contreras A, Chen C, Bakker I, Slots J. 1998. The utility of whole saliva to detect the oral presence of periodontopathic bacteria. *Journal of Periodontology* 69(7):828–833.

von Troil-Lindén B, Torkko H, Alaluusua S, Jousimies-Somer H, Asikainen S. 1995. Salivary levels of suspected periodontal pathogens in relation to periodontal status and treatment. *Journal of Dental Research* 74(11):1789–1795.

Wecke J, Kersten T, Madela K, Moter A, Göbel UB, Friedmann A, Bernimoulin J. 2000. A novel technique for monitoring the development of bacterial biofilms in human periodontal pockets. *Federation of European Microbiology Societies (FEMS) Microbiology Letters* 191(1):95–101.

Wilson KH, Wilson WJ, Radosevich JL, DeSantis TZ, Viswanathan VS, Kuczmarski TA, Andersen GL. 2002. High-density microarray of small-subunit ribosomal DNA probes. *Applied Environmental Microbiology.* 68(5):2535–2541.

Woolhouse MEJ. 2002. Population biology of emerging and re-emerging pathogens. *Trends in Microbiology* 10(10 Suppl):S3–S7.

Woolhouse MEJ. 2005 (March 17). *Session II: Ecology of the Host-Microbe Interactions.* Presentation at the Forum on Microbial Threats Workshop Ending the War Metaphor: The Changing for Unraveling the Host-Microbe Relationship, Washington, D.C., Institute of Medicine, Forum on Microbial Threats.

Woolhouse MEJ, Dye C. 2001. Population biology of emerging and re-emerging pathogens. *Philosophical Transactions of the Royal Society of London Series B, Biological Sciences* 356(Preface):981–982.

Woolhouse MEJ, Taylor LH, Haydon DT. 2001. Population biology of multi-host pathogens. *Science* 292(5519):1109–1112.

Woolhouse MEJ, Webster JP, Domingo E, Charlesworth B, Levin BR. 2002. Biological and biomedical implications of the coevolution of pathogens and their hosts. *Nature Genetics* 32(4): 569–577.

Woolhouse MEJ, Haydon DT, Antia R. 2005. Emerging pathogens: The epidemiology and evolution of species jumps. *Trends in Ecology and Evolution* 20:238–244.

WHO (World Health Organization). 1959. Zoonoses: Second report of the joint WHO/FAO expert committee. Geneva: The World Health Organization.

WHO. 2006. Emerging diseases. [Online]. Available: www.who.int/topics/emerging_diseases/en/ [accessed May 2, 2006].

Yershov G, Barsky V, Belgovskiy A, Kirillov E, Kreindlin E, Ivanov I, Parinov S, Guschin D, Drobishev A, Dubiley S, Mirzabekov A. 1996. DNA analysis and diagnostics on oligonucleotide microchips. *Proceedings of the National Academy of Sciences USA* 93(10):4913–4918.

Zhou J. 2003. Microarrays for bacterial detection and microbial community analysis. *Current Opinions in Microbiology* 6(3):288–294.

6

Manipulating Host-Microbe Interactions: Probiotic Research and Regulations

OVERVIEW

As defined by an expert panel convened in 2002 by the Food and Agriculture Organization of the United Nations (FAO) and the World Health Organization (WHO), probiotics are "live microorganisms administered in adequate amounts that confer a beneficial health effect on the host." (FAO/WHO, 2002). Contributors to this chapter discuss the meaning of "beneficial health effects" in this context, and more importantly, how such overtly qualitative notions can be replaced by quantifiable variables. The first two papers explore genetic and molecular mechanisms specific to interactions between probiotic bacteria and their hosts; two additional papers describe how the health benefits of probiotic bacteria are currently understood and how their safety and efficacy could be characterized in the future.

Recently developed genomic technologies provide a promising route to evaluating the effects of probiotics on the host-microbe relationship, according to Michiel Kleerebezem of the Wageningen Centre for Food Sciences in the Netherlands. In the first contribution to this chapter, he notes that comparative genomic studies of probiotic bacteria may lead to insights on the nature of molecular mechanisms that confer probiotic effects—findings that could be complemented by DNA microarray technology that analyzes host responses to probiotic microbes. Further, Kleerebezem describes how techniques previously used to elucidate in vivo responses of pathogenic bacteria to environmental parameters in such complex niches as the gastrointestinal (GI) tract, and that are currently being applied to probiotic bacteria, may permit the construction of site-directed bacterial vehicles for delivering beneficial molecules to the human GI tract: the next generation of probiotics.

Research in Suzanne Cunningham-Rundles' lab concerns the possible role of probiotic bacteria in the modulation of the host immune response. In their contributed paper, Cunningham-Rundles and coworkers describe recent studies characterizing the initial formation of mucosal immunity through interaction with the GI microflora—an interaction that may induce specific and persistent immune response patterns in the host, and which could potentially be manipulated with probiotics. In particular, they explore the potential of probiotic lactic acid bacteria to enhance systemic, as well as mucosal, immune response in infants and young children and the use of probiotic bacteria as antigen delivery vehicles or adjuvants in HIV-1-positive patients.

Based on the results of their efforts, Cunningham-Rundles noted in workshop discussion that she and her coworkers are preparing an investigational new drug (IND) application for probiotic-fortified formula intended for use in low birth-weight infants. The IND application process and its implications for probiotic development are described in the subsequent essay on U.S. probiotics regulatory issues by workshop participant Julienne Vaillancourt of the FDA's Office of Vaccine Research and Review in the Center for Biologics Evaluation and Research, which has regulatory authority over the development and marketing of probiotics for clinical treatment indications.

To date, all probiotics on the U.S. market fit the FDA definition of a dietary supplement ("a product taken by mouth that contains a dietary ingredient intended to supplement the diet"). Although this situation is expected to change, there is little incentive for manufacturers of probiotics—currently marketed as dietary supplements—to develop them as biotherapeutics given the rigors and expense of the associated review and regulation process. A similar situation currently exists in Europe, where several countries are currently considering legislation to require proof for health claims by manufacturers of dietary supplements. In the United States, the dietary supplement/biotherapeutic dichotomy is likely to remain a part of probiotic regulations for some time. However, as Vaillancourt notes, the regulatory process for biotherapeutics is likely to expand and change to reflect new knowledge; she identifies several issues that need to be addressed through collaborative efforts between all involved parties.

It is not only clear that guidelines and regulations governing probiotics must be revised to reflect recent research findings, but also that this goal is a fast-moving target. In the final contribution to this chapter, workshop presenter Lorenzo Morelli and coworkers describe the process and considerations that produced the recent FAO/WHO guidelines for the evaluation of probiotics in food and raise a variety of cutting-edge issues that need to be addressed in subsequent guidelines, including:

- new genomic techniques that allow enhanced characterization of the gut microbiota,
- evaluation of emerging methods that allow assessment of bacteria-epithelial interactions,

- potential for targeted probiotic or biotherapeutic methods, such as to enhance the production of a specific cytokine or to suppress a specific pathogen.

The authors emphasize the need for such guidelines to be flexible and to reflect ongoing communication between regulatory bodies and the scientific community.

MOLECULAR ANALYSIS OF PROBIOTIC-HOST INTERACTIONS IN THE GASTROINTESTINAL TRACT

Michiel Kleerebezem[1]

Abstract

Recent years have seen an explosion in the number of complete, and almost complete, genome sequences of lactic acid and other food-grade bacteria, including probiotic strains that are applied as functional food ingredients to increase the health of the consumer. This information is crucial for the development of functional, comparative, and other postgenomic approaches to unravel the in situ functionality of these bacteria in the human intestinal tract and how they affect consumer health at the molecular level. These advances can ultimately be exploited to develop novel and designer probiotics with a predestined impact on consumer gut health.

Introduction

The term *probiotics* was coined in the 1960s, although, the probiotic concept has existed for a much longer time. The definition of the term has changed through the years, but perhaps the most appropriate definition was published by an expert consultation at a meeting convened by the FAO and the WHO in October 2001, which states, "probiotics are live microorganisms which when administered in adequate amounts confer a health benefit on the host" (FAO/WHO, 2001). Although relatively simple, it defines six aspects that must be fulfilled by probiotic culture applications, while it encompasses probiotic applications outside the food market (Sanders, 2003):

- Probiotics must be alive, which redirects reference to physiological effects in hosts of the administration of dead cells or cellular fractions to an alternative term.
- Probiotics must deliver a measured physiological benefit that requires substantiation by studies performed in the target host organism.

---

[1]Wageningen Centre for Food Sciences, NIZO Food Research. P.O. Box 20, 6710 BA Ede, The Netherlands, Phone: 31-318-659629, Fax: 31-318-650400, E-mail: Michiel.Kleerebezem@nizo.nl.

- Probiotics are not necessarily administered as food products via the oral route, but could encompass other applications.
- Pharmaceutical and therapeutic applications of probiotics are not excluded.
- Restrictions in terms of mode of action are not defined; therefore, aspects such as survival of the gastrointestinal (GI) tract passage or affect on the normal microflora are not required.
- Because it is scientifically untenable to envision validated host-physiology effects convened by undefined microbial preparations, the definition also implies that probiotics are defined strains.

Despite this definition of the term *probiotics*, regulatory restrictions for the use of the term in specific applications are lagging. Moreover, probiotic health claims on products in general tend to be vaguely phrased. As a consequence, in most cases it is virtually impossible for consumers to perceive what to expect from a product carrying the probiotic designation.

Most probiotic preparations currently marketed aim at functional modulation of specific physiological aspects of the GI tract of the consumer. In this respect, it is important to note that these probiotic cultures are to exert their effects on host physiology within this highly complex ecosystem that is colonized by a myriad of endogenous microbes (*microbiota*, as described below). The species most commonly encountered in these products are specific strains of bifidobacteria and lactobacilli. The health benefit(s) attributed to these products is highly diverse, and the quality of the scientific evidence underlying these benefits is highly variable. The evidence is mostly descriptive and frequently lacks comparison of different strains of bacteria to validate the probiotic's specificity. In addition, the molecular basis of the effects on host physiology of specific probiotics remains largely unexplored. Therefore, correlating specific physiological effects measured in the target host to a specific characteristic of a bacterial strain is not yet possible. Such correlations could provide avenues toward second-generation probiotics with predestined or improved health effects.

Probiotics and the Human GI Tract Microbiota

The human GI tract is colonized by a vast and complex consortium of mainly bacterial cells. This microbiota consists of at least 10^{13} microbes, dominated by anaerobic bacteria, comprising over 1,000 species, of which the majority cannot yet be cultured under laboratory conditions (Vaughan et al., 2000; Zoetendal et al., 2004). Culture-independent molecular approaches that utilize the 16S ribosomal RNA (rRNA) genes as a universal bacterial biomarker have been used to monitor the composition of the dominant GI tract microbiota in different individuals at different time points in their lives. These approaches revealed a relatively stable composition in individual adults, but appeared to vary considerably when different individuals were compared (Zoetendal et al., 1998). Moreover, host development, host genotype, and environmental factors influence the composition of the microbiota, illustrating how microbiologically challenging this environmental niche is (Zoetendal et al., 2004). Many functions are associated with the bacterial GI tract communities and their interaction with the host system including roles in host nutrition, intestinal epithelial development and activity, education of the immune system, maintenance of the integrity of the mucosal barrier, and contribution to drug and xenobiotic metabolism. However, we are only beginning to understand the dimensions of these activities and interactions.

Next to the global microbiota-composition profiling efforts described above, dedicated 16S rRNA-based methods have been developed to track and trace specific species within the GI tract (Vaughan et al., 2005). These studies not only enable profiling the microbiota at the level of a specific species that is endogenously present in the GI tract, but also allow more detailed analyses of the fate of orally administered (probiotic) bacteria during their transit through this complex system. Nevertheless, these technologies do not allow the study of microbiota or probiotic in situ activity, and thus do not provide insight in their mode of action in relation to host functionality. In contrast, genomics-based approaches should allow the functional evaluation of host and microbe interactions at the molecular level. Such molecular studies should reveal the molecules involved in these interactions, which would allow the development of molecular models that underlie host-microbe interactions. Such mechanistic insight into the way probiotic bacteria affect health will not only contribute to novel, improved functional foods but also to the support of their health claims that will most likely be subject to an increased scientific scrutiny in the future. Therefore, these developments will not only provide benefits for the scientific or industrial community, but will also meet the interest of the consumer (de Vos et al., 2004) (Figure 6-1).

Bacterial Genomics

Over the past decade, the sequences of more than 200 bacterial genomes have become available in the public domain. Considerable attention has focused on pathogenic bacteria, including food-borne pathogens. However, over the last years, sequencing the genomes of GI tract commensals and symbionts as well as food-grade bacteria has received considerable attention. This progress includes elucidation of the (partial) genome sequences of more than 20 lactic acid bacteria and bifidobacteria (Table 6-1; Klaenhammer et al., 2005). Among these are the published complete genome sequences of species associated with probiotic health effects in humans, including *Lactobacillus plantarum* (Kleerebezem et al., 2003; van Kranenburg et al., 2005), *Lactobacillus acidophilus* (Altermann et al., 2005), *Lactobacillus johnsonii* (Pridmore et al., 2004), and *Bifidobacterium longum* (Schell et al., 2002). Additionally, the release of genomic sequences of commensal human GI bacteria such as *Bacteroides thetaiotaomicron* (Xu et al., 2003)

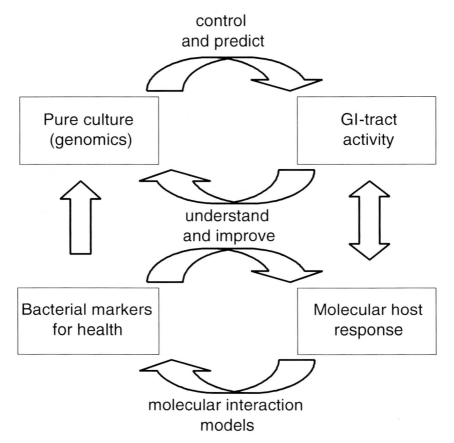

FIGURE 6-1 Schematic representation of pure culture genomics in relation to GI tract behavior, and corresponding molecular analyses of host responses. The molecular interaction models should allow the identification of bacterial and host markers involved in probiotic-mediated host health benefits. Such information can subsequently be employed to construct or select specific strains or mutants that have improved or enhanced health of the host, which would generate second-generation probiotic cultures with science-based health claims and validated modes of action.
SOURCE: Kleerebezem (2005).

will add valuable information to this field. Moreover, rapid expansion of this knowledge base is anticipated upon publication of the genomic sequences of several other species that can be categorized as (potential) probiotics (Table 6-1). The availability of these bacterial genome sequences and their annotated functions provides valuable clues towards the survival strategy of these bacteria during their residence in the human GI tract. Moreover, *in silico* comparative

TABLE 6-1 Overview of Genome Sequences of Food-Grade Bacteria. Adapted from Klaenhammer et al., 2005

Genus	Species	Strain(s)	Genome size (Mbp)
Bifidobacterium	longum	NCC2705, DJ010A	2.3, 2.4
	breve	NCIMB 8807	2.4
Brevibacterium	linens	ATCC9174	4.4
Enterococcus	faecalis	V583	3.2
Lactobacillus	acidophilus	NCFM	2.0
	gasseri	ATCC333323	1.8
	johnsonii	NCC533	2.0
	plantarum	WCFS1	3.3
	casei	ATCC334, BL23	2.5, 2.6
	rhamnosus	HN001	2.4
	helveticus	CM4, CNRZ32	2.0, 2.4
	sakei	23K	1.9
	delbrueckii	ATCCBAA365, ATCC11842, DN-100107	2.3, 2.3, 2.1
	reuteri		2.0
	salivarius	UCC118	
	brevus	ATCC367	2.0
Lactococcus	lactis spp. lactis	IL1403	2.3
	lactis spp. cremoris	SK11, MG1363	2.3, 2.6
Leuconostoc	mesenteroides	ATCC8293	2.0
Oenococcus	oeni	ATCCBAA331, IOEB84.13	1.8, 1.8
Pediococcus	pentacosus	ATCC25745	2.0
Propionibacterium	freundereichii	ATCC6207	2.6
Streptococcus	thermophilus	LMD9, LMG 18311, CNRZ1066	1.8, 1.9, 1.8

SOURCE: Kleerebezem, 2005.

genomics can provide important insight in diversity, evolutionary relationship, and functional variation between bacteria (Boekhorst et al., 2004, 2005), which might eventually generate a comprehensive prediction of microbe behavior during residence in the human GI tract. Based on the probiotic definition, it is postulated that probiotic features can be attributed to specific strains rather than to any particular species as a whole. This notion suggests that activities proposed to confer probiotic effects are expected to be variable among different strains of a species.

A clear example where this could experimentally be established is the mannose-specific adherence capacity observed in *L. plantarum* that is proposed to be involved in inhibition of pathogenic *Escherichia coli* infections via a mechanism of competitive exclusion (Adlerberth et al., 1996; Pretzer et al., 2005). It had been reported earlier that the capacity to adhere specifically to mannose moieties is a variable phenotype among *L. plantarum* strains. Nevertheless, thanks to the availability of the *L. plantarum* WCFS1 template genome and the corresponding DNA microarrays, this relevant phenotype could be correlated to a genotypic diversity that corresponded to a single gene that could subsequently be shown to encode the mannose-specific adhesion (therefore designated: *msa* gene) in this species by mutation analysis (Molenaar et al., 2005; Pretzer et al., 2005). The functional proof of the *E. coli* inhibitory, probiotic character mediated by this *msa* gene can now be established using isogenic variants that either lack or overexpress a functional copy of this gene. In analogy, application of host and microbe postgenomics tools in the actual in vivo setting enables new avenues towards more exploratory research aiming to unravel the molecular interactions between host and microbe that underly the health benefits mediated by consumption of probiotic bacteria (Figure 6-1).

Monitoring Bacterial Responses to Intestinal Conditions: In Vitro and In Vivo Approaches

Severe barriers are met by bacteria that we consume as part of our diet. These include several physical and chemical conditions, such as gastric acidity, the presence of bile salts, and stress conditions associated with oxygen gradients that are steep at the mucosal surface while the intestinal lumen is virtually anoxic. In addition, bacterial competition is high throughout the intestinal tract, but reaches a climax in the colon where bacterial densities are highest. Because the GI tract environment is highly complex and differs in different regions of this niche, many studies describe the in vitro response of bacteria to a simplified model that mimics a single host GI tract parameter. Most of these studies have focussed on intestinal pathogens, including studies describing the response toward acid and bile stress in bacteria such as *Salmonella* species, *Escherichia coli*, *Listeria monocytogenes*, and *Enterococcus faecalis*. More recent studies describe the molecular responses of food-grade and probiotic bacteria to similar stress conditions. Only a few studies describe genomewide approaches aiming at the identification of genes and proteins important for acid- and bile-resistance in lactobacilli or bifidobacteria. With *Lactobacillus plantarum*, a genetic screen resulted in the identification of more than 30 genes that are induced by bile-stress in vitro, and for a selection of these genes it could be established that induction of these genes also occurs in vivo in the duodenum of mice (Bron et al., 2004a). Additionally, a recent DNA microarray-based study in the same species revealed a number of genes and gene clusters of which the expression is significantly affected by the presence of bile acids (Bron et al., 2006). Many of these genes are predicted to play a role in the cell membrane or cell wall, which is in good agreement with several physiological studies in GI tract bacteria, including *Lactobacillus plantarum* and *Propionibacterium freudenreichii*, demonstrating how bile salts induce severe changes in the morphology of the cell membranes and/or cell walls of these organisms (Bron et al., 2004a; Leverrier et al., 2003). Overall, these in vitro studies have generated valuable insight in the responses of food-grade and probiotic bacteria to the individual parameters that are encountered in the host GI tract. However, the extrapolation of these results to the real-life situation in this highly complex niche is certainly not straightforward and requires a substantial amount of additional research to establish the importance of the in vitro responses in terms of the full response repertoire triggered in vivo (Bron et al., 2004a).

To experimentally approach the elucidation of in vivo responses of bacteria to environmental parameters in complex niches such as the GI tract, more sophisticated methods have been developed. Three main strategies have been employed for the identification of genes that are highly expressed in vivo as compared to laboratory conditions: in vivo expression technology (IVET) and recombination-based in vivo expression technology (R-IVET), signature-tagged mutagenesis (STM), and selective capture of transcribed sequences (SCOTS) (Bron et al., 2005). These in vivo gene-identification strategies were initially used exclusively in pathogenic bacteria, aiming at the identification of genes important to the virulence of these species. Recently, the first two reports appeared that describe the utilization of R-IVET strategies in food-grade or commensal microorganisms in order to determine the specific induction of gene expression in these bacteria after introduction in the GI tract of animal models. With *L. reuteri* an IVET strategy based on in vivo selection of an antibiotic-resistant phenotype led to the identification of three in vivo induced (*ivi*) genes during colonization of the GI tract of *Lactobacillus*-free mice (Walter et al., 2003). One of these genes encodes a peptide methionine sulfoxide reductase that has previously been identified using IVET in *Streptococcus gordonii* during endocarditis. Although not noticed by the authors at the time of publication, this finding already hinted at overlap in the genetic response triggered in the pathogenic and nonpathogenic bacteria upon contact with the host intestine. This notion was further exemplified by an R-IVET approach in *L. plantarum* (Bron et al., 2004b). This study revealed 72 *L. plantarum* genes that were *ivi* during passage of the GI tract of conventional mice. Functional classification of these genes indicated that prominent in vivo responses include functions associated with nutrient acquisition, intermediate and/or cofactor biosynthesis, stress response, and cell surface proteins. However, also a number of (conserved) hypothetical proteins were identified among the *L. plantarum ivi* genes (Bron et al., 2004b). Remarkably, one of the latter group of genes displayed significant homology (32 percent identity) to the conserved hypothetical protein that was identified with IVET in *L. reuteri* (Bron et al., 2004b; Walter et al., 2003), indicating conservation of GI tract responses in different lactobacilli. Moreover, a striking number of the *ivi* functions and pathways identified by R-IVET in *L. plantarum* were previously found among the *in vivo* response in pathogens, suggesting that survival rather than virulence is the explanation for the importance of these genes during host residence (Table 6-2; Bron et al., 2004b). Following the above-mentioned *ivi* gene-identification strategies, the actual in situ expression of a selection of the *L. plantarum ivi* genes could be obtained by quantitative reverse transcription polymerase chain reaction (qRT-PCR) using RNA preparations from mouse intestinal samples that had consumed

TABLE 6-2 Functional Classification of Predicted *ivi* Gene Functions in *L. plantarum* and Pathogenic Bacteria. Adapted from Bron et al., 2004b; de Vos et al, 2004

Functional Classes	Number of Functionally Classified *ivi* Genes Identified by R-IVET	
	L. plantarum	Pathogenic Bacteria
Transport and binding proteins	12	7
Regulatory functions	2	1
Energy metabolism	7	1
Cell envelope	4	0
Protein synthesis	3	0
Cellular processes	3	2
Purines, pyrimidines, nucleosides and nucleotides	2	1
DNA metabolism	1	1
Amino acid metabolism	1	2
Biosynthesis of co-factors, prosthetic groups and carriers	2	2
Fatty acid and phospholipid metabolism	3	0
Central intermediary metabolism	2	2
Protein fate	2	1
Transcription	0	0
Other categories	1	1

NOTE: The number of functionally classified *ivi* genes identified by R-IVET in *L. plantarum* during passage (left column) compared with those obtained in similar screening of pathogenic bacteria (right column). Hypothetical proteins are excluded in this comparison.

SOURCE: Kleerebezem, 2005.

L. plantarum containing food. Time-range analysis in a series of these mice revealed geographical differentiation of the induction patterns displayed by these *ivi* genes in the various regions of the mouse intestine (Unpublished observations, M. Marco, R. Bongers, and M. Kleerebezem. Wageningen Centre for Food Sciences, The Netherlands, 2005). This information could be exploited to construct dedicated, site-directed bacterial delivery vehicles aiming to deliver health beneficial (therapeutic) molecules in the GI tract of humans. The potential of lactic acid bacteria in this type of application has recently been reviewed by Hanniffy et al. (2004). In addition to in situ transcript detection, the importance for bacterial functionality in the host GI tract of the identified *ivi* genes can be established by comparative persistence and survival analysis of wild-type and isogenic mutant analysis in vivo. Such approaches have been performed in both lactobacilli. In *L. reuteri*, mutation of the methionine sulfoxide reductase-encoding *msrB* gene (one of the *ivi* genes) resulted in reduced ecological performance in the mouse GI tract as compared to the wild-type strain. Analogously, mutation of the *or*—the gene encoding the Lsp surface protein of *L. reuteri* that is implicated in adherence of this bacterium to epithelial cells—also resulted in similar in vivo performance defects (Walter et al., 2005). In *L. plantarum*, nine isogenic *ivi* mutants were constructed, mainly focusing on genes that encode proteins with a predicted role in cell envelope functionality, stress response, and regulation. Quantitative PCR experiments were performed to monitor the relative population abundance of the group of the *L. plantarum ivi* mutants in fecal samples after competitive passage through the GI tract of mice; the experiments revealed that the relative abundance of three of the *ivi* gene mutants was reduced by 100- to 1,000-fold compared to other mutant strains and the wild-type strain, suggesting a critical role for these *ivi* genes in GI tract survival and persistence (Bron et al., 2004c).

Global bacterial expression profiling of *Bacteroides thetaiotaomicron* residing in the cecum of monoassociated mice has recently been reported for the first time. By varying the mouse diet from a polysaccharide-rich diet to isocaloric diets that only contained simple sugars, this pioneering study revealed that *B. thetaiotaomicron* adapts its enzyme expression patterns to the sugars available; furthermore, upon paucity of the polysaccharides, the commensal microbe shifted its glycan-foraging behavior to the host mucous as a nutritive source, a property that aids its stability in the intestine (Sonnenburg et al., 2005). This work establishes that—although technically difficult—it is certainly feasible to monitor bacterial gene expression in the GI tract at a global level.

The experiments described above were all performed using mouse model systems, and an obvious question that should be raised is whether these bacterial responses to the residence in the mouse GI tract can be extrapolated to bacterial activities in the human GI tract. This question was addressed in a study aiming to measure *L. plantarum* gene expression in the human GI tract by analyzing RNA extracted from mucosa-associated cells and hybridising to *L. plantarum* WCFS1 microarrays or gene-specific qRT-PCR. Appropriate controls were performed and included the absence of specific hybridization in biopsies from a subject that had not consumed the *L. plantarum* cells, the absence of interference by human nucleic acids on the microarray, and confirmation of the specificity by sequence analysis of the gene-specific qRT-PCR (de Vries MC, Marco M, Kleerebezem M, Mangell P, Ahrne S, Molenaar D, de Vos Wm, Vaughan EE, Unpublished data). The ingested *L. plantarum* cells were found to be metabolically active in all subjects, and differences between gene expression between the individuals and intestinal location were apparent. Moreover, significant parallels were observed in the mouse intestine-induced *ivi* genes and those that were detected as being highly expressed in the human intestinal system. These findings support an at least partially conserved response of this bacterium to the GI tract conditions encountered in different host systems (de Vries et al., unpublished data).

The studies highlighted above give a first glimpse of what the near future could bring in terms of understanding probiotic activity in situ in the GI tract of host organisms. This information will be of critical importance to construct molecular host-microbe interaction models. However, the responses by the host to probiotic encounter should also be addressed to fill in both sides of the interaction model.

Monitoring Host Intestine Responses to Bacterial Encounters

There are not many studies available that detail the molecular response of the host intestinal system to the interaction with bacteria using a genomic-based approach. Studies in gnotobiotic mice have indicated that there is specific signalling between the commensal bacterium *B. thetaiotaomicron* and its host. Synthesis of host epithelial glycans is elicited by a *B. thetaiotaomicron* signal of which the expression is regulated by a fucose-binding bacterial transcription factor. This factor senses environmental levels of fucose and coordinates the decision to generate a signal for production of host fucosylated glycans when environmental fucose is limited or to induce expression of the bacteria's fucose utilization operon when fucose is abundant (Hooper et al., 1999).

Additional studies have evaluated the global intestinal response to colonization of gnotobiotic mice with *B. thetaiotaomicron*. This colonization dramatically affected the host's gene expression, including several important intestinal functions such as nutrient absorption, mucosal barrier fortification, and postnatal intestinal maturation (Hooper et al., 2001). From the in situ global transcription profiles mentioned above and follow-up experiments, it could be established that the production of a previously uncharacterised angiogenin is induced when gnotobiotic mice are colonized with *B. thetaiotaomicron*, revealing a mechanism whereby intestinal commensal bacteria influence GI tract bacterial ecology and shape innate immunity (Hooper et al., 2003). In addition, the cellular origin of the angiogenin response was investigated when different intestinal cell types were separated by laser-capture microdissection and analysed by qRT-PCR, revealing that angiogenin-3 mRNA is specifically induced only in crypt epithelial cells. Hence, these experiments strongly suggest an intestinal tissue-specific response of the host during colonization (Hooper et al., 2001). Interestingly, comparison of the changes in global host gene expression in mice after colonization with *B. thetaiotaomicron*, *Bifidobacterium infantis*, or *E. coli* led to the observation that part of this host response was only induced in mice by colonization with *B. thetaiotaomicron* (Hooper et al., 2001). However, analysis of a broader range of members of the intestinal microbiota will reveal what the level of bacterial response specificity within the host's tissues actually is.

One such study is currently being performed with *L. plantarum* (Personal communication, Erik Peters, M. Marco, J.I. Gordon, and M. Kleerebezem, Wageningen Centre for Food Sciences, The Netherlands, 2005). Overall, the aforementioned studies on *B. thetaiotaomicron* colonization of gnotobiotic mice provided valuable information on the influence of one particular member of the microbiota on the host. However, the host response during colonization by more complex mixtures of microbes, and/or the host response in other animal systems, remained to be investigated at that time. Recently, it was found that conventionalization of adult gnotobiotic mice with normal microbiota harvested from the distal intestine of conventionally raised mice produced a 60 percent increase in body fat content and insulin resistance despite reduced food intake. Studies of gnotobiotic and conventionalized mice revealed that the microbiota promotes absorption of monosaccharides from the gut lumen, resulting in induction of *de novo* hepatic lipogenesis. Fastin-induced adipocyte factor (Fiaf), a member of the angiopoietin-like family of proteins, is selectively suppressed in the intestinal epithelium of normal mice by conventionalization. Analysis of gnotobiotic and conventionalized, and normal and Fiaf knockout mice established that Fiaf is a circulating lipoprotein lipase inhibitor and that its suppression is essential for the microbiota-induced deposition of triglycerides in adipocytes. These results suggest that the gut microbiota have a major impact on food-derived energy harvest and storage in the host (Bäckhed et al., 2004). Another recent study investigated the host response during colonization of a different animal model. DNA microarray comparison of gene expression in the digestive tracts of six days postfertilization gnotobiotic, conventionalized and conventionally raised zebrafish (*Danio rerio*) revealed 212 genes regulated by the microbiota. Notably, 59 of these genes were also found to be regulated in the mouse intestine during colonization, including genes that encode functions involved in stimulation of epithelial proliferation, promotion of nutrient metabolism, and innate immune response, indicating a substantial overlap in the genetic response of mice and zebrafish towards intestinal colonization (Rawls et al., 2004). Despite these recent developments, an important future challenge lies within the translation of these animal host response analyses to the human system.

Concluding Remarks and Future Perspectives

At present, a large part of the consortium of bacteria residing in the GI tract has not been cultured in vitro. Because most genetic approaches require the cultivability of the microbe under investigation, the expansion of our knowledge of this group of bacteria is highly challenging and very limiting at this stage. The development of effective and robust methods to assess microbiota activity in situ in a culture-independent manner combined with metagenomic approaches will be critical for our understanding of the large number of uncultivable bacteria in the GI tract.

Historically, research on the bacterial flora of the GI tract has concentrated on pathogenic bacteria. More recently, research has expanded to nonpathogenic bacteria, including symbionts, commensals, and food bacteria. One obvious reason for this is the accumulating evidence that certain bacteria, especially strains from the genera *Lactobacillus* and *Bifidobacterium*, may have probiotic effects in humans and animals. At present, we start to appreciate the complexity of microbial distribution of specific bacteria along the human colon and the variations that can occur between different individuals. Moreover, knowledge on the activity and response of specific species to the conditions encountered when they transit through this complex niche is starting to accumulate. A promising prospect from the increasing availability of complete genome sequences is the construction of

DNA microarrays in several laboratories working on food-associated microbes. Genomics-based global investigations of gene expression in food-grade microbes under various conditions will further detail our understanding of their behavior. Besides the application of DNA microarray technology to reveal the bacterial side of host-microbe interactions, this technology also allows host response analyses. Combination of these knowledge datasets should enable scientists to unravel the mechanisms that are underlying the effects of intestinal and food-derived bacteria on host physiology, and will provide the probiotic arena with new and more scientifically solid consumer health benefits.

In conclusion, the genomewide transcript-profiling approaches that have been performed to date have provided us with clues of the possible role of individual host and bacterial genes during host-microbe interactions. Bacterium and host transcriptome information should allow the construction of molecular models that describe host-microbe interactions, allowing more pinpointed experiments in the future, designed on the basis of a molecular interaction hypothesis. Because GI tract bacteria such as *L. plantarum* and *B. thetaiotaomicron* are genetically accessible, gene deletion and overexpression mutants can be employed to study the impact of a single bacterial gene on host gene expression. Alternatively, knockout mice and/or antisense RNA approaches might allow gene silencing on the host side of the spectrum, thereby enabling the study of single host gene mutations on the in situ functionality of microbes.

Acknowledgments

My WCFS colleagues that shared unpublished information are cordially acknowledged.

ROLE OF PROBIOTICS IN MODULATION OF HOST IMMUNE RESPONSE

Susanna Cunningham-Rundles, Siv Ahrne, John Peoples, Francesca Tatad, Mohamed Mohamed, and Mirjana Nesin[2]

Abstract

Mucosal immune response is primed at birth, and responses generated at this time support specific immunity in later life. Recent studies show that mucosal

---

[2]Host Defenses Program, Department of Pediatrics, Weill Cornell Medical College, New York, NY 10021. Sources of Support: NIH NCI 29502, NIH NCRR M01RR00047, NIH NCRR M01RR6020, Probi, and The Children's Blood Foundation. Address for correspondence: Susanna Cunningham-Rundles, Professor of Immunology, Department of Pediatrics. Cornell University Weill Medical College, 1300 New York Avenue, New York, NY 10021. Telephone: (212) 746 3414; fax: (212) 746 8512; e-mail: scrundle@med.cornell.edu.

immunity is initially formed through interaction with the GI microflora. The composition of the developing microbiota in the neonatal period may induce specific immune response patterns that persist in the host. Environmental antigens, dietary factors, and nutrition can alter this interaction. Dietary factors also stimulate the growth of flora and may have selective effects on the composition of the microbiota. Infections and expression of host modifier genes can block or disrupt the establishment of controlled inflammation in the GI tract. Several lines of investigation suggest that alteration of gut microflora in association with lack of appropriate initial colonization, overuse of antibiotics, chronic infection, or malnutrition has a negative effect on host immune response. Probiotic lactic acid bacteria offer a possible approach for stimulating the GI immune system thereby enhancing systemic as well as mucosal immune response. Rigorous studies are needed to assess whether the microbial microenvironment can be modulated by the introduction of defined probiotic bacteria and to analyze the long-term potential for host defense.

Introduction

Mucosal membrane surfaces provide the strategic interface between the internal and external world and contain a large and variable antigenic load (Didierlaurent et al., 2002). In addition to the indigenous mucosal microbiota, the mucosal immune system must respond to potential microbial pathogens, food antigens, and environmental allergens (Eberl, 2005). Most infectious diseases are acquired by, or affect, mucosal surfaces such that preventive and protective host defenses require mucosal response. The gut immune system contains the highest numbers of macrophages, plasma cells, and T lymphocytes in the body. This highly specialized immune system is based on anatomical separation of inductive and effector sites, compartmentalization of pattern recognition receptors, and distinctive cellular functions that bridge innate and adaptive immune response (Hall et al., 1994; Macdonald and Monteleone, 2005; Pabst, 1987). Mucosal immune response is characteristically skewed towards a T helper type2 (Th2) cytokine pattern dominated by production of interleukin 4 (IL-4) and IL-5, which supports B-cell differentiation and the development of antibodies. Response to infection is mediated by secretory IgA antibodies and mucosal cytotoxic T cells and a highly developed innate immune response (Kelly and Conway, 2005; Knight et al., 2004; Rakoff-Nahoum et al., 2004).

The presence of large populations of commensal bacteria has a major influence on the development of immune response that is only now beginning to be studied in detail. Commensal flora directly activate the mucosal immune system leading to the development of Peyer's patches and to IgA plasma cells and CD4+T cells in the lamina propria. Maturation of the mucosal immune system and establishment of protective immunity varies between individuals but is usually fully developed in the first year of life, regardless of gestational age at birth. Experimental studies have shown that mucosal immune response is primed in the neonate and that responses generated at this time are retained in later life (Harrod et al., 2001). Host response exerts a selective pressure on colonizing species, as shown by longitudinal study of secretory immune response in saliva to colonizing bacteria in infants during tooth eruption (Cole et al., 1998). The evolution of bacterial species in the gut microflora over a lifetime has not been studied extensively, but preliminary studies indicate a possible increase in the species diversity of the dominant microflora with aging (Blaut et al., 2002; Saunier and Dore, 2002). One study indicates that a general reduction in specific serum IgM antibody to commensals may occur in old age, which could lead to relaxation of selective pressure and outgrowth of less benign bacterial populations. This may have relevance for increasing infections and decreased immune response in older people (Percival et al., 1996). A relationship between altered microflora and cancer may also exist, for example, through effects on levels of isothiocyanates, which mediate the cancer-protective effects of cruciferous vegetables (Rouzaud et al., 2003). Generally, microflora influence maintenance of intestinal homeostasis through direct effects on the development of organized lymphoid tissue (Rhee et al., 2004) and prevention of inflammation.

Recent studies show that gut bacteria induce cross-talk between epithelial cells and dendritic cells that leads to the release of IL-10 and IL-6 and, therefore, drive the polarization of T cells toward a noninflammatory Th2 response that is maintained even after exposure to Th1-inducing pathogens (Rimoldi et al., 2005). Intestinal immune stability depends upon the function of toll-like receptors (TLRs) and the nucleotide oligomerization domain NOD1 and NOD2 pattern-recognition receptors to convert the recognition of pathogen-associated molecules expressed by enteric bacteria in the gut into signals for antimicrobial peptide expression, barrier fortification, and proliferation of epithelial cells. This process can be blocked or disrupted by infections, or by the expression of certain host polymorphisms in the TLR or NOD genes that lead to uncontrolled gut inflammation, as in inflammatory bowel disease (IBD) (Abreu et al., 2005). Other critical influences on gut microflora include environmental antigens, dietary factors, and nutrients (Cunningham-Rundles, 2001; Macdonald and Monteleone, 2005; Pacha, 2000). Nondigestible dietary factors stimulate the growth of flora and have selective effects on the composition of the microbiota (Roller et al., 2004). The gut microbiota as a whole is essential for production of short-chain fatty acids from polysaccharides and has been shown to regulate host metabolism through direct effects on fat storage (Bäckhed et al., 2004). The interaction of host immune response and the microbiota may, therefore, indirectly influence metabolism.

How the gut immune system distinguishes between pathogenic and commensal bacteria is unclear. A pathogenic immune response in the gut wall characterized by a highly polarized Th1 response is the hallmark of Crohn's disease, and this response is probably directed against antigens of the commensal flora

(Macdonald et al., 2005). Commensal flora interact with the gut epithelium to stimulate the development of gut barrier function and this mutualism nonspecifically regulates inflammation (Macdonald and Monteleone, 2005). Development of immune tolerance towards food and environmental antigens, including commensal bacteria, is a central requirement for gut homeostasis. The primary mediators now appear to be regulatory T cells and dendritic cells that down regulate inflammatory response through production of IL-10 and transformation of growth factor beta-1 (Bilsborough and Viney, 2004; Caramalho et al., 2003). Tolerance to commensal antigens involves active suppression of T cell response has not been established.

Host-bacterial interaction has general implications for the development of adaptive immune response to environmental antigens and allergens in early childhood. A functional relationship between the composition of microflora and presence or absence of allergies and atopic disease in children has been shown by several well-constructed and thorough studies. These include a report of reduced colonization with lactobacilli and higher counts of aerobic bacteria in a large study of allergic children (Bjorksten et al., 1999) and the demonstration that characteristic differences in neonatal gut flora precede development of allergic responses (Kalliomaki et al., 2001a). In particular the microbiota of allergic children were less often colonized with lactobacilli and bifidobacteria. These findings led to a definitive study in which perinatal administration of probiotic lactobacilli was shown to decrease presentation of eczema in high-risk children (Kalliomaki et al., 2001b).

The concept that supplementation with some bacteria would lead to elective colonization and would prevent outgrowth of more pathogenic bacteria was originally proposed by Metchnicoff (1907). The term *probiotic* is generally accepted to include, "live microorganisms which when administered . . . confer a health benefit on the host" (Reid et al., 2003). Probiotic bacterial supplementation has shown consistent effects on resolution of antibiotic-associated diarrhea (Arvola et al., 1999) and recovery from acute diarrhea caused by rotavirus infection (Guandalini et al., 2000). In addition, combinations of lactobacilli, bifidobacteria, and *Streptococcus salivarius* prevent relapse of recurrent pouchitis, and may decrease the initial onset of pouch inflammation. Also, *Escherichia coli* strain Nissle 1917 is reported to maintain remission in ulcerative colitis (Sartor, 2005). These effects may be mediated by production of antimicrobial substances, local competition for adhesion receptors and nutrients, and stimulation of intestinal antigen-specific and nonspecific-immune responses. However, efforts to improve IBD and irritable bowel syndrome with probiotic bacterial supplementation have only had limited success, perhaps because the central mechanism of these disorders appears to involve altered host response to commensal flora (Schultz et al., 2004b). With the exception of prophylactic treatment of children at risk for atopic disease that clearly involves direct immunoregulatory effects, probiotic bacteria appear to stimulate enhancement of recovery through acute effects on the microbiota. It is possible that in adults the resident flora and interactive host response compose a formidable barrier that is not as readily affected by short-term colonization. Adult human flora appear to have a constrained diversity as only a limited number of bacterial divisions have been identified (Bäckhed et al., 2005). One study suggests that gut populations are fairly stable within individuals over time (Bäckhed et al., 2005; Zoetendal et al., 2004). However, another report, also on a few subjects, suggests marked variability over time (Barcenilla et al., 2000).

In summary, current studies suggest that host interaction with the microbiota shapes mucosal immune response. These studies also support the concept that probiotic bacteria could influence host response, as well as composition of the microbiota, at least transiently. Because host microbial cross-talk is initiated at birth and the immune system is primed by this exposure over the first year of life, studies in children may have unique potency. Settings of interest, including the low birth-weight infant and the immune compromised child, are discussed in the following sections.

Neonatal Response to Commensal Microbes

After birth, bacteria are always present in great abundance on skin and in the GI tract, and critical development of immune function occurs in early neonatal life in response to microbial colonization. Th2-skewed immune response prevails systemically in the neonate, and contact with microbial antigens acts to repolarize this orientation gradually during the first months of life (Prescott et al., 1998). Studies strongly suggest that absence of exposure to appropriate microbial signals and lack of a Th2 to Th1 switch is associated with allergic disease in high-risk children. Generally infants are initially colonized with *Escherichia coli* and streptococci and then by anaerobes belonging to *Bacteroides*, *Bifidobacterium*, and *Clostridia*. In contrast to formula-fed infants, bifidobacteria and lactobacilli predominate in the breast-fed infant. Breast-fed infants have higher levels of lactic acid bacteria and enhanced mucosal immune response (Martin et al., 2003). Our recent studies in healthy infants show that certain lactobacillus species, especially *L. rhamnosus*, thrive in the intestinal flora of breast-fed infants. After weaning, they are replaced by other lactobacillus species found in food (Ahrne et al., 2005).

Neonates usually acquire bacterial pathogens transplacentally. Most commonly these are Group B beta-hemolytic *Streptococcus* (GBBS), and gram-negative flora, *E. coli*, and *Listeria monocytogenes*. Premature neonates can acquire nosocomial infections and develop staphylococcal, enterococcal, and *P. aeruginosa* infections in association with hospitalization. Because the neonate is born with an immature immune system, there is a critical period when encounter with microbes may cause serious infection. Exposure to pathogens in association with prematurity adds an additional stress that can alter the development of normal immune response and is also likely to affect the composition of the microbiota. Some microorganisms, like coagulase negative staphylococci, rarely enter an uninterrupted mucosal barrier, although they can colonize it. Others, like GBBS, are actively transferred into cytoplasm of respiratory epithelial cells. Because maternal IgG antibodies acquired passively drop in the first days of life, pathogen-specific antibodies are decreased or absent, and neonates must depend upon the innate immune system (Cunningham-Rundles and Nesin, 2000).

Probiotic bacteria have been given to infants primarily for prophylaxis and alleviation of diarrheal disease, reduction in atopic disease, reduction in necrotizing enterocolitis, and reduction in infection, with generally beneficial effects (Kliegman, 2005; Schrezenmeir et al., 2004). In addition, there is increasing interest in the possible use of probiotics to promote the development of immune response (Huang et al., 2003). Immaturity of the neonatal immune response contributes significantly to the severity and morbidity of response to infections and to bacterial antigens. Recent studies indicate that both term and preterm infants have an increased capacity to produce inflammatory cytokines (Schultz et al., 2004a) and a decreased compensatory anti-inflammatory response syndrome that may predispose preterm infants to harmful effects of proinflammatory cytokines (Schultz et al., 2004a). The consequences of enhanced proinflammatory responses are implicated in the pathogenesis of neonatal disease (Goepfert et al., 2004; Huang et al., 2004). Although probiotic bacteria are generally regarded as safe and benefits from treatment are substantial, translocation of indigenous lactobacillus from a catheter is possible, and two cases of lactobacillus bacteremia from probiotic treatment in short bowel syndrome have been reported (Kunz et al., 2004; Thompson et al., 2001).

In previous studies, we observed that premature infants had a heightened proliferative response in vitro to *S. epidermidis* compared to adults in the first weeks of life suggesting a strong modulatory effect postbirth (Veber et al., 1991). Although *S. epidermidis* is a normal colonizer of human skin, rarely causing disease in term infants, this is the most common cause of late-onset sepsis in preterm infants. To ascertain if the neonate has a stereotypical response to microbes, we are analyzing the relative response of memory and naive T cells from cord blood of healthy term infants to specific microbial activators, *L. plantarum*, *S. epidermidis*, GBBS, and *E. coli* to determine if lack of memory T cells might be a barrier to response. Both CD4+ and CD8+RA+ cord blood T cells responded to *L. plantarum* and *S. epidermidis*, but only CD8+RA+ cells showed significant response to GBBS. Data in Figure 6-2 show the response of CD8+T cells as detected by the up-regulation of CD69 expression. Although memory response was essentially absent, as there are very few memory T cells in cord blood, naive cells were strongly activated by all tested microbial antigens. In addition, we are evaluating the specificity of cytokine response at the level of the producer cell using intracellular cytokine detection by flow cytometry. As shown in Figure 6-3, *E. coli* induced higher levels of both IL-6 and IL-8 production in cord blood monocytes compared to levels induced by *L. plantarum*. Insignificant production

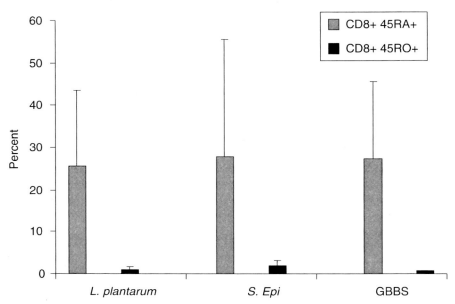

FIGURE 6-2 Response of CD8+ naive (CD45RA+) and CD8+ memory (CD45 RO+) cord blood T cells to bacterial antigens. Data are shown as percent of gated populations expressing CD69 after 18 hours of culture with whole inactivated bacterial cells. The three microbial activators on the x axis are L. plantarum, S. epidermidis, and Group B beta-hemolytic Streptococcus (GBBS).
SOURCE: Cunningham-Rundels (2005).

of either mediator was observed in T cells. These results indicate that the innate immune response in newborns to commensal bacteria is strong, and they also suggest that specific bacterial strains may have differential effects on the maturation of the immune system.

Response to Lactobacillus in HIV-1 Immune Deficiency

Primary immune deficiency is associated with sinopulmonary or GI infections, autoimmunity, and neoplasia (Kalha and Sellin, 2004, Cunningham-Rundles, 1994). Selective IgA deficiency carries an increased risk of celiac disease, IBD, and perhaps also GI malignancy. Recent studies suggest that IgA-deficient individuals carry an increased frequency of *E. coli* with potentially inflammatory properties in their microflora, which may contribute to the development of GI disorders such as IBD (Friman et al., 2002). Secondary immune deficiency caused by HIV-I infection is associated with increased risk of

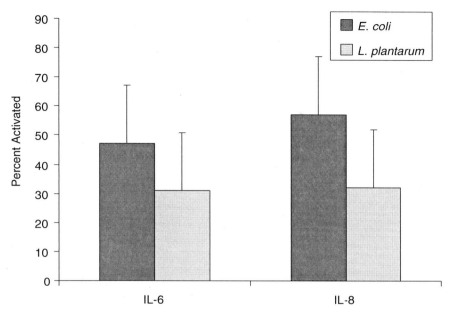

FIGURE 6-3 Intracellular cytokine response of cord blood monocytes from term infants to bacterial antigens. Data are shown as percent of monocytes producing the denoted cytokines after 18 hours of culture.
SOURCE: Cunningham-Rundels (2005).

GI malignancy (Crump et al., 1999). CD4+ T cell depletion during all stages of HIV disease occurs predominantly in the GI tract (Brenchley et al., 2004). The introduction of highly active antiretroviral therapy has resulted in a significant decrease in the incidence of opportunistic enteric pathogens as a consequence of immune recovery. Nonetheless, patients with advanced HIV-1 disease who were recently diagnosed or have a poor response to HAART can still suffer from a wide range of enteric pathogens. Bacterial vaginosis is associated with human immunodeficiency virus (HIV) acquisition, and this condition is associated with reduction of lactobacilli. Interestingly, inhibition of HIV infectivity has been shown with a natural human isolate of lactobacilli engineered to express functional 2-domain CD4 9 (Chang et al., 2003).

HIV-1 may play a direct enteropathogenic role and is implicated in both diarrhea and intestinal dysfunction. HIV-1-associated failure to thrive was a relatively common presentation in congenital HIV infection before the introduction of HAART, yet less severe growth problems still persist (Nachman et al., 2005; Watson and Counts, 2004). We have studied the effect of *L. plantarum* 299v in

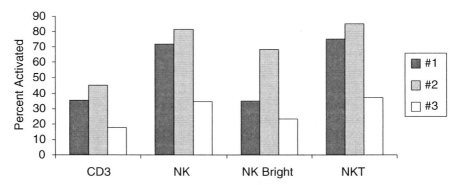

FIGURE 6-4 Differential response of T cells (CD3+) and natural killer (NK) subpopulations defined as NK (CD3–CD56+), NK bright (CD3–CD56+bright), and NKT (CD56+ CD3+) lymphocytes from HIV-positive children to bacterial antigens. Data are shown as percent of activated cells identified by up-regulation of CD69 after 18 hours of culture.
SOURCE: Cunningham-Rundles (2005).

the HIV-1-positive child for impact on growth and on specific systemic immune response following oral supplementation and found a growth benefit in advanced HIV-1 infection (Cunningham-Rundles et al., 2000). The level of immune response in vitro in HIV-1-positive children was essentially independent of percentage of CD4+ T cells unlike response to any other activator where level of response is strongly associated with CD4 T cell level (Cunningham-Rundles and Nesin, 2000). Comparison of T cell and natural killer (NK) cell subset responses to *L. plantarum* are shown in Figure 6-4. Although intersubject variation is evident, the NK and NKT responses are distinctly increased compared to the CD3+ T cell responses in HIV-1-positive children. These studies support current interest in commensal bacteria as antigen delivery vehicles as well as potential adjuvants in the immunocompromised host.

In summary, commensal bacteria have a modulatory effect on GI immune function that is critical for host interaction with neoantigens and also for the development and maintenance of systemic immune response. Probiotic bacteria have been shown to support gut defense through immune exclusion, immune elimination, and immune regulation in several settings and have potential future use as immune modulators. Further studies addressing critical mechanisms of action, specificity, and long-term consequences are warranted.

REGULATING PRE- AND PROBIOTICS: A U.S. FDA PERSPECTIVE

Julienne Vaillancourt[3]

Introduction

Probiotics is a term applied to microorganisms that are administered with the intention of providing a health benefit. Probiotic preparations are usually administered orally, and in some cases intravaginally or topically, as they are thought to act locally or regionally rather than systemically. Probiotic products typically contain bacteria that are considered nonpathogenic and commensal in humans, such as lactic-acid producing strains of *Lactobacillus* and *Bifidobacterium*. Many probiotic organisms have been traditionally used in food preparation, particularly as fermenting agents in dairy products. With the increased interest in alternative and complementary medicine, there has been a surge in the marketing and availability of these agents as dietary supplements. As dietary supplements, probiotics may be marketed in the United States based on "structure/function" claims or health claims, rather than on treatment claims. The latter would apply to market-approved drugs. However, recently there has been active interest across many medical disciplines in the use of probiotics for a myriad of clinical indications. Such proposed and investigated uses for these products exceed the definition of a dietary supplement and instead meet the definition of a drug per the Food, Drug, and Cosmetic Act of 1938. Probiotics used for clinical indications also meet the definition of a biological product per the Public Health Service Act of 1944 and are regulated overall as such. The Office of Vaccines Research and Review (OVRR) at the Center for Biologics Evaluation and Research (CBER) at the U.S. Food and Drug Administration (FDA) has regulatory authority over the development and marketing of probiotics for clinical treatment indications.

FDA/CBER's Experience in Regulating Probiotics as Biological Drug Products

As interest has grown in the United States over the last few years in studying the effects of probiotics on specific diseases and conditions, CBER/OVRR has provided much regulatory advice to individuals including practitioners interested in conducting clinical research to evaluate probiotics, recipients of government funding for such research, as well as probiotic manufacturers. These regulatory interactions have focused on a variety of proposed uses for probiotics, most of

---

[3]Division of Vaccines and Related Products Applications, Office of Vaccines Research and Review, Center for Biologics Evaluation and Research, U.S. Food and Drug Administration. 1401 Rockville Pike, Suite 370N, Rockville, MD 20852. Phone: 301-827-3070; Fax: 301-827-3532, e-mail: Julienne.Vaillancourt@fda.hhs.gov

which have been gastrointestinal in nature. Intended study populations have varied from premature neonates to older adults, and from healthy individuals who may be at risk for specific diseases to individuals afflicted with particular diseases or conditions. Single strain and multistrain probiotic products have been proposed for investigation. Also, most probiotic products that have been the subject of regulatory interaction with CBER have been intended for oral administration, which is logical given the GI nature of most proposed diseases of study and the intended local effect of these products. However, some products have been intended for other routes of administration, such as intravaginal. Finally, proposed indications have varied with respect to prevention versus treatment, as well as with respect to stand-alone therapy versus use of a probiotic preparation as adjunct therapy to antimicrobial or other therapy. The discussion that follows will reflect CBER/OVRR's experience and perspective on the regulation and clinical development of these products as biological drug products.[4]

Prebiotic substances, such as those that are available as food ingredients, are typically regulated by the FDA's Center for Food Safety and Nutrition (CFSAN) unless a prebiotic substance is formulated in a biological drug product intended to treat or prevent disease. In this case, the prebiotic substance is subject to regulation by CBER as a component or ingredient of a biological drug product.

Nonregulatory Product Terms

It is important to clarify for regulatory purposes that currently *probiotic*, *prebiotic*, and *live biotherapeutic* are not regulatory terms, even though these terms are used to describe particular products that if introduced into interstate commerce within the United States would be regulated by the FDA. Specifically, these terms are not used or defined in any law or regulation that pertains to food and drugs. Nonetheless, a brief description of these terms is provided for the purpose of this discussion.

Probiotic. There is wide and varied use of the term *probiotic* in the medical literature, lay literature, and product advertising. Frequently it is used to describe an oral preparation containing live, lactic acid-producing bacteria for intended GI benefits. A commonly cited definition from a report of a joint working group of the FAO and the WHO on guidelines for the evaluation of probiotics in food refers to probiotics as live microorganisms, which when administered in adequate amounts confer a health benefit on the host (FAO/WHO, 2002). A more inclusive

---

[4]The recommendations provided in this document do not reflect official U.S. FDA policy. As FDA guidance in this area is under development, the reader is encouraged to contact the OVRR in the CBER at FDA for particular pre- and probiotics candidate products to support investigational new drug applications. In addition, specific guidance on regulatory requirements for a particular product should be sought from the FDA.

definition that considers nonviable forms of probiotics (e.g., dead cells and bacterial cell fragments) has been proposed and defines probiotics as microbial cell preparations or components of microbial cells that have a beneficial effect on the health and well-being of the host (Salminen et al., 1999). The term *probiotic* has also been proposed to describe microorganisms that have general beneficial effects on the health of animals or humans, whereas the term *biotherapeutic agent* has been proposed to describe microorganisms having therapeutic effects in humans (Elmer et al., 1999).

Prebiotic. As with the term *probiotic*, different definitions have been used and proposed for the term *prebiotic*. A prebiotic may simply be defined as a substance that serves as nutrition or fermentation media for probiotic organisms. The International Scientific Association for Probiotics and Prebiotics (ISAPP) defines a prebiotic as a nondigestible substance that provides a beneficial physiological effect on the host by selectively stimulating the favorable growth or activity of a limited number of indigenous bacteria (Reid et al., 2003). A prebiotic may be administered on its own, usually as an oral preparation, as a food ingredient, or as a component of a product containing probiotic organisms to enhance their growth. Oligosaccharides are commonly used as prebiotics.

Live Biotherapeutic. Currently CBER/OVRR uses the term *live biotherapeutic* in a working manner to refer to those products under its regulatory jurisdiction that contain whole, live microorganisms (e.g., bacteria, yeast) with an intended therapeutic effect in humans. As noted above in this section, this term is not currently used or defined in any law or regulation pertaining to food and/or drugs. Live biotherapeutic products differ from traditional vaccine products because their dosing regimens more closely resemble those of drugs (i.e., they are typically administered on a daily basis for a given period of time or indefinitely), the postulated effects are frequently local rather than systemic, and the intended therapeutic effect is typically not induction of an adaptive immune response to a pathogenic organism but rather an effect that may be directly attributable to component organisms in the product (e.g., production of antibacterial substances). Probiotics intended for clinical or therapeutic use are categorized as live biotherapeutic products by CBER/OVRR.

Regulatory Definitions

The key to understanding how the FDA regulates probiotics (or any product under its jurisdiction) is summarized by the following statement: *Intended use determines how a substance is regulated.* If a probiotic product is intended to be used as a drug, it is regulated as a drug. If a probiotic product is intended to be used as a food or dietary supplement, it is regulated as such. The Food, Drug, and Cosmetic Act defines a drug and a dietary supplement, whereas the Public Health

Service Act defines a biological product. A set of corresponding regulations exists for each of these distinct areas, and these regulations are found in Part 21 of the Code of Federal Regulations (CFR), which is updated annually. For the purpose of this discussion, simplified regulatory definitions for these terms are provided below. A definition for the acronym *GRAS* (generally recognizable as safe), which CBER/OVRR has encountered in a number of regulatory submissions concerning probiotic products, is also provided. Of note, GRAS has been frequently misused as a regulatory term, concerning probiotic products that are considered biological drug products, because use of the term GRAS is limited to food regulation.

- ***Drug.*** An article intended for use in the diagnosis, cure, mitigation, treatment, or prevention of disease.[5]
- ***Dietary Supplement.*** A product taken by mouth that contains a "dietary ingredient" intended to supplement the diet.[6]
- ***Biological product.*** Includes any product containing microorganisms applicable to the prevention, treatment, or cure of a disease or condition of human beings,[7] and to which the Federal Food, Drug and Cosmetic Act applies.[8]
- ***GRAS (generally recognizable as safe).*** A food ingredient classification that distinguishes a substance from a food additive on the basis of common knowledge about safety for its intended use.[9]

---

[5] FD&C Act (Federal Food, Drug, and Cosmetic Act), June 25, 1938, as amended through December 31, 2004, codified at Title 21 United States Code (U.S.C.) available online at http://www.access.gpo.gov/uscode/title21/chapter9_.html.

[6] The current definition of a dietary supplement is a result of the Dietary Supplement Health Education Act of 1994 (DSHEA), P.L. 103-417, 21 U.S.C. 321 which amended the FD&C Act to provide standards for dietary supplements. The actual definition as written in the FD&C Act is more detailed than presented here and discusses claims and labeling. The full text of the DSHEA is available online at http://www.fda.gov/opacom/laws/dshea.html).

[7] The actual definition of a biological product per the Public Health Service Act, uses the term *virus* rather than *microorganism*. According to 21 CFR 600.3(h) a *virus* is interpreted to be a product containing the minute living cause of an infectious disease and includes, for example, bacteria and fungi. As use of the term *virus* might cause confusion, the term *microorganism* is used instead in an attempt to simplify the definition. According to 21 CFR 600.3(h)(5)(i) a product is considered "analogous to a virus," if it is prepared from or with a virus or agent actually or potentially infectious, without regard to the degree of virulence or toxicogenicity of the specific strain used.

[8] PHS Act (Public Health Service Act), July 1, 1944, Chap. 373, Title III, Sec. 351, 58 Stat. 702, currently codified at 42 U.S.C., Sec. 262 indicates that a biological product is a drug by definition. Therefore, biological products are subject to both drug and biological product regulations. See http://www.fda.gov/opacom/laws/phsvcact/sec262.htm); 21 CFR (Code of Federal Regulations, Title 21) Parts 1–1299. Washington, DC, Office of the Federal Register, National Archives and Records Administration, 2004.

[9] Use of the term *GRAS* is appropriate in the context of food regulation but not in the context of drug and biologic regulation. GRAS pertains to the *use* of a food substance, rather than the substance itself. Information about GRAS, 21 CFR 170.3 and 170.30, is available from FDA/CFSAN at http://www.cfsan.fda.gov/~dms/grasguid.html.

U.S. FDA Regulation of Probiotics:
Dietary Supplements Versus Biological Products

Probiotic products for ingestion may be lawfully marketed in the United States as dietary supplements under the Dietary Supplement Health and Education Act of 1994 (DSHEA) based on limited claims such as those that pertain to affecting the structure and function of the human body or general well-being,[10] but not based on drug or disease claims. Probiotic products intended for intravaginal or topical use are not dietary supplements by definition, because they are not intended for ingestion. If a probiotic product is intended to be used in a manner that meets the definition of a drug per the Food, Drug, and Cosmetic Act as indicated above, it cannot be introduced into interstate commerce unless it is either approved for such use by the U.S. FDA or an investigational new drug application (IND) is in effect with the U.S. FDA for that specific use. Most proposed uses of probiotics for clinical investigation meet the definition of a drug from a regulatory perspective.

The OVRR at the CBER has regulatory jurisdiction over most probiotic products intended for use as drugs. Because probiotic products intended for use as drugs are regulated as biological products under section 351 of the Public Health Service Act (PHS Act), they are subject to the biologics regulations (21 CFR 600).[11] For example, a probiotic for an intended clinical use must be marketed under an approved biologics license application (BLA) (21 CFR 601)[12] unless the product is excluded from the definition of a *new drug* under section 201(p) of the Food, Drug, and Cosmetic Act. Probiotic products intended for use as drugs are also subject to pertinent drug regulations. For example, when a probiotic product is proposed for evaluation in a clinical study, it may be viewed as an unapproved biological product and an investigational drug product, and thus would be subject to the regulations for an IND (21 CFR 312).[13] FDA reviews INDs to assure the safety and rights of patients in all clinical studies and to assure that studies to evaluate both safety and effectiveness are adequately designed to do so [21 CFR 312.22(a)].[14]

Any clinical investigator or probiotic manufacturer interested in evaluating a probiotic product for clinical use is encouraged to request a pre-IND meeting

---

[10]Section 403 (r)(6)(A) of the Food, Drug, and Cosmetic Act, 21 U.S.C. 343(r)(6)(A).

[11]21 CFR 600 stands for the Code of Regulations, Title 21 Food and Drugs, Part 600 refers to Biological Products- General.

[12]Part 601 refers to Licensing.

[13]Part 312 refers to Investigational New Drug Application.

[14]Subpart 22 refers to General principles of the IND submission. (a) FDA's primary objectives in reviewing an IND.

with CBER prior to submitting an IND.[15] A pre-IND meeting is an opportunity for a potential IND sponsor to obtain useful regulatory advice from FDA that, if heeded, might prevent regulatory delays (e.g., clinical holds) in the conduct of a proposed clinical trial (Miller and Ross, 2005).

In light of the current trend whereby practitioners recommend probiotics to their patients as a therapeutic modality for particular diseases or clinical indications, it is important to keep in mind the following:

- Biological products require premarket review and approval by the FDA. Dietary supplements do not.
- The safety, purity, and potency, as well as efficacy, of a biological product must be demonstrated for approval. Dietary supplements need not demonstrate any of these to be marketed.
- A probiotic product that is marketed or promoted as a treatment, prevention, or cure for a specific disease or condition without an approved indication for such is considered an unapproved and, thus, illegal drug.
- A probiotic manufacturer who intends to market a probiotic product based on a drug claim must seek approval for that claim.

The Biological Drug Development Pathway for Live Biotherapeutics

Data to support approval of a biological product are provided in a BLA to CBER for review. Clinical data for inclusion in a BLA are generated during the investigational stage of drug development. Adequate preclinical and chemistry, manufacturing, and controls (CMC) data are needed to support the initial clinical evaluation of a live biotherapeutic in human subjects. Figure 6-5 presents the typical stages of product development and regulatory review for live biotherapeutic products including probiotics for therapeutic uses. As with traditional pharmaceutical development, a live biotherapeutic product is expected to be evaluated in phase 1, 2, and 3 studies, which progressively build upon each other to provide supportive data for a license application. Safety is evaluated in all phases of investigational biological drug development. Other parameters such as colonization, which has yet to be consistently defined, may be important in live biotherapeutic development and recommended for evaluation during all three phases as well. Typically, dose selection for phase 3 efficacy studies—and often the proposed dose for marketing—are based on the results of phase 2 dose ranging studies. Pivotal phase 3 studies should be adequately designed to provide safety and efficacy data to support a licensed indication.

---

[15]The following FDA/CBER website provides many informational resources concerning how to submit an IND and how to conduct a clinical trial under IND. See http://www.fda.gov/cber/ind/ind.htm. Also, CBER's Office of Communication, Training, and Manufacturer's Assistance (OCTMA) may be contacted directly at (301) 827-1800 for assistance in the process.

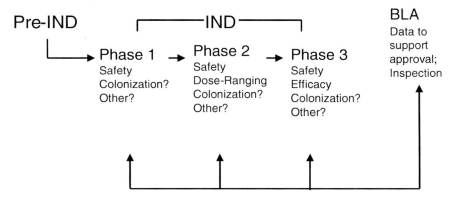

FIGURE 6-5 Stages of premarket review and regulation for live biotherapeutics.
SOURCE: Vaillancourt (2005).

Issues for Consideration
in the Development of Live Biotherapeutic Products

The CBER/OVRR has identified the following eight issues that merit consideration in the development of live biotherapeutic products:

1. The term *probiotic* is inconsistently used and lacks a standard definition.
2. The regulatory food ingredient term *GRAS* is inappropriately used to describe component microorganisms of live biotherapeutic products.
3. Submitted INDs frequently lack adequate chemistry, manufacturing, and controls (CMC) data that are required to support the clinical evaluation of a live biotherapeutic product in human subjects.[16] In this regard, probiotic manufacturers may not be familiar with biological product manufacturing requirements, which greatly exceed those for foods or dietary supplements.
4. There is a need for education among investigators and sponsors concerning how to prepare INDs and master files and submit them to CBER, and drug and biologics regulations in general.

---

[16]When the IND sponsor is not the manufacturer of the product, the IND sponsor must rely on obtaining CMC data from the manufacturer for submission in the IND, or alternatively, the manufacturer may submit such proprietary data directly to CBER for review in a master file (21 CFR 314.420) to support a proposed clinical study. A guideline on drug master files is available from FDA's Center for Drug Evaluation and Research at http://www.fda.gov/cder/guidance/dmf.htm. Prior to submitting a master file, a manufacturer is strongly advised to contact the Division of Vaccines and Related Products Applications at CBER/OVRR at (301) 827-3070.

5. Live biotherapeutic product development for any given clinical indication should focus on demonstrating a measurable treatment effect that reflects a meaningful clinical benefit.

6. Colonization should be explored as a valid function of the intended treatment effect and/or a postulated mechanism of action. In this regard, discussion is necessary on how it should be defined and how and when it should be evaluated in the clinical development of live biotherapeutic products.

7. There is a need for scientifically sound approaches to defining and evaluating the potency of live biotherapeutic products.[17]

8. With regard to the safety of live biotherapeutic products, there is a need for effective evaluation and management of the potential pathogenicity of product strains, particularly in targeted patient populations. Some factors to consider include virulence, host translocation, environmental persistence and the concomitant risk of infection to others, alterations in normal flora that may increase disease risk or susceptibility, and gene transfer in the therapeutic niche.

If these issues can be addressed, perhaps progress can be made in the overall development and regulatory evaluation of live biotherapeutic products, including probiotics for therapeutic uses, as a promising new class of biological drug products. However, efforts in addressing these issues should be collaborative and include funding institutions, manufacturers of live biotherapeutic products, clinical investigators, and regulatory agencies such as the U.S. FDA.

Conclusions

Although many probiotic products are marketed and available in the United States as dietary supplements, interest in the therapeutic use of probiotic products for a variety of clinical diseases and conditions is growing. Despite extensive retail and research experience with probiotics, there is a need for medical and scientific validation of their value in disease management. This may well require rigorous clinical trials and regulatory evaluation (Shanahan, 2003; Tannock, 2003). The FDA's CBER has regulatory jurisdiction over probiotic products intended for therapeutic use and refers to them as *live biotherapeutic products*. Specifically, CBER's OVRR has gained tremendous experience in this area in recent years. In general, the development of a live biotherapeutic product as a biological drug product should proceed along the established product and clinical development pathway for drugs and biologics, with safety being continuously

---

[17]Possible approaches to defining and evaluating the potency of live biotherapeutic products might include the quantitation of specific, live organisms or the production of particular substances (e.g., lactic acid).

evaluated. Many resources are available from FDA's CBER for guidance on U.S. regulatory standards for biological products and clinical study design that can be applied to the development of live biotherapeutic products. Finally, in its recent experience in regulating these products, CBER's OVRR has encountered numerous challenges and issues that impact valid evaluation of these products for therapeutic uses. Collaborative efforts in addressing these challenges and issues appear to be necessary.

FROM RESEARCH IN MICROBIOLOGY TO GUIDELINES

Lorenzo Morelli and Elena Bessi[18]

New Aspects of the War Metaphor: Good Bacteria as Potential Allies

From the point of view of a microbial ecologist the war metaphor describing the fight between humans and bacterial pathogens could still be useful if widened to include not only the human body and bacterial pathogens, but also potential bacterial allies already inhabiting, or parachuted into, the battleground to ensure support to the body.

A dramatic increase worldwide in research efforts (hundreds of papers are published every year with the key words *probiotics* or *prebiotics*), as well as a booming market of drugs, dietary supplements, and food claiming "contains good bacteria" or "good for feeding your good bacteria," urged the FAO and the WHO to hold two expert consultations to both review the state of the field and prepare guidelines for assessing probiotics (FAO/WHO, 2001; FAO/WHO, 2002). This overview will try to establish a link between cutting-edge research and regulatory efforts, with special attention paid to FAO/WHO documents[19] that are in progress.

In the following sections, some points of this potential new war strategy will be addressed by focusing on items that have been considered by the joint FAO/WHO consultations held in Argentina during 2001 and in Canada during 2002 (FAO/WHO, 2001; FAO/WHO, 2002). In addition to these documents, it could be worthwhile to recall the excellent documents prepared by the European Society for Paediatric Gastroenterology Hepatology and Nutrition (ESPGHAN) (Agostoni et al., 2004a,b), the French Food Safety Authority (AFSSA, 2005), and the Italian Ministry of Health (Ministero della Salute, 2006). These documents altogether provide a state-of-the-art assessment of this field as well as some guidelines for assessing safety and efficacy of pre- and probiotics.

---

[18]L. Morelli and E Bessi are from the Istituto di Microbiologia, UCSC; Via Emilia Parmense 84, 29100, Piacenza, Italy. Phone: +39-523-599248 Fax: +39-523-599246. E-mail: lorenzo.morelli @unicatt.it E Bessi is also with AAT, Srl, a spin-off company of UCSC; Via Emilia Parmense 84, 29100, Piacenza, Italy. E-mail: aat@libero.it.

[19]All paragraphs marked with this symbol are taken from documents (FAO/WHO, 2001) or (FAO/WHO, 2002).

Why FAO/WHO Issued Guidelines on Probiotics

A joint FAO/WHO expert consultation on health and nutritional properties of powdered milk with live lactic acid bacteria was held in Córdoba, Argentina, October 1–4, 2001. The consultation focused on the evaluation of the scientific evidence available on the properties, functionality, benefits, safety, and nutritional features of probiotic foods. Following are the reasons to convene such a consultation:

> The beneficial effects of food with added live microbes (probiotics) on human health, and in particular of milk products for children and other high-risk populations, are being increasingly promoted by health professionals. It has been reported that these probiotics can play an important role in immunological, digestive, and respiratory functions and could have a significant effect in alleviating infectious disease in children. As there is no current international consensus on the methodology to assess the efficacy and safety of these products it was considered necessary to convene an Expert Consultation to evaluate and suggest general guidelines for such assessments.

Bacterial Armies of the Gut

In order to assess the properties of probiotics, the joint FAO/WHO consultation suggested that (FAO/WHO, 2001):

> Probiotic microorganisms should not only be capable of surviving passage through the digestive tract, but also have the capability to proliferate in the gut. This means they must be resistant to gastric juices and be able to grow in the presence of bile under conditions in the intestines, or be consumed in a food vehicle that allows them to survive passage through the stomach and exposure to bile. They are gram-positive bacteria and are included primarily in two genera, *Lactobacillus* and *Bifidobacterium* (Holzapfel et al., 1998; Klein et al., 1998).

A microbial ecologist has to add that probiotic microorganisms, to be successful, have to take their place among the bacterial population already inhabiting the gut. To evaluate the potential of good bacterium to proliferate into a gut already heavily inhabited is not an easy task. Technical difficulties abound in analysing the gut microbiota as a whole. If we do not have a clear picture of what we are going to impact, then it is difficult to prepare guidelines or to regulate.

Composition of the vast and complex ecosystem formed by bacteria inhabiting the various sites of the intestine is only beginning to be understood due to the availability of molecular tools that allow culture independent assessment. However, the complexity of this research effort must be considered. It is generally estimated that each of us has about 10^{11} viable bacteria per gram of large bowel content. This multitude comprises at least 400–500 different species. The physiological, and also the clinical, potential of this bacterial organ is underlined when we consider that the total number of genes contained in the microbiota is about

50–100 times greater than in the human genome. A further level of complexity is the spatial and temporal diversity of the microbiota. The bacterial distribution varies greatly at different levels of the GI tract, ranging from less than 10^3 colony-forming units/mL (CFU/mL) in the stomach, where the number of ingested bacteria is dramatically reduced by the hostile gastric environment, to 10^{11} CFU/mL within the colon, where anaerobes outnumber aerobes by a ratio of 1000:1. Environmental conditions of the colon seem to favour the growth of selected bacterial groups; however, a clear picture of this complex process, in which ingested bacteria are greatly reduced by extremely hostile conditions and then survivors are hosted in a kind of bacterial luxury resort is not yet available. This could be a first suggestion for developing a strategy of alliance between humans and "good enteric bugs" to unravel the mechanisms used by the human gut for sorting out some bacterial groups to be favoured for reproduction in this environment.

Selection of Probiotic Strains for Human Use

Probiotics must be able to exert their benefits on the host through growth and/or activity in the human body (Collins et al., 1998; Morelli, 2000). However, it is the specificity of the action, not the source of the microorganism, that is important. Indeed, it is very difficult to confirm the source of a microorganism. Infants are born with none of these bacteria in the intestine, and the origin of the intestinal microbiota has not been fully elucidated. It is the ability to remain viable at the target site and to be effective that should be verified for each potentially probiotic strain (FAO/WHO, 2001).

This statement is in full opposition with "conventional wisdom," and even with many recent scientific reviews on the selection of probiotic bacteria stating that probiotic bacteria must be selected among "bacteria isolated from human beings." Even acknowledging the difficulty with determining the natural source of a particular strain, species including *Saccharomyces boulardii* and *Bifidobacterium animalis*, which are not considered to have humans as their natural habitat, are documented as very effective probiotics (see also comments on the efficacy of *Saccharomyces boulardii*, in the section "Good Bugs: Data with Consensus"). The assertion that probiotics must be of human origin should be laid to rest.

There is a general agreement that the term *dominant* bacteria is used to indicate species that are present at a level not less than one percent of the total fecal microbiota. As such, bacteria at a minimum concentration of 10^8 could be considered the likely players in gut health (Ducluzeau, 1988). To what extent exogenous bacteria can influence the microbe-associated characteristics is key to the probiotic concept. Some authors suggest that each person has his or her own rather stable profile of dominant (therefore more than 10^8 CFU/g) species. These observations still need to be confirmed by studies involving larger numbers of individuals. This is not a trivial task as the assessment of the ecological composition of the gut microbiota will depend on (1) the section of the GI tract sampled, (2) the "layer" of the GI pipeline, (3) age of the considered individual, (4) diet, and (5) the analytical methodology used.

Disproportionately, our knowledge of microbiota composition of human beings has been determined investigating the stool microbiota by means of microbiological plating techniques. However, this approach is laborious, time consuming, and limited in scope as a majority of the bacterial species present in feces are not culturable using standard microbiologic techniques (Blaut et al., 2002; Langendijk et al., 1995; Suau et al., 1999) or could become unviable during sample handling. Among those microorganisms that are culturable, species identification by traditional biochemical identification methods is often difficult. Assessment of gut microbiota using genetic techniques, applicable also to unviable bacterial cells, is a relatively new approach able to overcome at least some of these problems.

Molecular tools based on 16S rDNA sequence similarities such as fluorescent in situ hybridization (FISH), denaturing gradient gel electrophoresis (DGGE), quantitative dot blot hybridization, restriction fragment length polymorphism, and large scale 16S rDNA sequencing have helped to overcome limitations of conventional microbiological plating methods in studying the fecal microbiota composition (Suau, 2003). In addition, DNA microchips that allow for more efficient identification of bacterial species present in complex communities are currently under development in various laboratories. However, bias introduced through PCR or subcloning might affect such analyses (McCartney, 2002); the extent of such potential distortions has not been thoroughly investigated.

Both FAO/WHO documents strongly recommend the use of molecular biology techniques. In the 2001 document, section 11, you find "Potential probiotic strains must be identified by methods including internationally accepted molecular techniques." This should be taken as a strong recommendation that assessment of the identity of bacteria potentially used to promote health must be done by means of the best techniques available, which may be a combination of classical and DNA-based techniques. But new identification techniques are providing a novel assessment of the composition of the intestinal microbiota, suggesting that bacterial populations of the gut are not a single body. At the moment, these observations have not evolved into a new regulatory framework.

The Dominant Bacterial Population

Studies based on plating and cultivating reveal a fecal microbiota dominated by *Bacteroides*, *Eubacterium*, *Ruminococcus*, *Clostridium*, and *Bifidobacterium* (Finegold and Rolfe, 1983; Moore and Holdeman, 1974), but recent investigations based on genetic tools suggest that 70–80 percent of fecal bacteria are unculturable or extremely fastidious in their cultivation requirements (Blaut et al., 2002; Langendijk et al., 1995; Suau et al., 1999; Suau, 2003). It is possible that a new understanding of the bacterial composition of the intestinal microbiota will emerge given time. For example, in past investigations, *Fusobacterium prausnitzii* was reported either as one of the most frequent and numerous species or was seldom retrieved. A specific rRNA-targeted oligonucleotide probe (Suau et al., 2001) showed that *F. prausnitzii* and phylogenetically related species represent a dominant group within the human fecal microbiota, ranging from 5 percent to 16 percent of the total microbiota.

Anaerobes are the dominant component of the stool microbiota and very possibly of the colon. These groups of bacteria seem to be quite stable over time in healthy adults allowing for a bacterial species profile typical of each individual. Differences among individuals seem to be at the species, but not at the genus, level. Compositional changes of the dominant microbiota are rarely reflected by changes in metabolic activities generally assigned to the microbiota. However, the particular species responsible for specific metabolic activities is largely unknown.

Another puzzling observation is that genetic analysis will probably move some bacterial groups, now allotted among the dominant population on the basis of cultivation techniques, to a lower ranking in the list of the bacterial armies of the gut. They may move from the threshold between the large, "heavy infantry," and the highly specialized, parachuted corps. One example could be bifidobacteria, up to now considered a dominant population, but perhaps simply because they are less common among anaerobes.

The Subdominant Population

If human beings are looking for allies in the war against pathogens, they should not forget the so-called subdominant population bacteria that are detected at levels below 10^8 per gram of faeces. Among these groups we can encounter the most studied and used "healthy bacteria," the lactic acid bacteria, mainly belonging to the genus *Lactobacillus*. This bacterial population is always a subdominant one, but it is credited with an impressive number of positive actions (FAO/WHO, 2001), but meta-analysis has revealed a puzzling similarity among the efficacy of products containing bacteria of different origin and species. (Further details will be provided in the "Probiotic Activities with Consensus" section). As microbiologists, there are opportunities for new selection criteria and more potent allies to be used as biotherapeutics pharmaceuticals. If it were possible to identify mechanisms used by the human gut to sort out some ingested bacteria, favour their reproduction, and adopt them as "indigenous" we could have in our hands better companions in our fight against pathogens (Vinderola et al., 2004).

Mucosa-Associated Bacteria

If we are engaged in combat, the location of potential allies is another relevant aspect. The subdominant bacterial population may play a specific role by adhering to mucosa. Few data are available, but genetic analysis and biopsy samples clearly suggest that mucosa-associated bacteria differ from those recovered from feces. Even more interesting is that, for each individual, the same bacterial strains are uniformly distributed along the colon (Morelli, 2005a; Nelsen et al., 2003; Zoetendal et al., 2002).

Zoetendal et al. (2002) investigated the distribution of mucosa-associated bacteria in the ascending, transverse, and descending colon of 10 individuals and found that the predominant bacterial community was host specific and uniformly distributed along the colon. *Lactobacillus* community was dominated by a single species, *Lactobacillus gasseri*, in all sampling sites. In 7 out of the 10 subjects, no variation in the *Lactobacillus* population was detected, whereas minor differences among sampling sites were observed in the other three individuals.

Nielsen et al. (2003) investigated 10 volunteers for the presence of mucosa-associated lactobacilli and bifidobacteria. They confirmed that mucosa-associated bacterial communities are clearly different in composition from those recovered from fecal samples of the same subjects. High similarity between bacterial communities from different locations of the colon was also confirmed.

In our laboratory, we have focused our attention on the *Lactobacillus* population adhering to biopsies obtained from six individuals from the same three sites of the large bowel and the ileum. In all cases, *Lactobacillus fermentum* was isolated. These data suggest that the bacterial profile of mucosa-associated bacteria is much less complex than the profile obtained by fecal samples. In addition, we have recently characterised the *Lactobacillus* biota of seven adults; biopsies were obtained from the terminal ileum and from the ascending, descending, and transverse colon. From all subjects stool samples were also obtained. Results are summarized in Table 6-3.

TABLE 6-3 *Lactobacillus* Species Recovered and Genetically Identified from Biopsies of Seven Adults

Subjects	*Lactobacillus* species
A	*L. rhamnosus;* all sites
B	*L. rhamnosus; L. paracasei; L. fermentum*
C	*L. rhamnosus; L. paracasei; L. fermentum*
D	*L. rhamnosus; L. fermentum; L. gasseri; L. paracasei; L. salivarius*
E	*L. rhamnosus; L. fermentum; L. gasseri;*
F	*L. fermentum; a new species of the genus Lactobacillus*
G	*L. fermentum* all sites

SOURCE: Morelli, 2005.

Puzzling is that the species *L. fermentum* has been found in six out the seven subjects studied but only in biopsy samples and never in stools. This species of *Lactobacillus* species has been recovered from human stools, but it is not one of the most commonly isolated species.

Caution is to be exerted, as available data are still scarce (limited number of individuals sampled), but what is becoming evident is that strains stably entrapped into mucus or adhering to deeper layer intestinal tissues are different from those living as planktonic cells sometimes associated with food particles and found in stool.

It may be relevant to have a more clear picture of the biota established near the intestinal tissues, as these bacteria are probably in a better position to exert positive action for the human hosts such as the interaction with the gut associated lymphoid tissue (GALT), the competition for receptor sites of pathogens, or as players in cross-talk with the genes of enterocytes.

These bacteria could be considered the real potential allies in our war against pathogens. It could be argued that their total number is much lower than those found in the stool or as planktonic, free-flowing cells in the colon, but they are in better position to establish interactions with GALT and intestinal tissues or to block pathogens in their struggle for adhesion.

An interesting observation is that the large majority of scientific evidence reviewed by the FAO/WHO consultation was obtained by papers dealing with probiotics isolated from human stools. Furthermore, according to the latest results obtained by molecular techniques, we have to assume that all—or nearly all—of them belong to the subdominant population. This could open a world of opportunities for new research and new biotherapeutic bacteria.

Good Bugs Meet Us and We Become Friends

To end this section devoted to the considerations on microbial ecology of the gut as reviewed in the FAO/WHO documents, it is interesting to note that becoming friends may be easy but remaining friends for a lifetime is definitely a hard task and requires specific feelings and attitudes. Genetic techniques allow us to learn a little more about the human host-bacteria relationship. For example, consider the species distribution of lactobacilli among a range of higher animals including, quite surprisingly, fish and insects (Table 6-4).

Recently we identified an abundant *Lactobacillus* microbiota in honeybees, and, reinforcing the concept of host specificity, the four *Lactobacillus* species identified were all new species never before isolated (Bessi and Morelli, 2005). This data strongly suggests that a specific link between some species and specific hosts exists. However, more needs to be known about the nature of this host specificity. If unique species with a true affinity for humans are discovered, this could lead to a new generation of probiotics which, in turn, might necessitate new

TABLE 6-4 Host Specificity of the *Lactobacillus* Species

Animal Source	Genetic Taxonomy	References
Pigs	*L. amylovorus*	Axelsson and Lingren, 1987
Pigs	*L. amylovorus*	Pryde et al., 1999
Calves	*L. johnsonii*	Sarra et al., 1980
Poultry	*L. crispatus*	Morelli et al., unpublished results; Sarra et al., 1986
Poultry	*L. johnsonii*	
Humans	*L. gasseri, L. rhamnosus,*	Dunne et al., 1999; Morelli et al., 1998
	L. paracasei, L. reuteri	Song et al., 1999, 2000; Tannock et al., 2000
Honeybees	*L. plantarum, L. cellobiosum*	Bessi et al., 2005 submitted; Kvasnicov et al., 1971
Fishes	*L. fermentum*	Kvasnicov et al., 1977; Rawls et al., 2004

SOURCE: Morelli, 2005.

safety considerations. For example, probiotic bacteria currently on the market persist for weeks, at a maximum, in the gut of fed volunteers. Probiotics able to persist long term in the human gut may need to be reassessed for safety (Fujiwara et al., 2001).

To summarize:

- The gut microbiota compose a complex ecosystem with an enormous potential for influencing the whole health status of human beings.
- The composition of this ecosystem requires further investigation, and available genetic techniques are promising, but further improvements are needed.
- The analysis of fecal microbiota alone is not sufficient for comprehension of the complex situation occurring in this body site.
- Stool bacteria do not reflect the composition of mucosa-associated bacteria, but the latter are probably the most interesting allies in the war against pathogens.
- It is of interest to distinguish between dominant and subdominant bacteria among the total gut microbiota.
- Guidelines available at the moment consider probiotic products based on a relatively "old" concept. New products and new guidelines are emerging.

Looking for Allies in the Gut Microbiota: From History to Guidelines

E. Metchnikoff, the Nobel Prize winner, is credited with being the first to suggest the value of ingestion of beneficial bacteria. He asserted, "the dependence of the intestinal microbes on the food makes it possible to adopt measures to modify the flora in our bodies and to replace the harmful microbes by useful microbes" (Metchnikoff, 1907). He put into practice his observations by commercializing fermented milk, as well as a pharmaceutical preparation containing the same *Lactobacillus* strain selected for the food product. This little piece of history is useful to point out that good microorganisms have been used either as healthy food ingredients or as therapeutic products since the very beginning of the probiotic story. After one century of research and development, this duality is creating not only opportunities but also problems.

Metchnikoff's observations were useful to the dairy food industry, and several fermented dairy products were marketed during the last century, claiming to favor a good microbial balance in the gut. The rationale, according to the Metchnikoff concept, was clearly an ecological one—to modify the ratio among some components of intestinal microbiota. For example, Metchnikoff favoured lowering the number of putrefactive bacteria by replacing them with acid-producing ones in order to protect the human body from noxious substances. Unfortunately, only carefully selected strains, and not those generally contained in yogurt, are able to colonize the gut. It is now established that some yogurt starter cultures can survive—albeit in low quantities—to the intestinal transit, but they are unable to actively reproduce themselves in the gut. The evolution from Metchnikoff's work to probiotic is reflected in changes that, over time, occurred in the meaning of the same word.

At first probiotics was used to name "substances produced by microorganisms which promoted the growth of other microorganisms" (Lilly and Stillwell, 1965). A few years later, Parker redefined the word as "organisms and substances that contribute to intestinal microbial balance" (Parker, 1974). Then Fuller specified that probiotics are "live microbial feed supplements that beneficially affect the host animal by improving its intestinal balance" (1989). In more recent years, the meaning of this word has been refined several times and today a widely accepted definition of *probiotics* is "live microorganisms, which when consumed in adequate amounts, confer a health effect on the host" (Guarner and Schaafsma, 1998).

Some notes on different wording of the various definitions could be helpful:

• In the first definition the subject of the definition was *substances* then *viable bacteria* appear, and *nowadays live microorganisms* remained alone.

• The probiotic activity was originally quite similar to a feed supplement for bacteria, then it turned into an ecological action towards the intestinal microbiota. Nowadays, there is increasing evidence that the presence of specific bacterial strains in the human gut could have a favourable action per se, without any detectable change in the overall composition of the gut microbiota.

• At the end, today the positive action is no more related to intestinal ecology but is simply a "health effect."

• In the more recent definitions, a dose effect is included.

If the above are definitions derived from the scientific community, here is the regulatory counterpart:

- Expert consultation held jointly by the FAO and the WHO redefined the term *probiotics* as "live microorganisms which when consumed in adequate amounts as part of food (water is included as a food) confer a health benefit on the host."
- The consultation agreed that the scope of the meeting would include probiotics and prebiotics in food and exclude reference to the term *biotherapeutic agents* and beneficial microorganisms not used in food.

Probiotic Activities with Consensus

The expert consultation reviewed

- disorders associated with the GI tract,
- prevention of diarrhea caused by certain pathogenic bacteria and viruses,
- *Helicobacter pylori* infection and complications,
- inflammatory diseases and bowel syndromes,
- cancer,
- constipation,
- mucosal immunity,
- allergy,
- cardiovascular disease,
- urogenital tract disorders,
- bacterial vaginosis,
- yeast vaginitis,
- urinary tract infections, and
- use of probiotics in otherwise healthy people.

What seems relevant to a microbiologist in this section of the presentation is that the above evidence of probiotic activities have been obtained with bacterial probiotic populations detected in fecal samples at a level less than 1/100 of the total bacterial population.

The same levels have been detected when probiotics were found active in

- significant reduction in atopic dermatitis in allergic children,
- treatment of pouch infections,
- gut-associated immune response modulation,
- lactose intolerance reduction,
- gastric inflammation in *H. pylori* disease reduction,
- urogenital infections prevention and treatment,
- intestinal transit modulation,
- IBD and Crohn's diseases symptom reduction,
- an active role in arthritis prevention and treatment, and
- an active role in autoimmune diseases treatment and incidence reduction.

All the above observations have led the FAO and the WHO to formulate these optimistic but prudent statements:

- The experts agreed that adequate scientific evidence exists to indicate that there is potential for the derivation of health benefits from consuming food containing probiotics. However, it was felt that additional research data are needed to confirm a number of these health benefits in humans, applying a systematic approach and following the guidelines for the assessment of probiotics suggested in this report.
- There is good evidence that specific strains of probiotics are safe for human use and able to confer some health benefits on the host, but such benefits cannot be extrapolated to other strains without experimentation.

If we look to the scientific literature produced after the two FAO/WHO documents were released, we can note that the attention is now focused on the bacteria actually present in the dominant population. Commensal dominant microbiota coevolved with their hosts and express a number of components able to activate innate and adaptive immunity (Vaarala, 2003); the mucosal immune system has developed specialized regulatory, anti-inflammatory mechanisms for eliminating or tolerating nondangerous food, antigens, and commensal microorganisms (Tlaskavola-Hogenova et al., 2004). The important role of commensal bacteria in mucosal immunity development was first demonstrated in a germ-free animal model; colonization of germ-free zebrafish with individual members of its microbiota revealed the bacterial species specificity of selected host responses. Rawls et al. 2004 studies revealed 212 genes regulated by the microbiota, and 59 responses that are conserved in the mouse intestine, including those involved in stimulation of epithelial proliferation, promotion of nutrient metabolism, and innate immune responses (2004).

These studies are elucidating the role of bacteria that form the vast majority of the gut microbiota. These studies are strategically different from all the scientific literature produced on subdominant probiotic bacteria. It could be speculated that when these studies are turned into applications, a new regulatory framework will be necessary.

Good Bugs: Data with Consensus

To reinforce the opinion that currently available guidelines have been generated by an initial, but still evolving, generation of probiotics, it is worthwhile to look at some more consensus analysis. At least five meta-analyses (Cremonini et al., 2002; D'Souza et al., 2002; Elmer et al., 1996; Szajewska and Mrukowicz, 2001; Van Niel et al., 2002) showed that some selected bacteria could be active in reducing the severity of antibiotic-associated diarrhea. Diarrhea associated with antibiotics is presumed to result from the antibiotics disrupting the normal biota in the gut of a healthy person. Such disruptions cause dysfunction of the gut's ecosystem, and they may allow pathogenic bacteria to colonize the gut and gain access to the mucosa. Whether probiotic supplements stop this process by reducing the disruption or by acting as substitutes for the healthy microbiota is unclear. It is also unclear if the mechanism of action is competition with pathogens for the nutrients, or adhesion sites, or pathogen inhibition by means of antimicrobial production, or something else. If we consider all meta-analyses supporting the efficacy of probiotics when applied to antibiotic-associated diarrhea, it is possible to point out some further observations.

All meta-analyses suggest that probiotics can be used to prevent antibiotic-associated diarrhea, while statistical comparison suggests that *S. boulardii* and *lactobacilli* have a similar potential to be used in this situation. On the contrary, the efficacy of probiotics in treating antibiotic-associated diarrhea remains to be proven. All meta-analyses include clinical trials in which a range of totally different antibiotics have been used, but it has been shown that the positive action of probiotics in preventing the onset of diarrhea is not influenced by the drug(s) used. Moreover, it is also interesting to note that the trial scored negative, in terms of odds ratio, in all meta-analyses performed with a daily dose of *S. boulardii* reduced to one-fifth of the recommended dosage. This could be a positive observation stressing the importance of the dosage. One recent study supporting this hypothesis is a controlled trial of three probiotic regimens (*Lactobacillus* GG, *Saccharomyces boulardii*, or a mixture of *Lactobacillus acidophilus* and *Bifidobacterium*) to prevent diarrhea associated with anti-*Helicobacter pylori* antibiotic treatments. Authors showed a 5 percent incidence of diarrhea with all probiotic used, compared to 30 percent with placebo. It is possible to speculate that all the above observations could be explained by some (still unknown) nonspecific mechanisms, possibly based on general ecological considerations more than on specific, strain-related activity.

This observation could also be reinforced by data presented on the efficacy of probiotics in prevention of recurrent *Clostridium difficile* disease. In this case the efficacy seems to be related to only some specific probiotic preparations; for at least one of them, there are also some suggestions about the mechanisms active against *C. difficile*. Here, we are probably crossing the boundaries between probiotics and biotherapeutics.

FAO/WHO constructed a decision tree (Figure 6-6) to obtain data with consensus for new probiotic products (FAO/WHO, 2002). A detailed characterization of the strain is required and at least one double blind, randomised efficacy trial is mandatory to use the term *probiotic* for a food product containing viable bacterial cells endowed with some specific properties beneficial for the consumers.

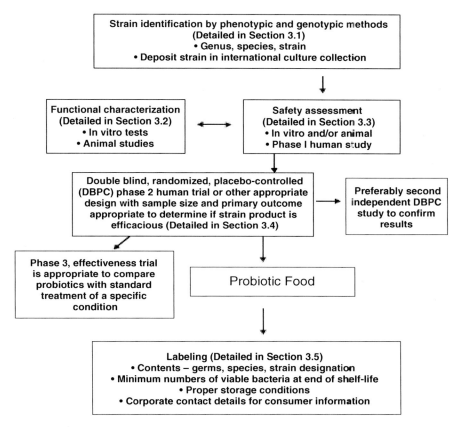

FIGURE 6-6 Guidelines for the evaluation of probiotics for food use.
SOURCE: FAO/WHO (2002).

Are These Allies Safe for Us?

When dealing with war, you need to be sure that your allies are true allies and not imposing undue risk. As far as the lactobacilli and bifidobacteria are concerned, there is a general consensus that they are "safe" but several new items have recently raised some worries.

- There is concern over the use in foods of probiotic bacteria that contain specific drug resistance genes.
- The consultation recognized the need for the development of standardized assays for the determination of drug insensitivity or resistance profiles in lactobacilli and bifidobacteria.

- Due to the relevance of this problem, further research is suggested for antibiotic resistance of lactobacilli and bifidobacteria.
- Research is required to relate the antibiotic resistance of lactobacilli and bifidobacteria and the potential for transmission of genetic elements to other intestinal and/or food-borne microorganisms.

The European Union has recently funded a research project, named ACE-ART (Assessment and Critical Evaluation of Antibiotic Resistance Transferability in Food Chain). The project (www.aceart.net) started one year ago and aims to provide a critical evaluation of the presence of antibiotic resistance genes in non-pathogenic bacteria belonging to *Lactobacillus*, *Bifidobacterium*, *Lactococcus*, and *Streptococcus thermophilus*. One of us (Morelli) is the coordinator of this project, involving 14 laboratories spread all over Europe. At the moment more than 1,300 strains belonging to 20 species have been studied; a little more that 100 strains with "atypical" profiles of antibiotic resistance have been detected.

Prebiotics or the Modification of the Host Nutritional Environment

Prebiotics were not assessed by FAO/WHO consultation and only the following remarks were made:

- Prebiotics are generally defined as "nondigestible food ingredients that beneficially affect the host by selectively stimulating the growth and/or activity of one or a limited number of bacterial species already established in the colon, and thus improve host health" (Gibson and Roberfroid, 1995).
- The concept of prebiotics essentially has the same aim as probiotics: to improve host health via modulation of the intestinal flora, although by a different mechanism. However, there are some cases in which prebiotics may be beneficial for the probiotic, especially with regard to bifidobacteria; that is the synbiotic concept. Synbiotics are defined as "mixtures of probiotics and prebiotics that beneficially affect the host by improving the survival and implantation of live microbial dietary supplements in the gastrointestinal tract of the host" (Andersson et al., 2001). If a synbiotic relationship is intended, then it should be verified scientifically, following the guidelines outlined in section 5 of this report.

Conclusion

More than a dozen years of intense microbiological, genetic, and clinical research have provided enough sound science to convince regulatory bodies that it is necessary to provide suggestions and guidelines for this evolving field; however, it is paramount to realize the difficulty in establishing guidelines for a field which is in fast progress. New techniques that allow enhanced characterization of the gut microbiota are now a long way from "culture and phenotype" and we are approaching a no-culture, genotype-only approach. Moreover, emerging methods that allow assessment of bacteria-epithelial interactions are also to be evaluated. As it is more a possibility that lifelong cross-talk between the host and the gut microbiota determines whether health is maintained or disease intervenes, it is clear that understanding of these bacteria-bacteria and bacteria-host immune and epithelial cell interactions is likely to lead to a greater insight of disease pathogenesis. It is highly possible that a new generation of probiotic or biotherapeutic could be used for obtaining a more targeted use, such as enhancing the production of a specific cytokine or suppressing a specific pathogen.

If guidelines are prepared to provide suggestions and regulatory boundaries, it is important to take note that flexibility as well as constant dialogue between regulatory bodies and the scientific community is necessary. To manage this new war we must look for new allies, but we need also to write down new "alliance treaties" or guidelines for an optimal use of these alliances.

Acknowledgments

We would like to thank Mary Ellen Sanders, president of the International Scientific Association for Probiotics and Prebiotics (ISAPP), for critically reading and editing the manuscript.

REFERENCES

Abreu MT, Fukata M, Arditi M. 2005. TLR signaling in the gut in health and disease. *Journal of Immunology* 174(8):4453–4460.

Adlerberth I, Ahrne S, Johansson ML, Molin G, Hanson LA, Wold AE. 1996. A mannose-specific adherence mechanism in Lactobacillus plantarum conferring binding to the human colonic cell line HT-29. *Applied Environmental Microbiology* 62(7):2244–2251.

AFSSA (Agence Francaise de Sécurité Sanitaire des Aliments/French Food Safety Agency). 2005 (February). Effects of probiotics and prebiotics on flora and immunity in adults. [Online]. Available: http://www.usprobiotics.org/docs/AFFSA%20probiotic%20prebiotic%20flora%20immunity%2005.pdf [accessed January 12, 2006].

Agostoni C, Axelsson I, Braegger C, Goulet O, Koletzko B, Michaelsen KF, Rigo J, Shamir R, Szajewska H, Turck D, Weaver LT (ESPGHAN Committee on Nutrition). 2004a. Probiotic bacteria in dietetic products for infants: A commentary by the ESPGHAN Committee on Nutrition. *Journal of Pediatric Gastroenterology and Nutrition* 39(4):365–374.

Agostoni C, Axelsson I, Goulet O, Koletzko B, Michaelsen KF, Puntis JW, Rigo, J, Shamir R, Szajewska H, Turck D (ESPGHAN Committee on Nutrition). 2004b. Prebiotic oligosaccharides in dietetic products for infants: A commentary by the ESPGHAN Committee on Nutrition. *Journal of Pediatric Gastroenterology and Nutrition* 39(5):465–473.

Ahrne S, Lonnermark E, Wold AE, Aberg N, Hesselmar B, Saalman R, Strannegard IL, Molin G, Adlerberth I. 2005. Lactobacilli in the intestinal microbiota of Swedish infants. *Microbes and Infection* 7(11–12):1256–1262.

Altermann E, Russell WM, Azcarate-Peril MA, Barrangou R, Buck BL, McAuliffe O, Souther N, Dobson A, Duong T, Callanan M, Lick S, Hamrick A, Cano R, Klaenhammer TR. 2005. Complete genome sequence of the probiotic lactic acid bacterium *Lactobacillus acidophilus* NCFM. *Proceedings of the National Academy of Sciences USA* 102(11):3906–3912.

Andersson H, Asp N-G, Bruce A, Roos S, Wadstrom T, Wold AE. 2001. Health effect of probiotics and prebiotics: A literature review on human studies. *Scandanavian Journal of Nutrition* 45: 58–75.

Arvola T, Laiho K, Torkkeli S, Mykkanen H, Salminen S, Maunula L, Isolauri E. 1999. Prophylactic *Lactobacillus* GG reduces antibiotic-associated diarrhea in children with respiratory infections: A randomized study. *Pediatrics* 104(5):e64.

Axelsson L, Lindgren S. 1987. Characterization and DNA homology of *Lactobacillus* strains isolated from pig intestine. *Journal of Applied Bacteriology* 62(5):433–440.

Bäckhed F, Ding H, Wang T, Hooper LV, Koh GY, Nagy A, Semenkovich, CF, Gordon JI. 2004. The gut microbiota as an environmental factor that regulates fat storage. *Proceedings of the National Academy of Sciences USA* 101(44):15718–15723.

Bäckhed F, Ley RE, Sonnenburg JL, Peterson DA, Gordon JI. 2005. Host-bacterial mutualism in the human intestine. *Science* 307(5717):1915–1920.

Barcenilla A, Pryde SE, Martin JC, Duncan SH, Stewart CS, Henderson C, Flint HJ. 2000. Phylogenetic relationships of butyrate-producing bacteria from the human gut. *Applied Environmental Microbiology* 66(4):1654–1661.

Bessi E, Morelli L. 2005. *Lactobacillus apis, Lactobacillus alvei, Lactobacillus larvae* and *Lactobacillus insectis* spp. nov., isolated from larvae, faeces and guts of healthy honeybees. *Systematic and Applied Microbiology.* In press.

Bilsborough J, Viney JL. 2004. In vivo enhancement of dendritic cell function. *Annals of the New York Academy of Sciences* 1029:83–87.

Bjorksten B, Naaber P, Sepp E, Mikelsaar M. 1999. The intestinal microflora in allergic Estonian and Swedish 2-year-old children. *Clinical and Experimental Allergy* 29(3):342–346.

Blaut M, Collins MD, Welling GW, Dore J, van Loo J, de Vos W. 2002. Molecular biological methods for studying the gut microbiota: The EU human gut flora project. *British Journal of Nutrition* 87(Suppl 2):S203–S211.

Boekhorst J, Siezen RJ, Zwahlen MC, Vilanova D, Pridmore RD, Mercenier A, Kleerebezem M, de Vos WM, Brussow H, Desiere F. 2004. The complete genomes of *Lactobacillus plantarum* and *Lactobacillus johnsonii* reveal extensive differences in chromosome organization and gene content. *Microbiology* 150(pt 11):3601–3611.

Boekhorst J, de Been MW, Kleerebezem M, Siezen RJ. 2005. Genome-wide detection and analysis of cell wall-bound proteins with LPxTG-like sorting motifs. *Journal of Bacteriology* 187(14):4928–4934.

Brenchley JM, Schacker TW, Ruff LE, Price DA, Taylor JH, Beilman GJ, Nguyen PL, Khoruts A, Larson M, Haase AT, Douek DC. 2004. CD4+ T cell depletion during all stages of HIV disease occurs predominantly in the gastrointestinal tract. *Journal of Experimental Medicine* 200(6): 749–759.

Bron PA, Marco M, Hoffer SM, Van Mullekom E, de Vos WM and Kleerebezem M. 2004a. Genetic characterization of the bile salt response in *Lactobacillus plantarum* and analysis of responsive promoters in vitro and in situ in the gastrointestinal tract. *Journal of Bacteriology* 186(23): 7829–7835.

Bron PA, Grangette C, Mercenier A, de Vos WM, Kleerebezem M. 2004b. Identification of *Lactobacillus plantarum* genes that are induced in the gastrointestinal tract of mice. *Journal of Bacteriology* 186(17):5721–5729.

Bron PA, Meijer M, Bongers RS, De Vos WM, Kleerebezem M. 2004c. In: *The Molecular Response of Lactobacillus plantarum to Intestinal Passage and Conditions* [thesis]. (Ponsen en Looijen, Wageningen, Wageningen University). Pp. 129–153.

Bron PA, De Vos WM, Kleerebezem M. 2005. In: Vaughan EE, Ouwehand A, eds. *Gastrointestinal Microbiology.* New York: Marcel Dekker, Inc. In press.

Bron PA, Molenaar D, De Vos WM, Kleerebezem M. 2006. DNA micro-array-based identification of bile-responsive genes in Lactobacillus plantarum. *Journal of Applied Microbiology* 100(4): 728–738.

Caramalho I, Lopes-Carvalho T, Ostler D, Zelenay S, Haury M, Demengeot J. 2003. Regulatory T cells selectively express toll-like receptors and are activated by lipopolysaccharide. *Journal of Expimental Medicine* 197(4):403–411.
Chang TL, Chang CH, Simpson DA, Xu Q, Martin PK, Lagenaur LA, Schoolnik GK, Ho DD, Hillier SL, Holodniy M, Lewicki JA, Lee PP. 2003. Inhibition of HIV infectivity by a natural human isolate of *Lactobacillus jensenii* engineered to express functional two-domain CD4. *Proceedings of the National Academy of Sciences USA* 100(20):11672–11677.
Cole MF, Bryan S, Evans MK, Pearce CL, Sheridan MJ, Sura PA, Wientzen R, Bowden GH. 1998. Humoral immunity to commensal oral bacteria in human infants: Salivary antibodies reactive with *Actinomyces naeslundii* genospecies 1 and 2 during colonization. *Infection and Immunity* 66(9):4283–4289.
Collins K, Salminen S, von Wright A, Morelli L, Marteau P, Brassart D, de Vos WM, Fonden R, Saxelin M, Mogensen G, Birkeland SE, Mattila-Sandholm T. 1998. Demonstration of safety of probiotics, a review. *International Journal of Food Microbiology* 44(1–2):93–106.
Cremonini F, Di Caro S, Santarelli L, Gabrielli M, Candelli M, Nista EC, Lupascu A, Gasbarrini G, Gasbarrini A. 2002. Probiotics in antibiotic-associated diarrhoea. *Digest of Liver Diseases* 34(suppl 2):S78–S80.
Crump M, Gospodarowicz M, Shepherd FA. 1999. Lymphoma of the gastrointestinal tract. *Seminars in Oncology* 26(3):324–337.
Cunningham-Rundles C. 1994. Clinical and immunologic studies of common variable immunodeficiency. *Current Opinion in Pediatrics* 6(6):676–681.
Cunningham-Rundles S. 2001. Nutrition and the mucosal immune system. *Current Opinion in Gastroenterology* 17(2):171–176.
Cunningham-Rundles S. 2005 (March 17). *Session IV: Novel Approaches for Mitigating the Development of Resistance*. Presentation at the Forum on Microbial Threats Workshop Ending the War Metaphor: The Changing for Unraveling the Host-Microbe Relationship, Washington, D.C., Institute of Medicine, Forum on Microbial Threats.
Cunningham-Rundles S, Nesin MC. 2000. Bacterial infections in the immunologically compromised host In: Nataro JP, Blaser MJ, Cunningham-Rundles S, eds. *Persistent Bacterial Infections*. Washington, DC: American Society of Microbiology Press. Pp.145–164
Cunningham-Rundles S, Ahrne S, Bengmark S, Johann-Liang R, Marshall F, Metakis L, Califano C, Dunn AM, Grassey C, Hinds G, Cervia J. 2000. Probiotics and immune response. *American Journal of Gastroenterology* 95(1 Suppl):S22–S25.
de Vos WM, BronPA, Kleerebezem M. 2004. Post-genomics of lactic acid bacteria and other food-grade bacteria to discover gut functionality. *Current Opinion in Biotechnology* 15(2):86–93.
Didierlaurent A, Sirard JC, Kraehenbuhl JP, Neutra MR. 2002. How the gut senses its content. *Cell Microbiology* 4(2):61–72.
D'Souza AL, Rajkumar C, Cooke J, Bulpitt CJ. 2002. Probiotics in prevention of antibiotic associated diarrhoea: Meta-analysis. *British Medical Journal* 324(7350):1361.
Ducluzeau R. 1988. Role of experimental microbial ecology in gastroentrology. In: Bergogne-Berezin E, ed. *Microbial Ecology and Intestinal Infection*, Springer-Verlag, France. Pp. 7–26.
Dunne C, Murphy L, Flynn S, O'Mahony L, O'Halloran S, Feeney M, Morrissey D,Thornton G, Fitzgerald G, Daly C, Kiely B, Quigley EM, O'Sullivan GC, Shanahan F, Collins JK. 1999. Probiotics: From myth to reality. Demonstration of functionality in animal models of disease and in human clinical trials [review]. *Antonie Van Leeuwenhoek* 76(1–4):279–292.
Eberl G. 2005. Inducible lymphoid tissues in the adult gut: Recapitulation of a fetal developmental pathway? *Nature Reviews Immunology* 5(5):413–420.
Elmer GW, Surawicz CM, McFarland LV. 1996. Biotherapeutic agents. A neglected modality for the treatment and prevention of selected intestinal and vaginal infections. *Journal of the American Medical Association* 275(11):870–876.

Elmer GW, McFarland LV, Surawicz CM. 1999. *Biotherapeutic Agents and Infectious Diseases.* Totowa, NJ: Humana Press.

FAO/WHO (Food and Agriculture Organization/World Health Organization). 2001 (October). Expert Consultation on Evaluation of Health and Nutritional Properties of Probiotics in Food Including Powder Milk with Live Lactic Acid Bacteria. Córdoba, Argentina. [Online]. Available: http://www.who.int/foodsafety/publications/fs_ management/en/probiotics.pdf [accessed January 3, 2005].

FAO/WHO. 2002 (April 30, May 1). Guidelines for the evaluation of probiotics in food. Report of a Joint FAO/WHO Working Group on Drafting Guidelines for the Evaluation of Probiotics in Food. Ontario, Canada.

Finegold SM, Rolfe RD. 1983. Susceptibility testing of anaerobic bacteria. *Diagnostic Microbiology and Infectious Disease* 1(1):33–40.

Friman V, Nowrouzian F, Adlerberth I, Wold AE. 2002. Increased frequency of intestinal *Escherichia coli* carrying genes for *S. fimbriae* and haemolysin in IgA-deficient individuals. *Microbial Pathogenesis* 32(1):35–42.

Fujiwara S, Seto Y, Kimura A, Hashiba H. 2001. Establishment of orally administered *Lactobacillus gasseri* SBT2055SR in the gastrointestinal tract of humans and its influence on intestinal microflora and metabolism. *Journal of Applied Microbiology* 90(3):343–345.

Fuller R. 1989. Probiotics in man and animals. *Journal of Applied Bacteriology* 66:365–378.

Gibson GR, Roberfroid MB. 1995. Dietary modulation of the human colonic microbiota: Introducing the concept of prebiotics. *Journal of Nutrition* 125(6):1401–1412.

Goepfert AR, Andrews WW, Carlo W, Ramsey PS, Cliver SP, Goldenberg RL, Hauth JC. 2004. Umbilical cord plasma interleukin-6 concentrations in preterm infants and risk of neonatal morbidity. *American Journal of Obstetrics and Gynecology* 191(4):1375–1381.

Guandalini S, Pensabene L, Zikri MA, Dias JA, Casali LG, Hoekstra H, Kolacek S, Massar K, Micetic-Turk D, Papadopoulou A, de Sousa JS, Sandhu B, Szajewska H, Weizman Z. 2000. *Lactobacillus* GG administered in oral rehydration solution to children with acute diarrhea: A multicenter European trial. *Journal of Pediatric Gastroenterology and Nutrition* 30(1):54–60.

Guarner F, Schaafsma GJ. 1998. Probiotics. *International Journal of Food Microbiology* 39(3):237–238.

Hall PA, Coates PJ, Ansari B, Hopwood D. 1994. Regulation of cell number in the mammalian gastrointestinal tract: The importance of apoptosis. *Journal of Cell Science* 107(pt 12):3569–3577.

Hanniffy S, Wiedermann U, Repa A, Mercenier A, Daniel C, Fioramonti J, Tlaskolova H, Kozakova H, Israelsen H, Madsen S, Vrang A, Hols P, Delcour J, Bron P, Kleerebezem M, Wells J. 2004. Potential and opportunities for use of recombinant lactic acid bacteria in human health. *Advanced Applications in Microbiology* 56:1–64.

Harrod T, Martin M, Russell MW. 2001. Long-term persistence and recall of immune responses in aged mice after mucosal immunization. *Oral Microbiology and Immunology* 16(3):170–177.

Holzapfel WH, Haberer P, Snel J, Schillinger U, Huis in't Veld JH. 1998. Overview of gut flora and probiotics [review]. *International Journal of Food Microbiology* 41(2):85–101.

Hooper LV, Xu J, Falk PG, Midtvedt T, Gordon JI. 1999. A molecular sensor that allows a gut commensal to control its nutrient foundation in a competitive ecosystem. *Proceedings of the National Academy of Sciences USA* 96(17):9833–9838.

Hooper LV, Wong MH, Thelin A, Hansson L, Falk PG, Gordon JI. 2001. Molecular analysis of commensal host-microbial relationships in the intestine. *Science* 291(5505):881–884.

Hooper LV, Stappenbeck TS, Hong CV, Gordon JI. 2003. Angiogenins: A new class of microbicidal proteins involved in innate immunity. *Nature Immunology* 4(3):269–273.

Huang Y, Shao XM, Neu J. 2003. Immunonutrients and neonates. *European Journal of Pediatrics* 162(3):122–128.

Huang HC, Wang CL, Huang LT, Chuang H, Liu CA, Hsu TY, Ou CY, Yang KD. 2004. Association of cord blood cytokines with prematurity and cerebral palsy. *Early Human Development* 77(1–2):29–36.

Kalha I, Sellin JH. 2004. Common variable immunodeficiency and the gastrointestinal tract. *Current Gastroenterology Reports* 6(5):377–383.

Kalliomaki M, Kirjavainen P, Eerola E, Kero P, Salminen S, Isolauri E. 2001a. Distinct patterns of neonatal gut microflora in infants in whom atopy was and was not developing. *Journal of Allergy and Clinical Immunology* 107:129–134.

Kalliomaki M, Salminen S, Arvilommi H, Kero P, Koskinen P, Isolauri E. 2001b. Probiotics in primary prevention of atopic disease: A randomised placebo-controlled trial. *Lancet* 357(9262):1076–1079.

Kelly D, Conway S. 2005. Bacterial modulation of mucosal innate immunity. *Molecular Immunology* 42(8):895–901.

Klaenhammer TR, Barrangou R, Buck BL, Azcarate-Peril MA, Altermann E. 2005. Genomic features of lactic acid bacteria effecting bioprocessing and health. *FEMS Microbiology Reviews* 29(3):393–409.

Kleerebezem M. 2005 (March 17). *Session IV: Novel Approaches for Mitigating the Development of Resistance*. Presentation at the Forum on Microbial Threats Workshop Ending the War Metaphor: The Changing Agenda for Unraveling the Host-Microbe Relationship, Washington, D.C., Institute of Medicine, Forum on Microbial Threats.

Kleerebezem M, Boekhorst J, van Kranenburg R, Molenaar D, Kuipers OP, Leer R, Tarchini R, Peters SA, Sandbrink HM, Fiers MW, Stiekema W, Lankhorst RM, Bron PA, Hoffer SM, Groot MN, Kerkhoven R, de Vries M, Ursing B, de Vos W M, Siezen RJ. 2003. Complete genome sequence of *Lactobacillus plantarum* WCFS1. *Proceedings of the National Academy of Sciences USA* 100(4):1990–1995.

Klein G, Pack A, Bonaparte C, Reuter G. 1998. Taxonomy and physiology of probiotic lactic acid bacteria. *International Journal of Food Microbiology* 41(2):103–125.

Kliegman RM. 2005. Oral probiotics reduce the incidence and severity of necrotizing enterocolitis in very low birth weight infants. *Journal of Pediatrics* 146(5):710.

Knight PA, Pemberton AD, Robertson KA, Roy DJ, Wright SH, Miller HR. 2004. Expression profiling reveals novel innate and inflammatory responses in the jejunal epithelial compartment during infection with Trichinella spiralis. *Infection and Immunity* 72(10):6076–6086.

Kunz AN, Noel JM, Fairchok MP. 2004. Two cases of *Lactobacillus bacteremia* during probiotic treatment of short gut syndrome. *Journal of Pediatric Gastroenterology and Nutrition* 38(4):457–458.

Kvasnikov EI, Kovalenko NK, Nesterenko OA. 1971. *Lactobacilli* of bees. *Veterinariia* 8:38–39.

Kvasnikov EI, Kovalenko NK, Materinskaia LG. 1977. *Lactobacilli* of freshwater fishes. *Mikrobiologiia* 46(4):755–760.

Langendijk PS, Schut F, Jansen GJ, Raangs GC, Kamphuis GR, Wilkinson MH, Welling GW. 1995. Quantitative fluorescence in situ hybridization of *Bifidobacterium* spp. with genus-specific 16S rRNA-targeted probes and its application in fecal samples. *Applied Environmental Microbiology* 61(8):3069–3075.

Leverrier P, Dimova D, Pichereau V, Auffray Y, Boyaval P, Jan G. 2003. Susceptibility and adaptive response to bile salts in *Propionibacterium freudenreichii*: Physiological and proteomic analysis. *Applied Environmental Microbiology* 69(7):3809–3818.

Lilly DM, Stillwell RH. 1965. Probiotics: Growth-promoting factors produced by microorganisms. *Science* 147:747–748.

Macdonald TT, Monteleone G. 2005. Immunity, inflammation, and allergy in the gut. *Science* 307(5717):1920–1925.

Macdonald TT, Disabatino A, Gordon JN. 2005. Immunopathogenesis of Crohn's disease. *Journal of Parenteral and Enteral Nutrition* 29(4 Suppl):S118–S125.

Martin R, Langa S, Reviriego C, Jiminez E, Marin ML, Xaus J, Fernandez L, Rodriguez JM. 2003. Human milk is a source of lactic acid bacteria for the infant gut. *Journal of Pediatrics* 143(6):754–758.

McCartney AL. 2002. Application of molecular biological methods for studying probiotics and the gut flora. *British Journal of Nutrition* 88(Suppl 1):S29–S37.

Metchnikoff E. 1907. The prolongation of life. In *Optimistic Studies* Heinemann W. ed., London: G. P. Putnam & Sons. Pp. 1–100.

Miller D, Ross J. 2005. Vaccine INDs: Review of clinical holds. *Vaccine* 23(9):1099–1101.

Ministero della Salute. 2006. Ministero della Salute homepage. [Online]. Available: http://www.ministerosalute.it/ [accessed January 12, 2006].

Molenaar D, Bringel F, Schuren FH, de Vos WM, Siezen RJ, Kleerebezem M. 2005. Exploring *Lactobacillus plantarum* genome diversity by using microarrays. *Journal of Bacteriology* 187(17):6119–6127.

Moore WE, Holdeman LV. 1974. Human fecal flora: The normal flora of 20 Japanese-Hawaiians. *Applied Microbiology* 27(5):961–979.

Morelli L. 2000. In vitro selection of probiotic lactobacilli: A critical appraisal [review]. *Current Issues in Intestinal Microbiology* 1(2):59–67.

Morelli L. 2005 (March 17). *Session IV: Novel Approaches for Mitigating the Development of Resistance*. Presentation at the Forum on Microbial Threats Workshop Ending the War Metaphor: The Changing for Unraveling the Host-Microbe Relationship, Washington, D.C., Institute of Medicine, Forum on Microbial Threats.

Morelli L, Cesena C, de Haen C, Gozzini L. 1998. Taxonomic *Lactobacillus* composition of feces from human newborns during the first few days. *Microbial Ecology* 35(2):205–212.

Nachman SA, Lindsey JC, Moye J, Stanley KE, Johnson GM, Krogstad PA, Wiznia AA. 2005. Growth of human immunodeficiency virus-infected children receiving highly active antiretroviral therapy. *Pediatric Infectious Disease Journal* 24(4):352–357.

Nielsen DS, Moller PL, Rosenfeldt V, Paerregaard A, Michaelsen KF, Jakobsen M. 2003. Case study of the distribution of mucosa-associated *Bifidobacterium* species, *Lactobacillus* species, and other lactic acid bacteria in the human colon. *Applied Environmental Microbiology* 69(12):7545–7548.

Pabst R. 1987. The anatomical basis for the immune function of the gut. *Anatomy and Embryology* 176(2):135–144.

Pacha J. 2000. Development of intestinal transport function in mammals. *Physiological Reviews* 80(4):1633–1667.

Parker RB. 1974. Probiotics: The other half of the antibiotic story. *Animal Nutrition and Health* 29:4–8.

Percival RS, Marsh PD, Challacombe SJ. 1996. Serum antibodies to commensal oral and gut bacteria vary with age. *FEMS Immunology and Medical Microbiology* 15(1):35–42.

Prescott SL, Macaubas C, Holt BJ, Smallacombe TB, Loh R, Sly PD, Holt PG. 1998. Transplacental priming of the human immune system to environmental allergens: Universal skewing of initial T cell responses toward the Th2 cytokine profile. *Journal of Immunology* 160(10):4730–4737.

Pretzer G, Snel J, Molenaar D, Wiersma A, Bron PA, Lambert J, de Vos WM, van der Meer R, Smits MA, Kleerebezem M. 2005. Biodiversity-based identification and functional characterization of the mannose-specific adhesin of *Lactobacillus plantarum*. *Journal of Bacteriology* 187(17): 6128–6136.

Pridmore RD, Berger B, Desiere F, Vilanova D, Barretto C, Pittet AC, Zwahlen MC, Rouvet M, Altermann E, Barrangou R, Mollet B, Mercenier A, Klaenhammer T, Arigoni F, Schell MA. 2004. The genome sequence of the probiotic intestinal bacterium *Lactobacillus johnsonii* NCC 533. *Proceedings of the National Academy of Sciences USA* 101(8):2512–2517.

Pryde SE, Richardson AJ, Stewart CS, Flint HJ. 1999. Molecular analysis of the microbial diversity present in the colonic wall, colonic lumen, and cecal lumen of a pig. *Applied Environmental Microbiology* 65(12):5372–5327.

Rakoff-Nahoum S, Paglino J, Eslami-Varzaneh F, Edberg S, Medzhitov R. 2004. Recognition of commensal microflora by toll-like receptors is required for intestinal homeostasis. *Cell* 118(6): 229–241.
Rawls JF, Samuel BS, Gordon JI. 2004. Gnotobiotic zebrafish reveal evolutionarily conserved responses to the gut microbiota. *Proceedings of the National Academy of Sciences USA* 101(13): 4596–4601.
Reid G, Sanders ME, Gaskins HR, Gibson GR, Mercenier A, Rastall R, Roberfroid M, Rowland I, Cherbut C, Klaenhammer TR. 2003. New scientific paradigms for probiotics and prebiotics. *Journal of Clinical Gastroenterology* 37(2):105–118.
Rhee KJ, Sethupathi P, Driks A, Lanning DK, Knight KL. 2004. Role of commensal bacteria in development of gut-associated lymphoid tissues and preimmune antibody repertoire. *Journal of Immunology* 172(2):1118–1124.
Rimoldi M, Chieppa M, Salucci V, Avogadri F, Sonzogni A, Sampietro GM, Nespoli A, Viale G, Allavena P, Rescigno M. 2005. Intestinal immune homeostasis is regulated by the crosstalk between epithelial cells and dendritic cells. *Nature Immunology* 6(5):507–514.
Roller M, Rechkemmer G, Watzl B. 2004. Prebiotic inulin enriched with oligofructose in combination with the probiotics *Lactobacillus rhamnosus* and *Bifidobacterium lactis* modulates intestinal immune functions in rats. *Journal of Nutrition* 134(1):153–156.
Rouzaud G, Rabot S, Ratcliffe B, Duncan AJ. 2003. Influence of plant and bacterial myrosinase activity on the metabolic fate of glucosinolates in gnotobiotic rats. *British Journal of Nutrition.* 90(2):395–404.
Salminen S, Ouwehand A, Benno Y, Lee YK. 1999. Probiotics: How are they defined? *Trends in Food Science and Technology* 10:107–110.
Sanders ME. 2003. Probiotics: Considerations for human health. *Nutrition Reviews* 61(3):91–99.
Sarra PG, Magri M, Bottazzi V, Dellaglio F. 1980. Genetic heterogeneity among *Lactobacillus acidophilus* strains. *Antonie Van Leeuwenhoek* 46(2):169–176.
Sarra PG, Vescovo M, Fulgoni M. 1986. Study on crop adhesion genetic determinant in *Lactobacillus reuteri. Microbiologica* 9(3):279–285.
Sartor RB. 2005. Probiotic therapy of intestinal inflammation and infections. *Current Opinion in Gastroenterology* 21(1):44–50.
Saunier K, Dore J. 2002. Gastrointestinal tract and the elderly: Functional foods, gut microflora and healthy ageing. *Digest of Liver Diseases* 34(Suppl 2):S19–S24.
Schell MA, Karmirantzou M, Snel B, Vilanova D, Berger B, Pessi G, Zwahlen MC, Desiere F, Bork P, Delley M, Pridmore RD, Arigoni F. 2002. The genome sequence of *Bifidobacterium longum* reflects its adaptation to the human gastrointestinal tract. *Proceedings of the National Academy of Sciences USA* 99(22):14422–14427.
Schrezenmeir J, Heller K, McCue M, Llamas C, Lam W, Burow H, Kindling-Rohracker M, Fischer W, Sengespeik HC, Comer GM, Alarcon P. 2004. Benefits of oral supplementation with and without synbiotics in young children with acute bacterial infections. *Clinical Pediatrics* 43(3):239–249.
Schultz C, Temming P, Bucsky P, Gopel W, Strunk T, Hartel C. 2004a. Immature anti-inflammatory response in neonates. *Clinical and Experimental Immunology* 135:130–136.
Schultz M, Timmer A, Herfarth HH, Sartor RB, Vanderhoof JA, Rath HC. 2004b. Lactobacillus GG in inducing and maintaining remission of Crohn's disease. *BMC Gastroenterology* 4:5.
Shanahan F. 2003. Probiotics: A perspective on problems, pitfalls. *Scandinavian Journal of Gastroenterology* 237(Suppl):34–36.
Song YL, Kato N, Matsumiya Y, Liu CX, Kato H, Watanabe K. 1999. Identification of *Lactobacillus* species of human origin by a commercial kit, API50CHL. *Rinsho Biseibutshu Jinsoku Shindan Kenkyukai Shi* 10(2):77–82.

Song Y, Kato N, Liu C, Matsumiya Y, Kato H, Watanabe K. 2000. Rapid identification of 11 human intestinal *Lactobacillus* species by multiplex PCR assays using group- and species-specific primers derived from the 16S-23SrRNA intergenic spacer region and its flanking 23S rRNA. *FEMS Microbiology Letters* 187(2):167–173.

Sonnenburg JL, Xu J, Leip DD, Chen CH, Westover BP, Weatherford J, Buhler JD, Gordon JI. 2005. Glycan foraging in vivo by an intestine-adapted bacterial symbiont. *Science* 307(5717):1955–1959.

Suau A. 2003. Molecular tools to investigate intestinal bacterial communities. *Journal of Pediatric Gastroenterology and Nutrition* 37(3):222–224.

Suau A, Bonnet R, Sutren M, Godon JJ, Gibson GR, Collins MD, Dore J. 1999. Direct analysis of genes encoding 16S rRNA from complex communities reveals many novel molecular species within the human gut. *Applied Environmental Microbiology* 65(11):4799–4807.

Suau A, Rochet V, Sghir A, Gramet G, Brewaeys S, Sutren M, Rigottier-Gois L, Dore J. 2001. *Fusobacterium prausnitzii* and related species represent a dominant group within the human fecal flora. *Systematic and Applied Microbiology* 24(1):139–145.

Szajewska H, Mrukowicz JZ. 2001. Probiotics in the treatment and prevention of acute infectious diarrhea in infants and children: A systematic review of published randomized, double-blind, placebo-controlled trials. *Journal of Pediatric Gastroenterology and Nutrition* 33(Suppl 2):S17–S25.

Tannock GW. 2003. Probiotics: Time for a dose of realism. *Current Issues in Intestinal Microbiology* 4(2):33–42.

Tannock GW, Munro K, Harmsen HJ, Welling GW, Smart J, Gopal PK. 2000. Analysis of the fecal microflora of human subjects consuming a probiotic product containing *Lactobacillus rhamnosus* DR20. *Applied Environmental Microbiology* 66(6):2578–2588.

Thompson C, McCarter YS, Krause PJ, Herson VC. 2001. *Lactobacillus acidophilu*s sepsis in a neonate. *Journal of Perinatology* 21(4):258–260.

Tlaskalova-Hogenova H, Stepankova R, Hudcovic T, Tuckova L, Cukrowska B, Lodinova-Zadnikova R, Kozakova H, Rossmann P, Bartova J, Sokol D, Funda DP, Borovska D, Rehakova Z, Sinkora J, Hofman J, Drastich P, Kokesova A. 2004. Commensal bacteria (normal microflora), mucosal immunity and chronic inflammatory and autoimmune diseases [review]. *Immunology Letters* 93(2–3):97–108.

Vaarala O. 2003. Immunological effects of probiotics with special reference to lactobacilli [Review]. *Clinical and Experimental Allergy* 33(12):1634–1640.

Vaillancourt R. 2005 (March 17). *Session IV: Novel Approaches for Mitigating the Development of Resistance*. Presentation at the Forum on Microbial Threats Workshop Ending the War Metaphor: The Changing Agenda for Unraveling the Host-Microbe Relationship, Washington, D.C., Institute of Medicine, Forum on Microbial Threats.

van Kranenburg R, Golic N, Bongers R, Leer RJ, de Vos WM, Siezen RJ, Kleerebezem M. 2005. Functional analysis of three plasmids from *Lactobacillus* plantarum. *Applied Environmental Microbiology* 71(3):1223–1230.

Van Niel CW, Feudtner C, Garrison MM, Christakis DA. 2002. *Lactobacillus* therapy for acute infectious diarrhea in children: A meta-analysis. *Pediatrics* 109(4):678–684.

Vaughan EE, Schut F, Heilig HG, Zoetendal EG, de Vos WM, Akkermans AD. 2000. A molecular view of the intestinal ecosystem. *Current Issues of Interest in Microbiology* 1(1):1–12.

Vaughan EE, Heilig HG, Ben-Amor K, de Vos WM. 2005. Diversity, vitality and activities of intestinal lactic acid bacteria and bifidobacteria assessed by molecular approaches. *FEMS Microbiology Review* 29(3):477–490.

Veber MB, Cunningham-Rundles S, Schulman M, Mandel F, Auld PA. 1991. Acute shift in immune response to microbial activators in very-low-birth-weight infants. *Clinical and Experimental Immunology* 83(3):391–395.

Vinderola CG, Medici M, Perdigon G. 2004. Relationship between interaction sites in the gut, hydrophobicity, mucosal immunomodulating capacities and cell wall protein profiles in indigenous and exogenous bacteria. *Journal of Applied Microbiology* 96(2):230–243.

Walter J, Heng NC, Hammes WP, Loach DM, Tannock, GW, Hertel C. 2003. Identification of *Lactobacillus reuteri* genes specifically induced in the mouse gastrointestinal tract. *Applied Environmental Microbiology* 69(4):2044–2051.

Walter J, Chagnaud P, Tannock GW, Loach DM, Dal Bello F, Jenkinson HF, Hammes WP, Hertel C. 2005. A high-molecular-mass surface protein (Lsp) and methionine sulfoxide reductase B (MsrB) contribute to the ecological performance of *Lactobacillus reuteri* in the murine gut. *Applied Environmental Microbiology* 71(2):979–986.

Watson DC, Counts DR. 2004. Growth hormone deficiency in HIV-infected children following successful treatment with highly active antiretroviral therapy. *Journal of Pediatrics* 145(4): 549–551.

Xu J, Bjursell MK, Himrod J, Deng S, Carmichael LK, Chiang HC, Hooper LV, Gordon JI. 2003. A genomic view of the human-*Bacteroides thetaiotaomicron* symbiosis. *Science* 299(5615):2074–2076.

Zoetendal EG, Akkermans AD, de Vos WM. 1998. Temperature gradient gel electrophoresis analysis of 16S rRNA from human fecal samples reveals stable and host-specific communities of active bacteria. *Applied Environmental Microbiology* 64(10):3854–3859.

Zoetendal EG, von Wright A, Vilpponen-Salmela T, Ben-Amor K, Akkermans AD, de Vos WM. 2002. Mucosa-associated bacteria in the human gastrointestinal tract are uniformly distributed along the colon and differ from the community recovered from feces. *Applied Environmental Microbiology* 68(7):3401–3407.

Zoetendal EG, Collier CT, Koike S, Mackie RI, Gaskins HR. 2004. Molecular ecological analysis of the gastrointestinal microbiota: A review. *Journal of Nutrition and Dietetics* 134(2):465–472.

APPENDIX A

Forum on Microbial Threats

Board on Global Health

Institute of Medicine

The National Academies

Ending the War Metaphor: The Changing Agenda
for Unraveling the Host-Microbe Relationship

March 16–March 17, 2005
KECK 100
National Academies
500 Fifth Street, N.W.
Washington, D.C. 20001

AGENDA

WEDNESDAY, MARCH 16, 2005

8:30–9:00	**Continental Breakfast**
9:00	**Welcome and Opening Remarks**

Stanley Lemon, The University of Texas Medical Branch, Galveston; Chair, Forum on Microbial Threats

9:15	**Arms Races with Evolving Diseases: "We've Met the Enemy and He Is Us"**
	Joshua Lederberg, Rockefeller University **Stanley Falkow**, Stanford University
10:15	Discussion
10:30	Break

Session I: Host-Pathogen Interactions: Defining the Concepts of Pathogenicity, Virulence, Colonization, Commensalism, and Symbiosis

Moderator:	P. Frederick Sparling, University of North Carolina Vice-chair, Forum on Microbial Threats
10:45	Colonization
	Jeffrey I. Gordon, Washington University School of Medicine, or, **Karen Guillemin**, University of Washington
11:45	Discussion
12:15	**Lunch—Welcoming Remarks by Dr. Harvey Fineberg, President, Institute of Medicine**
1:00–2:30	**Commensalism and Symbiosis—Host, Microbial, and Environmental Factors**
	Abigail Salyers, University of Illinois, Champaign-Urbana **Jo Handelsman**, Department of Plant Pathology, University of Wisconsin, Madison
2:30–2:45	Discussion
2:45–3:00	Break
3:00–4:15	**Pathogenicity and Virulence**
	Martin Blaser, New York University School of Medicine **BJ Staskawicz**, University of California, Berkeley
4:15–5:45	**Open Discussion of Day 1**
Moderator:	David Relman, Stanford University
	Balfor Sartor, University of North Carolina **Maria G. Dominguez-Bello**, University of Puerto Rico, Rio Piedras
5:45	**Adjournment of the first day**

APPENDIX A

6:00	Reception
7:15	Dinner Meeting of the Forum on Microbial Threats [location TBD]

THURSDAY, MARCH 17, 2005

8:00–8:30	Continental Breakfast
8:30	Opening Remarks/Summary of Day 1

P. Frederick Sparling, University of North Carolina
Vice-chair, Forum on Microbial Threats

Session II: Ecology of Host-Microbe Interactions

Moderator: Stephen S. Morse, Columbia University

8:40–9:25	Endogenous Microbial Communities

David Stahl, University of Washington
Mark E.J. Woolhouse, Centre for Tropical Veterinary Medicine, University of Edinburgh

9:25–10:15	How the Host "Sees" and Responds to Pathogens

Marian Neutra, Harvard Medical School and Children's Hospital
David Relman, Stanford University

10:15–10:30	Discussion
10:30–10:45	Break

Session III: Understanding the Dynamic Relationships of Host-Microbe Interactions—Discussion Panel

Moderator:	David Relman, Stanford University
10:45–12:15	Lonnie King, Michigan State University Stanley Falkow, Stanford University Jeffrey I. Gordon, Washington University School of Medicine
12:15–12:45	Lunch

Session IV: Novel Approaches for Mitigating the Development of Resistance

Moderator: **James Hughes**, Emory University

12:45–1:30 **Using Pre- and Probiotics to Modify Host-Environmental Factors to Promote Health and Mitigate Disease**

Michiel Kleerebezem, Holland
Suzanne Cunningham-Rundles, Cornell University

1:30–2:00 **Governmental Approaches to Regulating Pre- and Probiotics**

Lorenzo Morelli, Istituto di Microbiologia UCSC—Italy
Julienne Vaillancourt, CBER, FDA

2:00–2:15 Discussion

Session V: Challenges and Opportunities to Developing a New Paradigm to Replace the "War Metaphor"

Moderator: **Fredrick Sparling**, University of North Carolina, Chapel Hill

2:15–4:00 With the backdrop of the previous days' presentations and discussion, Forum members, panel discussants, and the audience will comment on the issues and next steps that they would identify as priority areas for consideration within industry, academia, public health organizations, and other government sectors. The discussion of priorities will summarize the issues surrounding emerging opportunities for more effective collaboration as well as the remaining research and programmatic needs. The confounding issues of the major obstacles to preparing an optimal response, particularly as it relates to the complexities of interaction between private industry, research and public health agencies, regulatory agencies, policy makers, academic researchers, and the public, will be explored with an eye toward innovative responses to such challenges.

Panel Discussants:

Joshua Lederberg, Rockefeller University
David Stahl, University of Washington

4:00 Adjourn

APPENDIX B

Acronyms

ACE-ART	Assessment and Critical Evaluation of Antibiotic Resistance Transferability
AFSSA	French Food Safety Authority
AIDS	acquired immunodeficiency syndrome
AOM	azoxymethane
BLA	biologics license application
CBER	Center for Biologics Evaluation and Research
CDC	Centers for Disease Control and Prevention
CFB	*Cytophaga-Flavobacterium-Bacteroides*
CFR	Code of Federal Regulations
CFSAN	Center for Food Safety and Applied Nutrition
CLL	chronic lymphocytic leukemia
CMC	chemistry, manufacturing, and controls
CONV-R	conventionally raised
CPS	capsular polysaccharide synthesis
DGGE	denaturing gradient gel electrophoresis
DLCL	diffuse large B-cell lymphomas
DNA	deoxyribonucleic acid
DPF	day post-fertilization
DSHEA	Dietary Supplement Health and Education Act
DSS	dextran sodium sulfate

ESPGHAN	European Society for Paediatric Gastroenterology Hepatology and Nutrition
FAE	follicle-associated epithelium
FAO	Food and Agriculture Organization
FDA	Food and Drug Administration
Fiaf	fastin-induced adipocyte factor
FISH	fluorescent in-situ hybridization
FLS	flagellin sensitivity
GALT	gut-associated lymphoid tissue
GBBS	Group B beta-hemolytic *Streptococcus*
GE	gastroesophageal
GERD	gastroesophageal reflux disease
GF	germ-free
GI	gastrointestinal
GPI	glycosylphatidylinositol
GRAS	generally recognizable as safe
HAART	highly active antiretroviral therapy
HIV	human immunodeficiency virus
HLA	human lymphocyte antigen
IBD	inflammatory bowel disease
IgA	immunoglobulin A
IgG	immunoglobulin G
IFN	interferon
IL	interleukin
IND	investigational new drug
IOM	Institute of Medicine
ISAPP	International Scientific Association for Probiotics and Prebiotics
IVET	in vivo expression technology
LPL	lipoprotein lipase
LPS	lipopolysaccharide
LRR-TM	leucine-rich repeat transmembrane
MALT	mucosa-associated lymphoid tissue
MEMS	microelectromechanical systems
NBS LRR	nucleotide-binding site plus leucine-rich repeat
NCBI	National Centre for Biotechnology Information

NK	natural killer
NSAID	nonsteroidal anti-inflammatory drug
OCTN	organic cation transporter genes
OVRR	Office of Vaccine Research and Review
PBMC	peripheral blood mononuclear cell
PCR	polymerase chain reaction
PRR	pattern recognition receptor
qRT	quantitative reverse transcription
RNA	ribonucleic acid
RPM	Resistance to *P. syringae* pv *maculicola*
RPS	Resistance to *P. syringae*
SARS	severe acute respiratory syndrome
SCID	severe combined immune deficient
SCOTS	selective capture of transcribed sequences
SLOTU	species-level operational taxonomic unit
SPF	specific pathogen free
STM	signature-tagged mutagenesis
T-DNA	transfer DNA
TGF	transforming growth factor
Th	T helper
TLR	toll-like receptor
TMV	tobacco mosaic virus
VTEC	verocytotoxigenic *E. coli*
WB	whole blood
WHO	World Health Organization

APPENDIX C

Forum Member Biographies

Stanley M. Lemon, M.D. (*Chair*), is the John Sealy Distinguished University Chair and Director of the Institute for Human Infections and Immunity at the University of Texas Medical Branch (UTMB) at Galveston. He received his undergraduate A.B. degree in biochemical sciences from Princeton University summa cum laude, and his M.D. with honor from the University of Rochester. He completed postgraduate training in internal medicine and infectious diseases at the University of North Carolina at Chapel Hill, and is board certified in both. From 1977 to 1983, he served with the U.S. Army Medical Research and Development Command, followed by a 14-year period on the faculty of the University of North Carolina School of Medicine. He moved to UTMB in 1997, serving first as chair of the Department of Microbiology and Immunology, then as dean of the School of Medicine from 1999 to 2004. Dr. Lemon's research interests relate to the molecular virology and pathogenesis of the positive-stranded RNA viruses responsible for hepatitis. He has had a long-standing interest in antiviral and vaccine development, and has served previously as chair of the Anti-Infective Drugs Advisory Committee of the U.S. Food and Drug Administration (FDA). He is the past chair of the Steering Committee on Hepatitis and Poliomyelitis of the World Health Organization (WHO) Programme on Vaccine Development. He presently serves as a member of the U.S. Delegation of the U.S.–Japan Cooperative Medical Sciences Program, and chairs the Board of Scientific Councilors of the National Center for Infectious Diseases (NCID) of the Centers for Disease Control and Prevention (CDC). He was co-chair of the Committee on Advances in Technology and the Prevention of their Application to Next Generation Biowarfare

Threats for the National Academy of Sciences and recently chaired an Institute of Medicine (IOM) study committee related to vaccines for the protection of the military against naturally occurring infectious disease threats.

P. Frederick Sparling, M.D. (*Vice-chair*), is the J. Herbert Bate Professor Emeritus of Medicine, Microbiology, and Immunology at the University of North Carolina (UNC) at Chapel Hill, and is director of the North Carolina Sexually Transmitted Infections Research Center. Previously, he served as chair of the Department of Medicine and chair of the Department of Microbiology and Immunology at UNC. He was president of the Infectious Disease Society of America from 1996–1997. He was also a member of the IOM's Committee on Microbial Threats to Health (1991–1992). Dr. Sparling's laboratory research is in the molecular biology of bacterial outer membrane proteins involved in pathogenesis, with a major emphasis on *gonococci* and *meningococci*. His current studies focus on the biochemistry and genetics of iron-scavenging mechanisms used by *gonococci* and *meningococci* and the structure and function of the *gonococcal porin* proteins. He is pursuing the goal of a vaccine for gonorrhea.

Margaret A. Hamburg, M.D. (*Vice-chair*), is vice president for Biological Programs at the Nuclear Threat Initiative (NTI), a charitable organization working to reduce the global threat from nuclear, biological, and chemical weapons. Dr. Hamburg is in charge of the biological program area. Before taking on her current position, Dr. Hamburg was the Assistant Secretary for Planning and Evaluation, U.S. Department of Health and Human Services, serving as a principal policy advisor to the Secretary of Health and Human Services with responsibilities including policy formulation and analysis, the development and review of regulations and/or legislation, budget analysis, strategic planning, and the conduct and coordination of policy research and program evaluation. Prior to this, she served for almost six years as the Commissioner of Health for the City of New York. As chief health officer in the nation's largest city, Dr. Hamburg's many accomplishments included the design and implementation of an internationally recognized tuberculosis control program that produced dramatic declines in tuberculosis cases, the development of initiatives that raised childhood immunization rates to record levels, and the creation of the first public health bioterrorism preparedness program in the nation. She completed her internship and residency in internal medicine at the New York Hospital/Cornell University Medical Center and is certified by the American Board of Internal Medicine. Dr. Hamburg is a graduate of Harvard College and Harvard Medical School. She currently serves on the Harvard University Board of Overseers. She has been elected to membership in the IOM, the New York Academy of Medicine, and the Council on Foreign Relations, and is a Fellow of the American Association for the Advancement of Science and the American College of Physicians.

David Acheson, M.D., is chief medical officer at the Center for Food Safety and Applied Nutrition, U.S. FDA. He received his medical degree at the University of London. After completing internships in general surgery and medicine, he continued his postdoctoral training in Manchester, England, as a Wellcome Trust Research Fellow. He subsequently was a Wellcome Trust Training Fellow in Infectious Diseases at the New England Medical Center and at the Wellcome Research Unit in Vellore, India. Dr. Acheson was associate professor of medicine, Division of Geographic Medicine and Infectious Diseases, New England Medical Center, until 2001. He then joined the faculties of the Department of Epidemiology and Preventive Medicine and Department of Microbiology and Immunology at the University of Maryland Medical School. Currently at the FDA, his research concentration is on food-borne pathogens and encompasses a mixture of molecular pathogenesis, cell biology, and epidemiology. Specifically, his research focuses on Shiga toxin-producing *E. coli* and understanding toxin interaction with intestinal epithelial cells using tissue culture models. His laboratory has also undertaken a study to examine Shiga toxin-producing *E. coli* in food animals in relation to virulence factors and antimicrobial resistance patterns. More recently, Dr. Acheson initiated a project to understand the molecular pathogenesis of *Campylobacter jejuni*. Other studies have undertaken surveillance of diarrheal disease in the community to determine causes, outcomes, and risk factors of unexplained diarrhea. Dr. Acheson has authored/coauthored over 72 journal articles, and 42 book chapters and reviews, and is coauthor of the book *Safe Eating* (Dell Health, 1998). He is reviewer of more than 10 journals and is on the editorial board of *Infection and Immunity* and *Clinical Infectious Diseases*. Dr. Acheson is a Fellow of the Royal College of Physicians, a Fellow of the Infectious Disease Society of America, and holds several patents.

Ruth L. Berkelman, M.D., is the Rollins Professor and director of the Center for Public Health Preparedness and Research at the Rollins School of Public Health, Emory University in Atlanta. She received her A.B. from Princeton University and her M.D. from Harvard Medical School. Board certified in pediatrics and internal medicine, she began her career at the CDC in 1980, and later became deputy director of the NCID. She also served as a senior advisor to the director, CDC, and Assistant Surgeon General in the U.S. Public Health Service. In 2001, she came to her current position at Emory University, directing a center focused on emerging infectious disease and other urgent threats to health, including terrorism. She has also consulted with the biologic program of the Nuclear Threat Initiative and is most recognized for her work in infectious diseases and disease surveillance. She was elected to the IOM in 2004. Currently a member of the IOM's Forum on Microbial Threats and the Board on Life Sciences of the National Academy of Science, she also chairs the Board of Public and Scientific Affairs at the American Society of Microbiology.

Enriqueta C. Bond, Ph.D., is president of the Burroughs Wellcome Fund. Dr. Bond received her undergraduate degree from Wellesley College, her M.A. from the University of Virginia, and her Ph.D. in molecular biology and biochemical genetics from Georgetown University. She is a member of the Institute of Medicine, the American Association for the Advancement of Science, the American Society for Microbiology, and the American Public Health Association. Dr. Bond serves on the Council of the IOM as its vice-chair; she chairs the Board of Scientific Counselors for the NCID at the CDC, and she chairs the IOM's Clinical Research Roundtable. She serves on the board and executive committee of the Research Triangle Park Foundation, and on the board of the Medicines for Malaria Venture. Prior to being named president of the Burroughs Wellcome Fund in 1994, Dr. Bond served on the staff of the IOM since 1979, becoming the Institute's executive officer in 1989.

Roger G. Breeze, Ph.D., received his veterinary degree (1968) and Ph.D. degree in veterinary pathology (1973) at the University of Glasgow, Scotland. He was engaged in teaching, diagnostic pathology, and research on respiratory and cardiovascular diseases at the University of Glasgow Veterinary School from 1968 to 1977 and at Washington State University College of Veterinary Medicine, where he was professor and chair of the Department of Microbiology and Pathology, from 1977 to 1987. From 1984 to 1987 he was deputy director of the Washington Technology Center, the state's high-technology sciences initiative, based in the College of Engineering at the University of Washington. In 1987, he was appointed director of the U.S. Department of Agriculture's (USDA's) Plum Island Animal Disease Center, a biosafety level 3 facility for research and diagnosis of the world's most dangerous livestock diseases. In that role, he initiated research into the genomic and functional genomic basis of disease pathogenesis, diagnosis, and control of livestock RNA and DNA virus infections. This work became the basis of U.S. defense against natural and deliberate infection with these agents and led to his involvement in the early 1990s in biological weapons defense and proliferation prevention. From 1995 to 1998 he directed research programs in 20 laboratories in the southeast for the USDA Agricultural Research Service before going to Washington D.C. to establish biological weapons defense research programs for USDA. He received the Distinguished Executive Award from President Clinton in 1998 for his work at Plum Island and in biodefense. Since 2004, he has been CEO of Centaur Science Group, which provides consulting services in biodefense. His main commitment is to the Defense Threat Reduction Agency's Biological Weapons Proliferation Prevention program in Europe, the Caucasus, and Central Asia.

Steven J. Brickner, Ph.D., is research advisor, antibacterials chemistry, at Pfizer Global Research and Development. He received his Ph.D. in organic chemistry from Cornell University and was a NIH Postdoctoral Research Fellow at the University of Wisconsin–Madison. Dr. Brickner is a medicinal chemist with nearly 20 years of research experience in the pharmaceutical industry, all focused on the discovery and development of novel antibacterial agents. He is an inventor/co-inventor on 21 U.S. patents and has published numerous scientific papers, primarily within the area of the oxazolidinones. Prior to joining Pfizer in 1996, he led a team at Pharmacia and Upjohn that discovered and developed linezolid, the first member of a new class of antibiotics to be approved in the last 35 years.

Joseph Bryan, M.D., graduated from Oklahoma Christian College in 1974 and from the University of Oklahoma College of Medicine in 1979. After completing a residency in internal medicine at the Alton Ochsner Medical Foundation in New Orleans in 1982, he participated in clinical trials in Salvador, Brazil. He completed a research fellowship in central nervous system infections at the University of Virginia in July 1984. Dr. Bryan became an officer in the medical corps of the U.S. Navy in October 1984 and completed a fellowship in infectious diseases at the National Naval Medical Center in Bethesda, Maryland, in November 1986. Dr. Bryan served at the Uniformed Services University of the Health Sciences, conducing clinical trials and epidemiologic studies in Pakistan, Zambia, and Belize. In 1997, he became the course director for military tropical medicine and participated in other tropical and preventive medical courses through the Naval School of Health Sciences in Bethesda. In July 2000, Dr. Bryan joined the Office of Medical Services of the Department of State as a consultant in infectious diseases and tropical and travel medicine. He has been elected a Fellow in the American College of Physicians and Infectious Disease Society of America. He has published 39 peer-reviewed papers, 9 invited articles, and 1 book chapter. He serves as an adjunct professor at the Uniformed Services University.

Nancy Carter-Foster, M.S.T.M., is senior advisor for health affairs for the U.S. Department of State, Assistant Secretary for Science and Health, and the Secretary's Representative on HIV/AIDS. She is responsible for identifying emerging health issues and making policy recommendations for the United States foreign policy concerns regarding international health, and coordinates the department's interactions with the nongovernmental community. She is a member of the IOM's Forum on Microbial Threats, the Infectious Diseases Society of America (IDSA), and the American Association of the Advancement of Science (AAAS). She has helped bring focus to global health issues in U.S. foreign policy and brought a national security focus to global health. In prior positions as director for congressional and legislative affairs for the Economic and Business Affairs Bureau of the U.S. Department of State, Foreign Policy Advisory to the majority whip U.S. House of Representatives, trade specialist advisor to the House of Representatives Ways and Means Trade Subcommittee, and consultant to the World Bank, Asia Technical Environment Division, Ms. Carter-Foster has worked on a wide variety of health, trade, and environmental issues amassing in-depth knowledge and experience in policy development and program implementation.

Gail H. Cassell, Ph.D., is vice president of Scientific Affairs, Distinguished Lilly Research Scholar for Infectious Diseases, Eli Lilly & Company. Previously, she was the Charles H. McCauley Professor and (since 1987) chair, Department of Microbiology, University of Alabama Schools of Medicine and Dentistry at Birmingham, a department which, under her leadership, has ranked first in research funding from the National Institutes of Health (NIH) since 1989. She is a member of the Director's Advisory Committee of the Centers for Disease Control and Prevention (CDC). Dr. Cassell is past president of the American Society for Microbiology (ASM) and is serving her third 3-year term as chair of the Public and Scientific Affairs Board of ASM. She is a former member of the National Institutes of Health (NIH) Director's Advisory Committee and a former member of the Advisory Council of the National Institute of Allergy and Infectious Diseases (NIAID). She has also served as an advisor on infectious diseases and indirect costs of research to the White House Office on Science and Technology and was previously chair of the Board of Scientific Counselors of the National Center for Infectious Diseases (NCID), CDC. Dr. Cassell served eight years on the Bacteriology-Mycology-II Study Section and served as its chair for three years. She serves on the editorial boards of several prestigious scientific journals and has authored over 275 articles and book chapters. She has been intimately involved in the establishment of science policy and legislation related to biomedical research and public health. Dr. Cassell has received several national and international awards and an honorary degree for her research on infectious diseases.

Mark Feinberg, M.D., Ph.D., is vice president for Policy, Public Health, and Medical Affairs in the Merck Vaccine Division of Merck & Co., Inc. He received his bachelor's degree magna cum laude from the University of Pennsylvania in 1978, and his M.D. and Ph.D. degrees from Stanford University School of Medicine in 1987. From 1985–1986, Dr. Feinberg served as a project officer for the Committee on a National Strategy for AIDS of the IOM and the National Academy of Sciences. Following receipt of his M.D. and Ph.D. degrees, Dr. Feinberg pursued postgraduate residency training in internal medicine at the Brigham and Women's Hospital of Harvard Medical School and postdoctoral fellowship research in the laboratory of Dr. David Baltimore at the Whitehead Institute for Biomedical Research. From 1991 to 1995, Dr. Feinberg was an assistant professor of medical and microbiology and immunology at the University of California, San Francisco (UCSF), where he also served as an attending physician in the AIDS/Oncology Division and as director of the Virology Research Laboratory at San Francisco General Hospital. From 1995 to 1997, Dr. Feinberg was a medical officer in the Office of AIDS Research in the Office of the director of the NIH, and chair of the NIH Coordinating Committee on AIDS Etiology and Pathogenesis Research. During this period, he also served as executive secretary of the NIH Panel to Define Principles of Therapy of HIV Infection. Prior to joining Merck in 2004, Dr. Feinberg served as professor of medicine and microbiology and immunology at the Emory University School of Medicine, and as an investigator at the Emory Vaccine Center. Dr. Feinberg also founded and served as the medical director of the Hope Clinic—a clinical research facility devoted to the clinical evaluation of novel vaccines and to translational research studies of human immune system biology. At UCSF and Emory, Dr. Feinberg and colleagues were engaged in the preclinical development and evaluation of novel vaccines for HIV and other infectious diseeases, and in basic research studies focused on revealing fundamental aspects of host-virus relationships that underlie the pathogenesis of HIV and simian immunodeficiency virus (SIV) infections. In addition to his other professional roles, Dr. Feinberg has also served as a consultant to, and member of, several committees of the IOM and the National Academy of Sciences.

J. Patrick Fitch, Ph.D., is a program leader for Chemical and Biological National Security (CBNP) at the University of California, Lawrence Livermore National Laboratory (LLNL). CBNP is a $54 million program (FY02) at LLNL with over 140 staff. CBNP activities include basic pathogen biology and materials sciences and deployed operational systems for counter terrorism support. Prior to CBNP, Dr. Fitch led several different LLNL divisions including genomics, bioengineering, and engineering research. His research interests include bioinstrumentation, computer modeling of pathogen biology and host response, and medical devices. In addition to journal, conference, and patent publications, Dr. Fitch has authored several books and book chapters including *An Engineering Introduction to Biotechnology* (SPIE Press, 2002). Dr. Fitch received a Ph.D. degree in electrical engineering from Purdue University in 1984 and B.S. degrees in physics and engineering science from Loyola College in 1981. Dr. Fitch is a senior member of the Institute of Electrical and Electronic Engineers (IEEE), Fellow of the American Society for Laser Medicine and Surgery, Member of the International Society for Optical Engineering (SPIE), editorial board member of *Biomedical Engineering*, advisor board member for the College of Engineering at Colorado State University, and former board member of the California State Breast Cancer Research Program. He received an IEEE Best Paper Award for nonlinear digital signal processing in 1988, national Federal Laboratory Consortium for Technology Transfer (FLC) awards for medical devices in both 1998 and 1999, and the 2002 LLNL Science and Technology Award. Dr. Fitch also successfully developed and marketed a medical device business strategy to venture investors.

S. Elizabeth George, Ph.D., is deputy director, Biological Countermeasures Portfolio Science and Technology Directorate, Department of Homeland Security.

Until merging into the new department on March 1, 2003, Dr. George was the program manager of the Chemical and Biological National Security Program in the Department of Energy's National Nuclear Security Administration's Office of Nonproliferation Research & Engineering. Significant accomplishments include the design and deployment of BioWatch, the nation's first civilian biological threat agent monitoring system and PROTECT, the first civilian operational chemical detection and response capability deployed in the Washington subway system. Previously, she spent 16 years at the U.S. Environmental Protection Agency (EPA), Office of Research and Development, National Health and Ecological Effects Research Laboratory, Environmental Carcinogenesis Division, where she was branch chief of the Molecular and Cellular Toxicology Branch. She received her B.S. in biology (1977) from Virginia Polytechnic Institute and State University and M.S. and Ph.D. in microbiology (1979 and 1984) from North Carolina State University. She was a National Research Council Fellow (1984–1986) in the laboratory of Dr. Larry Claxton at the U.S. EPA. Dr. George is the 2005 chair of the Chemical and Biological Terrorism Defense Gordon Research Conference. She has served as councilor for the Environmental Mutagen Society and president and secretary of the Genotoxicity and Environmental Mutagen Society. She holds memberships in the American Society for Microbiology and the American Association for the Advancement of Science and is an adjunct faculty member in the School of Rural Public Health, Texas A&M University. Dr. George is a recipient of the U.S. EPA Bronze Medal and Scientific and Technological Achievement Awards and Department of Homeland Security (DHS) Under Secretary's Award for Science and Technology. She is author on numerous journal articles and has presented her research at national and international meetings.

Jesse L. Goodman, M.D., M.P.H., was professor of medicine and chief of infectious diseases at the University of Minnesota, and is now serving as deputy director for the U.S. FDA's Center for Biologics Evaluation and Research, where he is active in a broad range of scientific, public health, and policy issues. After joining the FDA commissioner's office, he has worked closely with several centers and helped coordinate the FDA's response to the antimicrobial resistance problem. He was cochair of a recently formed federal interagency task force which developed the national Public Health Action Plan on antimicrobial resistance. He graduated from Harvard College and attended the Albert Einstein College of Medicine followed by internal medicine, hematology, oncology, and infectious diseases training at the University of Pennsylvania and University of California–Los Angeles, where he was also chief medical resident. He received his master's of public health from the University of Minnesota. He has been active in community public health activities, including creating an environmental health partnership in St. Paul, Minnesota. In recent years, his laboratory's research has focused on the molecular pathogenesis of tick-borne diseases. His laboratory isolated the etiological intracellular agent of the emerging tick-borne infection, human granulocytic ehrlichiosis, and identified its leukocyte receptor. He has also been an active clinician and teacher and has directed or participated in major multicenter clinical studies. He is a Fellow of the Infectious Diseases Society of America and, among several honors, has been elected to the American Society for Clinical Investigation.

Eduardo Gotuzzo, M.D., is principal professor and director at the Instituto de Medicina Tropical "Alexander von Humbolt," Universidad Peruana Cayetan Heredia (UPCH), in Lima, Peru, as well as chief of the Department of Infectious and Tropical Diseases at the Cayetano Heredia Hospital. He is also an adjunct professor of medicine at the University of Alabama—Birmingham School of Medicine. Dr. Gotuzzo has proven to be an active member in numerous international societies such as President of the Latin America Society of Tropical Disease (2000–2003), the Scientific Program of Infectious Diseases Society of America (2000–2003), the International Organizing Committee of the International Congress of Infectious Diseases (1994–Present), president elect of the International Society for Infectious Diseases (1996–1998), and president of the Peruvian Society of Internal Medicine (1991–1992). He has published over 230 articles and chapters as well as 6 manuals and 1 book. Recent honors and awards include being named an honorary member of American Society of Tropical Medicine and Hygiene (since 2002), associate member of the National Academy of Medicine (since 2002), honorary member of the Society of Internal Medicine (since 2000), distinguished visitor at the Faculty of Medical Sciences, University of Cordoba, Argentina (since 1999), and received the Golden Medal for "Outstanding Contribution in the field of Infectious Diseases," awarded by the Trnava University, Slovakia (1998), among many others.

Jo Handelsman, Ph.D., received her Ph.D. in molecular biology from the University of Wisconsin–Madison in 1984 and joined the faculty of the UW–Madison Department of Plant Pathology in 1985 where she is currently a Howard Hughes Medical Institute Professor. Her research focuses on the genetic and functional diversity of microorganisms in soil and insect gut communities. The Handelsman lab has concentrated on discovery and biological activity of novel antibiotics from cultured and uncultured bacteria and has contributed to the pioneering of a new technique, called metagenomics, which facilitates the genomic analysis of assemblages of uncultured microorganisms. Handelsman is studying the midgut of the gypsy moth to understand the basis for resistance and susceptibility of microbial communities to invasion, developing it as a model for the microbial community in the human gut. In addition to her passion for understanding the secret lives of bacteria, Dr. Handelsman is dedicated to improving science education and the advancement of women in research universities. She is director of the Howard Hughes Medical Institute New Generation Program for Scientific Teaching, which is dedicated to teaching graduate students and postdoctoral students the principles and practices of teaching and mentoring. She is codirector of the National Academies Summer Institute for Undergraduate Education in Biology, which is a collaborative venture between HHMI and the National Academies that aims to train a nationwide network of faculty who are outstanding teachers and mentors. Dr. Handelsman is codirector of the Women in Science and Engineering Leadership Institute (WISELI), at the University of Wisconsin–Madison, whose mission is to understand the impediments to the successful recruitment and advancement of women faculty in the sciences and develop and study interventions intended to reduce the barriers.

Carole A. Heilman, Ph.D., is director of the Division of Microbiology and Infectious Diseases (DMID) of the NIAID. Dr. Heilman received her bachelor's degree in biology from Boston University in 1972, and earned her master's degree and doctorate in microbiology from Rutgers University in 1976 and 1979, respectively. Dr. Heilman began her career at the NIH as a postdoctoral research associate with the National Cancer Institute where she carried out research on the regulation of gene expression during cancer development. In 1986, she came to NIAID as the influenza and viral respiratory diseases program officer in DMID and, in 1988, she was appointed chief of the respiratory diseases branch where she coordinated the development of acellular pertussis vaccines. She joined the Division of AIDS as deputy director in 1997 and was responsible for developing the Innovation Grant Program for Approaches in HIV Vaccine Research. She is the recipient of several notable awards for outstanding achievement. Throughout her extramural career, Dr. Heilman has contributed articles on vaccine design and development to many scientific journals and has served as a consultant to the World Bank and WHO in this area. She is also a member of several professional societies, including the Infectious Diseases Society of America, the American Society for Microbiology, and the American Society of Virology.

David L. Heymann, M.D., is currently the executive director of the WHO Communicable Diseases Cluster. From October 1995 to July 1998 he was director of the WHO Programme on Emerging and Other Communicable Diseases Surveillance and Control. Prior to becoming director of this program, he was the chief of research activities in the Global Programme on AIDS. From 1976 to 1989, prior to joining WHO, Dr. Heymann spent 13 years working as a medical epidemiologist in sub-Saharan Africa (Cameroon, Ivory Coast, the former Zaire, and Malawi) on assignment from the CDC in CDC-supported activities aimed at strengthening capacity in surveillance of infectious diseases and their control, with special emphasis on the childhood immunizable diseases, African hemorrhagic fevers, pox viruses, and malaria. While based in Africa, Dr. Heymann participated in the investigation of the first outbreak of Ebola in Yambuku (former Zaire) in 1976, then again investigated the second outbreak of Ebola in 1977 in Tandala, and in 1995 directed the international response to the Ebola outbreak in Kikwit. Prior to

1976, Dr. Heymann spent two years in India as a medical officer in the WHO Smallpox Eradication Programme. Dr. Heymann holds a B.A. from the Pennsylvania State University, an M.D. from Wake Forest University, and a Diploma in Tropical Medicine and Hygiene from the London School of Hygiene and Tropical Medicine. He has also completed practical epidemiology training in the Epidemic Intelligence Service (EIS) training program of the CDC. He has published 131 scientific articles on infectious diseases in peer-reviewed medical and scientific journals.

Phil Hosbach, Ph.D., is vice president of New Products and Immunization Policy at Sanofi Pasteur. The departments under his supervision are new product marketing, state and federal government policy, business intelligence, bids and contracts, medical communications, public health sales, and public health marketing. His current responsibilities include oversight of immunization policy development. Mr. Hosbach acts as Sanofi Pasteur's principle liaison with CDC. Mr. Hosbach graduated from Lafayette College in 1984 with a degree in biology. He has 20 years of pharmaceutical industry experience, including the last 17 years focused solely on vaccines. He began his career at American Home Products in Clinical Research in 1984. He joined Aventis Pasteur (then Connaught Labs) in 1987 as clinical research coordinator and has held research and development positions of increasing responsibility, including clinical research manager and director of clinical operations. Mr. Hosbach also served as project manager for the development and licensure of Tripedia, the first diphtheria, tetanus, and acellular pertussis (DTaP) vaccine approved by FDA for use in U.S. infants. During his clinical research career at Aventis Pasteur, he contributed to the development and licensure of seven vaccines and has authored or coauthored several clinical research articles. From 2000 through 2002, Mr. Hosbach served on the Board of Directors for Pocono Medical Center, in East Stroudsburg, Pennsylvania. Since 2003 he has actively served on the board of directors of Pocono Health Systems, which includes Pocono Medical Center.

James M. Hughes, M.D., received his B.A. in 1966 and M.D. in 1971 from Stanford University. He completed a residency in internal medicine at the University of Washington and a fellowship in infectious diseases at the University of Virginia. He is board certified in internal medicine, infectious diseases, and preventive medicine. He first joined CDC as an epidemic intelligence service officer in 1973. During his CDC career, he has worked primarily in the areas of foodborne disease and infection control in health care settings. He became director of the NCID in 1992. The center is currently working to address domestic and global challenges posed by emerging infectious diseases and the threat of bioterrorism. He is a member of the IOM and a fellow of the American College of Physicians, the Infectious Diseases Society of America, and the American Association for the Advancement of Science. He is an Assistant Surgeon General in the Public Health Service.

Stephen Johnston, Ph.D., is a professor and director at the University of Texas Southwestern Medical Center. A major focus of Dr. Johnston's lab has been technology development. His interest of late has been especially in the area of vaccine development. He was co-inventor with Dr. John Sanford of the hand-held, helium gene gun, and he and Dr. Sanford used the gene gun to first demonstrate gene (DNA) immunization. Genetic vaccines have revolutionized approaches to delivering and developing vaccines. In this regard, Johnston's group first published on a method, expression library immunization, that offers a systematic approach to searching genomic information for new vaccines. His group has also developed techniques for discovering peptides that target specific cells and is employing this to create more effective, targeted vaccines. Through the Center for Biomedical Inventions, his group with collaborators in immunology, instrumentation, genomics, and chemistry is attempting to forge a fully integrated approach to developing the best methods for delivery and discovering vaccines.

Gerald T. Keusch, M.D., is provost and dean for Global Health at Boston University and Boston University School of Public Health. He is a graduate of Columbia College (1958) and Harvard Medical School (1963). After completing a residency in internal medicine, fellowship training in infectious diseases, and two years as a NIH research associate at the SEATO Medical Research Laboratory in Bangkok, Thailand, Dr. Keusch joined the faculty of Mt. Sinai School of Medicine in 1970, where he established a laboratory to study the pathogenesis of bacillary dysentery and the biology and biochemistry of Shiga toxin. In 1979, he moved to Tufts Medical School and New England Medical Center in Boston to found the Division of Geographic Medicine, which focused on the molecular and cellular biology of tropical infectious disease. In 1986, he integrated the clinical infectious diseases program into the Division of Geographic Medicine and Infectious Diseases, continuing as division chief until 1998. He has worked in the laboratory and in the field in Latin America, Africa, and Asia on basic and clinical infectious diseases and HIV/AIDS research. From 1998 to 2003, he was associate director for International Research and Director of the Fogarty International Center at the NIH. Dr. Keusch is a member of the American Society for Clinical Investigation, the Association of American Physicians, the American Society for Microbiology, and the Infectious Diseases Society of America (IDSA). He is the recipient of the Squibb (1981), Finland (1997), and Bristol (2002) Awards of the IDSA. In 2002, he was elected to the IOM of the National Academies.

Rima F. Khabbaz, M.D., is director of the NCID at the CDC. She received her B.S. in 1975 and her MD in 1979 from the American University of Beirut in

Beirut, Lebanon. She trained in internal medicine and completed a fellowship in infectious diseases at the University of Maryland in Baltimore. She is board certified in internal medicine. She first joined CDC as an epidemic intelligence service officer in 1980. During her CDC career, she worked primarily in the areas of health care-associated infections and viral diseases. She is a fellow of the Infectious Diseases Society of America (IDSA) and an elected member of the American Epidemiologic Society. She served on the Blood Product Advisory Committee of the FDA, on the FDA's Transmissible Spongiform Encephalopathy Advisory Committee, and on IDSA's Annual Meeting Scientific Program Committee. She played a leading role in developing CDC's programs related to blood safety and food safety and in CDC's responses to outbreaks of new and/or re-emerging diseases.

Lonnie King, D.V.M., is dean of the College of Veterinary Medicine, Michigan State University. Dr. King's previous positions include both associate administrator and administrator of the USDA Animal and Plant Health Inspection Service (APHIS) and deputy administrator for USDA/APHIS/Veterinary Services. Before his government career, Dr. King was in private practice. He also has experience as a field veterinary medical officer, station epidemiologist, and staff assignments involving emergency programs and animal health information. Dr. King has also directed the American Veterinary Medical Association's Office of Governmental Relations, and is certified in the American College of Veterinary Preventive Medicine. He has served as president of the Association of American Veterinary Medicine Colleges, and currently serves as cochair of the National Commission on Veterinary Economic Issues, lead dean at Michigan State University for food safety with responsibility for the National Food Safety and Toxicology Center, the Institute for Environmental Toxicology, and the Center for Emerging Infectious Diseases. He is also codeveloper and course leader for science, politics, and animal health policy. Dr. King received his B.S. and D.V.M. degrees from Ohio State University and his M.S. degree in epidemiology from the University of Minnesota. He has also completed the Senior Executive Program at Harvard University, and received an M.P.A. from American University. Dr. King previously served on the Committee for Opportunities in Agriculture, the Steering Committee for a Workshop on the Control and Prevention of Animal Diseases, and the Committee to Ensure Safe Food from Production to Consumption.

George Korch, Ph.D., attended Boston University and earned a B.S. in Biology in 1974, followed by postgraduate study in mammalian ecology at the University of Kansas from 1975 to 1978. He earned his Ph.D. from the Johns Hopkins School of Hygiene and Public Health in Immunology and Infectious Diseases in 1985, followed by postdoctoral experience at Johns Hopkins from 1985 to 1986. His area of training and specialty is the study of the epidemiology of zoonotic viral pathogens and in medical entomology. For the past 15 years, he has also engaged in research and program management for medical defense against biological pathogens used in terrorism or warfare.

Joshua Lederberg, Ph.D., is professor emeritus of molecular genetics and informatics and Sackler Foundation Scholar at the Rockefeller University in New York City. His lifelong research, for which he received the Nobel Prize in 1958, has been in genetic structure and function in microorganisms. He has a keen interest in international health and was cochair of a previous IOM Committee on Emerging Microbial Threats to Health (1990–1992) and currently is cochair of the Committee on Emerging Microbial Threats to Health in the 21st Century. He has been a member of the National Academy of Sciences since 1957 and is a charter member of the IOM.

Joseph Malone, M.D., the director of the Department of Defense Global Emerging Infection System (DoD-GEIS), completed the CDC's Epidemic Intelligence Service (EIS) program in June 2003. He graduated from Boston University School of Medicine in 1980, and trained in internal medicine and infectious diseases at Naval Hospitals in San Diego, California, and Bethesda, Maryland, leading to board certification. He was a staff physician at the Naval Hospitals in San Diego and Bethesda. He deployed to Guantanamo Bay, Cuba, in support of Operation Safe Harbor and was attached to Surgical Team 1 during Operation Desert Shield. He later directed the Infectious Disease Division and HIV unit at the Naval Medical Center at Portsmouth, Virginia in 1996. In 1999 he worked for the Disease Surveillance Program (in affiliation with DoD-GEIS) at the U.S. Naval Medical Research Unit No. 3 in Cairo, Egypt. While at CDC's EIS program he was deployed to New York City to assist in the emergency public health response after the attacks on September 11, 2001, assisted in the public health response to documented anthrax contamination in Kansas City, and was the acting state epidemiologist for the State of Missouri from February to June 2003. CAPT Malone has several military awards, including the HHS/USPHS Crisis Response Service Award. He is an associate professor at the Uniformed Services University of Health Sciences and holds the Certificate of Knowledge in Travelers' Health and Tropical Medicine from the American Society of Tropical Medicine and Hygiene. He has over 20 publications.

Lynn Marks, M.D., is board certified in internal medicine and infectious diseases. He was on faculty at the University of South Alabama College of Medicine in the Infectious Diseases department focusing on patient care, teaching, and research. His academic research interest was on the molecular genetics of bacterial pathogenicity. He subsequently joined SmithKline Beecham's (now GlaxoSmithKline) anti-infectives clinical group and later progressed to global head of the Consumer Healthcare division Medical and Regulatory group. He then returned to pharmaceutical research and development as global head of the Infectious Diseases Therapeutic Area Strategy Team for GlaxoSmithKline.

Edward McSweegan, Ph.D., is a program officer at the NIAID. He graduated from Boston College in 1978 (B.S.) and has degrees in microbiology from the University of New Hampshire (M.S.) and the University of Rhode Island (Ph.D.). He was a National Research Council Associate from 1984 to 1986 and did postdoctoral research at the Naval Medical Research Institute in Bethesda, Maryland. Dr. McSweegan served as an American Association for the Advancement of Science (AAAS) Diplomacy Fellow in the U.S. State Department from 1986 to 1988 and negotiated science and technology agreements with Poland, Hungary, and the former Soviet Union. After moving to the NIH, he continued to work on international health and science projects in Egypt, Israel, India, and Russia. Currently, Dr. McSweegan manages NIAID's bilateral program with India, the Indo–U.S. Vaccine Action Program, and represents NIAID in the DHHS Biotechnology Engagement Program (BTEP) with Russia and related countries. He is a member of AAAS, the American Society for Microbiology, and the D.C. Science Writers Association. He is the author of numerous journal articles and science articles.

Stephen S. Morse, Ph.D., is director of the Center for Public Health Preparedness at the Mailman School of Public Health of Columbia University, and a faculty member in the epidemiology department. Dr. Morse recently returned to Columbia from four years in government service as program manager at the Defense Advanced Research Projects Agency (DARPA), where he codirected the Pathogen Countermeasures Program and subsequently directed the Advanced Diagnostics Program. Before coming to Columbia, he was assistant professor (virology) at the Rockefeller University in New York, where he remains an adjunct faculty member. Dr. Morse is the editor of two books, *Emerging Viruses* (Oxford University Press, 1993; paperback, 1996) (selected by *American Scientist* for its list of 100 Top Science Books of the 20th Century), and *The Evolutionary Biology of Viruses* (Raven Press, 1994). He currently serves as a section editor of the CDC journal *Emerging Infectious Diseases* and was formerly an editor-in-chief of the Pasteur Institute's journal *Research in Virology*. Dr. Morse was chair and principal organizer of the 1989 NIAID/NIH Conference on Emerging Viruses (for which he originated the term and concept of emerging viruses/infections); served as a member of the IOM-NAS Committee on Emerging Microbial Threats to Health (and chaired its Task Force on Viruses), and was a contributor to its report, *Emerging Infections* (1992); was a member of the IOM's Committee on Xenograft Transplantation; currently serves on the Steering Committee of the IOM's Forum on Emerging Infections, and has served as an adviser to WHO, the Pan-American Health Organization, the FDA, the Defense Threat Reduction Agency (DTRA), and other agencies. He is a Fellow of the New York Academy of Sciences and a past chair of its microbiology section. He was the founding chair of ProMED (the nonprofit international Program to Monitor Emerging Diseases) and was one of the originators of ProMED-mail, an international network inaugurated by ProMED in 1994 for outbreak reporting and disease monitoring using the Internet. Dr. Morse received his Ph.D. from the University of Wisconsin–Madison.

Michael T. Osterholm, Ph.D., M.P.H., is director of the Center for Infectious Disease Research and Policy at the University of Minnesota where he is also professor at the School of Public Health. Previously, Dr. Osterholm was the state epidemiologist and chief of the acute disease epidemiology section for the Minnesota Department of Health. He has received numerous research awards from the NIAID and the CDC. He served as principal investigator for the CDC-sponsored Emerging Infections Program in Minnesota. He has published more than 240 articles and abstracts on various emerging infectious disease problems and is the author of the best selling book, *Living Terrors: What America Needs to Know to Survive the Coming Bioterrorist Catastrophe.* He is past president of the Council of State and Territorial Epidemiologists. He currently serves on the NAS-IOM Forum on Emerging Infections. He has also served on the IOM Food Safety, Production to Consumption, the IOM Committee on the Department of Defense Persian Gulf Syndrome Comprehensive Clinical Evaluation Program, and as a reviewer for the IOM report on chemical and biological terrorism.

George Poste, Ph.D., D.V.M., is director of the Arizona Biodesign Institute and Dell E. Webb Distinguished Professor of Biology at Arizona State University. From 1992 to 1999, he was chief science and technology officer and president, Research and Development of SmithKline Beecham (SB). During his tenure at SB, he was associated with the successful registration of 29 drug, vaccine, and diagnostic products. He is chairman of diaDexus and Structural GenomiX in California and Orchid Biosciences in Princeton. He serves on the board of directors of AdvancePCS and Monsanto. He is an advisor on biotechnology to several venture capital funds and investment banks. In May 2003, he was appointed as director of the Arizona Biodesign Institute at Arizona State University. This is a major new initiative combining research groups in biotechnology, nanotechnology, materials science, advanced computing, and neuromorphic engineering. He is a Fellow of Pembroke College at Cambridge and Distinguished Fellow at the Hoover Institution and Stanford University. He is a member of the Defense Science Board of the U.S. Department of Defense and in this capacity he chairs the Task Force on Bioterrorism. He is also a member of the National Academy of Sciences Working Group on Defense Against Bioweapons. Dr. Poste is a board certified pathologist, a Fellow of the Royal Society, and a Fellow of the Academy of Medical Sciences. He was awarded the rank of Commander of the British Empire by Queen Elizabeth II in 1999 for services to medicine and for the advancement of biotechnology. He has published over 350 scientific papers, co-edited 15 books on cancer, biotechnology, and infectious diseases and serves on the editorial board of multiple technical journals. He is invited routinely to be the keynote speaker at a wide variety of academic, corporate, investment, and government meetings to discuss the impact of biotechnology and genetics on health care and the challenges posed by bioterrorism.

David A. Relman, M.D., Ph.D., is an associate professor of medicine (infectious diseases and geographic medicine) and of microbiology and immunology at Stanford University School of Medicine, Stanford, California, and chief of the infectious disease section at the Veterans Affairs Palo Alto Health Care System, Palo Alto, California. Dr. Relman received his B.S. in biology from Massachusetts Institute of Technology, Cambridge, Massachusetts, and his M.D. from Harvard Medical School. He completed his residency in internal medicine and a clinical fellowship in infectious diseases at Massachusetts General Hospital, Boston, after which he moved to Stanford in 1994. His major focus is laboratory research directed toward characterizing the human endogenous microbial flora, host-microbe interactions, and identifying previously unrecognized microbial pathogens using molecular and genomic approaches. He has described a number of new human microbial pathogens. Dr. Relman's lab (*http://relman.stanford.edu*) is currently exploring human oral and intestinal microbial ecology, sources of variation in host genomewide expression responses to infection and during states of health, and how *Bordetella* species (including the agent of whooping cough) cause disease. He has published over 150 peer-reviewed articles, reviews, editorials, and book chapters on pathogen discovery and bacterial pathogenesis. Dr. Relman has served on scientific program committees for the American Society of Microbiology (ASM); the Infectious Diseases Society of America (IDSA); and advisory panels for NIH, CDC, the departments of Energy and Defense, and National Aeronautics and Space Administration (NASA). He was co-chair of the Committee on Advances in Technology and the Prevention of their Application to Next Generation Biowarefare Threats for the NAS. He is a member of the board of directors of the IDSA and the Board of Scientific Counselors at National Institute of Dental and Craniofacial Research (NIDCR) at the NIH. He received the Squibb Award from IDSA in 2001, the Senior Scholar Award in Global Infectious Diseases from the Ellison Medical Foundation in 2002, and is a Fellow of the American Academy of Microbiology.

Gary A. Roselle, M.D., received his M.D. from Ohio State University School of Medicine in 1973. He served his residency at Northwestern University School of Medicine and his Infectious Diseases fellowship at the University of Cincinnati School of Medicine. Dr. Roselle is the program director for infectious diseases for the VA Central Office in Washington, D.C., as well as the chief of the medical service at the Cincinnati VA Medical Center. He is a professor of medicine in the Department of Internal Medicine, Division of Infectious Diseases at the University of Cincinnati College of Medicine. Dr. Roselle serves on several national advisory committees. In addition, he is currently heading the Emerging Pathogens Initiative for the Department of Veterans Affairs. Dr. Roselle has received commendations from the Cincinnati Medical Center Director, the Under Secretary for Health for the Department of Veterans Affairs, and the Secretary of Veterans Affairs for his work in the infectious diseases program for the Department of Veterans Affairs. He has been an invited speaker at several national and international meetings, and has published over 80 papers and several book chapters.

Janet Shoemaker is director of the American Society for Microbiology's Public Affairs Office, a position she has held since 1989. She is responsible for managing the legislative and regulatory affairs of this 42,000-member organization, the largest single biological science society in the world. She has served as principal investigator for a project funded by the National Science Foundation (NSF) to collect and disseminate data on the job market for recent doctorates in microbiology and has played a key role in American Society for Microbiology (ASM) projects, including the production of the ASM *Employment Outlook in the Microbiological Sciences* and *The Impact of Managed Care and Health System Change on Clinical Microbiology*. Previously, she held positions as assistant director of public affairs for ASM, as ASM coordinator of the U.S./U.S.S.R. Exchange Program in Microbiology, a program sponsored and coordinated by the NSF and the U.S. Department of State, and as a freelance editor and writer. She received her baccalaureate, cum laude, from the University of Massachusetts, and is a graduate of the George Washington University programs in public policy and in editing and publications. She has served as commissioner to the Commission on Professionals in Science and Technology, and as the ASM representative to the ad hoc Group for Medical Research Funding, and is a member of Women in Government Relations, the American Society of Association Executives, and the American Association for the Advancement of Science. She has co-authored published articles on research funding, biotechnology, biological weapons control, and public policy issues related to microbiology.

Terence Taylor is president and executive director of the International Institute for Strategic Studies–US (IISS–US). He is also assistant director of the IISS in London. He studies international security policy, risk analysis, scientific and technological developments, and their impact on political and economic stability worldwide. He is one of the Institute's leading experts on issues associated with nuclear, biological, and chemical weapons and their means of delivery. He has a particular responsibility for IISS on all issues affecting public safety and security in relation to biological risks and advances in the life sciences. He was one of the commissioners to the UN Special Commission on Iraq for which he also conducted missions as a chief inspector. He was a Research Fellow on the Science Program at the Center for International Security and Cooperation at Stanford University where he carried out, among other subjects, studies of the implications for government and industry of the weapons of mass destruction treaties and agreements. He has also carried out consultancy work for the International Committee of the Red Cross on the implementation and development of the laws of armed conflict and consultancy for private companies on political risk analysis (both regional and country specific). He is chairman of the Permanent Monitoring Panel on Risk Analysis for the World Federation of Scientists. He served as a career officer in the British Army on operations in many parts of the world, including counterterrorist operations and UN peacekeeping. His publications include monographs, book chapters and articles for, among others, Stanford University, the World Economic Forum, SIPRI, the Crimes of War Project, *International Herald Tribune*, *Wall Street Journal*, the *International Defence Review*, the *Independent* (London), *Tiempo* (Madrid), the *International and Comparative Law Quarterly*, the *Washington Quarterly*, and other scholarly journals including unsigned contributions to IISS publications.